MANUAL OF
Clinical Exercise
Testing, Prescription
and Rehabilitation

MANUAL OF
Clinical Exercise Testing, Prescription and Rehabilitation

ZIYA ALTUĞ, PT, MS
Physical Therapist/Exercise Physiologist
St. Francis Medical Center
Pittsburgh, Pennsylvania
Forbes Back Institute/WorkAgain Program
Pittsburgh, Pennsylvania

JANET L. HOFFMAN, MS
Exercise Physiologist
Forbes Back Insitute/WorkAgain Program
Pittsburgh, Pennsylvania

JEROME L. MARTIN, PhD, PT (editor)
Dean
John G. Rangos, Sr., School of Health Sciences
Duquesne University
Pittsburgh, Pennsylvania

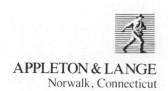

APPLETON & LANGE
Norwalk, Connecticut

0-8385-0241-5

Prentice-Hall International (UK) Limited, *London*
Prentice-Hall of Australia Pty. Limited, *Sydney*
Prentice-Hall Canada, Inc., *Toronto*
Prentice-Hall Hispanoamericana, S.A., *Mexico*
Prentice-Hall of India Private Limited, *New Delhi*
Prentice-Hall of Japan, Inc., *Tokyo*
Simon & Schuster Asia Pte. Ltd., *Singapore*
Editora Prentice-Hall do Brasil, Ltda., *Rio de Janeiro*
Prentice Hall, *Englewood Cliffs, New Jersey*

Library of Congress Cataloging-in-Publication Data

Altuğ, Ziya.
    Manual of clinical exercise testing, prescription, and
rehabilitation / Ziya Altuğ, Janet L. Hoffman : Jerome L. Martin
(editor).
      p. cm.
    Includes bibliographical references and index.
    ISBN 0-8385-0241-5
    1. Exercise therapy. 2. Exercise tests. I. Hoffman, Janet L.
II. Martin, Jerome L. (Jerome Lee) III. Title
    [DNLM: 1. Exercise Test--methods. 2. Exercise Therapy--methods.
WB 541 A469m]
RM725.A45 1992
615.8'2--dc20
DNLM/DLC
for Library of Congress   92-21898
                                                           CIP

Acquisitions Editor: Cheryl L. Mehalik
Production Editors: Sandra K. Huggard, Sasha K. Kintzler
Designer: Michael J. Kelly
Photography: Audio-Visual Communications, Forbes Health System, Pittsburgh, Pennsylvania

PRINTED IN THE UNITED STATES OF AMERICA

DEDICATIONS

*To Mom and Dad for their encouragement throughout the years
and to my brother Aykut, for his help in preparing this book.*
Z.A.

*Thanks to my family for love, support, and encouragement.
To "the farm"—thanks for all you have done for me.*
J.L.H.

Contributors

Aykut Altuğ, BS
Graduate Student in Mechanical Engineering
University of Pittsburgh
Pittsburgh, Pennsylvania
Appendix A—Abbreviations, Symbols, and Conversion Factors
Appendix B—Physical Science Formulas

Stephen M. Slane, MS, PT
Director
Forbes Back Institute/WorkAgain Program
Pittsburgh, Pennsylvania
Author: *Functional Capacities Assessment in Work Hardening*. Thorofare,
      NJ: SLACK, Inc; in prep.
Chapter 8—Work Performance Testing

Contents

Preface

This book provides clinically relevant components of exercise testing, prescription, and rehabilitation in one easy-to-read format. This format features tables, figures, lists, and charts.

The book is written primarily for physical therapists, occupational therapists, athletic trainers, exercise physiologists, and physical educators specializing in sports medicine or work hardening (ie, industrial rehabilitation). The book also serves as a reference guide for undergraduate physical therapy, occupational therapy, athletic training, exercise physiology, and physical education students studying the practical applications of exercise testing, exercise prescription, and therapeutic exercise. The book may also be used in graduate physical therapy classes focusing on sports medicine, exercise science, and work hardening (ie, industrial rehabilitation).

The book is divided into the following:

Section One—Clinical Principles of Exercise Testing, Prescription, and Rehabilitation

Section Two—Clinical Guidelines for Exercise Testing

Section Three—Clinical Guidelines for Exercise Prescription and Rehabilitation

Section One outlines various principles, concepts, guidelines, contraindications, and general standards for safety as they relate to exercise testing and prescription.

Section Two provides the reader with a comprehensive overview of the testing protocols used for flexibility, strength, cardiovascular endurance, kinanthropometry, sport performance, and work performance. Each chapter provides several clinically relevant exercise testing procedures with original source(s) referenced for each test. The original source(s), as well as sections pertaining to testing in the suggested readings, assist the clinician in obtaining **reliability measures**.

Finally, Section Three focuses on clinically relevant guidelines for prescribing and designing exercise and rehabilitation programs for flexibility, strength, cardiovascular endurance, and sport performance. Within each of these chapters, the clinician and student are given the specific exercise prescription parameters (ie, mode, intensity, frequency, and duration) for prescribing therapeutic exercises for flexibility, strength, cardiovascular endurance, and sport performance.

The following list outlines key features of this book:

1. References at the end of each chapter provide up-to-date and historically relevant material to assist the clinician in obtaining further information.

2. Suggested readings at the end of the book provide an up-to-date reading list for those clinicians seeking additional information on clinically relevant topics (eg, arthritis, ergogenic aids, nutrition).

3. Appendices at the end of the book feature abbreviations, conversion factors, formulas, sources of exercise science calculations, evaluation forms, a chart of laboratory tests affected by exercise, a vitamin and mineral chart, an organizations listing, and a journals listing.

4. A Glossary at the end of the book consists of definitions of specific terms and concepts used throughout the book. The terms and concepts defined in the glossary generally have been represented as they appear in the original source(s), with the original source(s) cited as a reference.

5. Illustrations at the end of Chapters 9, 10, and 12 display clinically relevant flexibility and strength exercises. The clinician may copy these photographs and design a specific flexibility or strength program specific to each client's needs.

6. Tables and figures are easy-to-read and comprehensive.

Throughout the book the term **exercise prescription** refers to the programing or organization of exercise or exercise sessions. The term **prescription** is not used in the medical context in this book. The term prescription typically refers to a written direction or order by a physician for dispensing and administering drugs, therapy, etc.[1] We have also used the term **client** instead of **patient** throughout the book. The term patient, however, may be substituted in appropriate clinical settings and situations.

Finally, the authors appreciate any comments from readers regarding suggestions for future editions.

Ziya Altuğ, PT, MS
Janet L. Hoffman, MS
Jerome L. Martin, PhD, PT (editor)
Pittsburgh, Pennsylvania

REFERENCE

1. Thomas CL, ed. *Taber's Cyclopedic Medical Dictionary*. 15th ed. Philadelphia, Pa: FA Davis Co; 1985.

Acknowledgments

We would like to thank the following for their assistance in the preparation of this book:

Stephany S. Scott (former medical editor at Appleton & Lange) for bringing our thoughts from a dream to a reality. Aykut Altuğ for typing, retyping, and proofreading the entire text. The Forbes Health System, Pittsburgh, Pennsylvania for sponsoring the photography for this text and to Ann Wetzel for her assistance in arranging for the sponsorship. Donald Selchan (director), Kristin Petersen, Robert Davis, and Claire Hamley of Audio-Visual Communications at the Forbes Health System, Pittsburgh, Pennsylvania for arranging all the photographs in the text. Joseph Gianoni, MS, PT, ATC (assistant director) of the Forbes Back Institute, Pittsburgh, Pennsylvania for critiquing the manuscript. Susan S. Biery, medical librarian at the University of Pittsburgh for her assistance in obtaining references. Stephen M. Slane, MS, PT (director) and Carol Huffman, PT (former assistant director) of the Forbes WorkAgain/Forbes Back Institute, Pittsburgh, Pennsylvania for supporting us in the clinic. Thomas Winner, PT (director) of St. Francis Medical Center, Physical Therapy Department for providing me (Z.A.) an opportunity to work in an excellent outpatient clinic and complete the final phases of this book. Finally, a special thanks to Cheryl L. Mehalik (senior editor), Sandra K. Huggard and Sasha Kintzler (production editors), Tracey Schelmetic (editorial assistant), and the Appleton & Lange team for their professionalism and support.

Section One 1

Clinical Principles of Exercise Testing, Prescription, and Rehabilitation

Chapter One 1

Principles of Exercise Testing

CONCEPTS OF TESTING

Purpose of Testing

The following list outlines the various purposes of testing:

1. Assess physical fitness and functional capacity in order to design an appropriate and safe conditioning or rehabilitation program.
2. Assess functional abilities in order to determine return-to work status.
3. Assess for potential imbalances (eg, strength, flexibility, cardiovascular, nutritional).
4. Assess the efficacy of interventions (eg, medical, nutritional, therapeutic).
5. Collect baseline information in order to establish a client profile.
6. Obtain follow-up and baseline data for research.
7. Test a research hypothesis.
8. Develop a normative data base.
9. Monitor training progress.
10. Monitor rehabilitation progress.
11. Develop clinical and home exercise programs.
12. Provide data contributing to the diagnosis of disease and dysfunction in asymptomatic and symptomatic individuals.
13. Screen and assess for deformities.
14. Compare the individual's fitness level to established norms.
15. Motivate individuals by comparing pre- and post-test results as a visible record of their progress.
16. To assess the following in sport-specific settings[4,19]:
    a. Physical maturity so that assignment to an appropriate group for sports participation is possible
    b. The athlete's knowledge regarding injury prevention, nutrition, ergogenic aids, and ergolytic substances
    c. Conditions that predispose the athlete to injury or death
    d. Growth spurt activity
    e. Alignment disorders (eg, scoliosis)

3

Types of Assessment

The following categories outline the various types of testing that may be taken into consideration when evaluating a client:

1. Demographic assessment (eg, age, gender)
2. Lifestyle assessment (eg, dietary patterns, exercise patterns, smoking history, drinking history)
3. Medical history screening (eg, verbal screening, written screening questionnaire)
4. General medical assessment (eg, evaluation by family physician, blood analysis, urinalysis, x-rays)
5. Special medical assessment (eg, evaluation by a specialized physician such as an orthopedic surgeon, blood analysis, urinalysis, computerized axial tomography, magnetic resonance imaging, myelography, electromyography)
6. Neurological assessment (eg, reflexes, sensation, cranial nerves, coordination, equilibrium, strength)
7. Muscular strength assessment (eg, manual, isometric, isotonic, isokinetic, functional)
8. Flexibility and range of motion assessment (eg, passive, active)
9. Cardiovascular assessment (eg, resting blood pressure and heart rate, resting and exercise ECGs, treadmill and bicycle ergometer testing, echocardiography, coronary angiography, Holter monitoring)
10. Kinanthropometric assessment (eg, height, weight, skinfolds, hydrostatic weighing, circumferences, diameters)
11. Nutritional assessment (eg, screening questionnaire, 24-hour recall, blood analysis, urinalysis)
12. Work-specific functional assessment (eg, sitting, standing, crawling, reaching, climbing, pushing, pulling)
13. Sport-specific skill assessment (eg, speed, balance, agility, power)

GUIDELINES FOR EXERCISE TESTING

Clinical Personnel and Certifications

Clinical specialists (see Table 1–1) within various professional organizations (eg, American Physical Therapy Association, American Occupational Therapy Association, National Athletic Trainers' Association) are expanding their range of clinical practice and, therefore, it is becoming apparent that standards need to be identified in order to assure quality of care. These organizations must be willing to work together and establish standards that are mutually agreed upon.

Each professional organization has its own standards for clinical competence through licensure and certification. Table 1–2 provides clinicians with a sampling

TABLE 1–1. CLINICAL SPECIALISTS INVOLVED IN EXERCISE TESTING AND PRESCRIPTION

1. Physician
2. Physical therapist
3. Exercise physiologist
4. Athletic trainer
5. Occupational therapist
6. Physical educator
7. Cardiovascular nurse specialist
8. Dietician
9. Certified exercise specialist (see Table 1–2)

TABLE 1–2. SPECIALTY CERTIFICATIONS FOR EXERCISE TESTING AND PRESCRIPTION

American College of Sports Medicine (ACSM)
1. Health and fitness track
   a. Health/fitness director
   b. Health/fitness instructor
   c. Exercise leader
2. Clinical track
   a. Preventive/rehabilitative program director
   b. Preventive/rehabilitative exercise specialist
   c. Exercise test technologist

American Physical Therapy Association (APTA)
1. Cardiopulmonary certified specialist
2. Sports certified specialist
3. Orthopedic certified specialist
4. Clinical electrophysiologic certified specialist
5. Neurologic certified specialist
6. Pediatric certified specialist

American Heart Association (AHA)
1. Basic cardiac life support
2. Advanced cardiac life support

Young Men's Christian Association (YMCA)
1. Physical fitness specialist
2. YMCArdiac therapy program specialist

National Strength and Conditioning Association (NSCA)
1. Certified strength and conditioning specialist

Institute for Aerobics Research
1. Physical fitness specialist certification
2. Group exercise leadership certification

of the types of certifications that are available from various professional organizations. For addresses of the organizations listed, please refer to Appendix G.

Testing Responsibilities of the Clinician

The following outlines various pre-test, test, and post-test responsibilities of a clinician:

PRE-TEST RESPONSIBILITIES

1. Obtain an accurate medical history.
2. Identify absolute and relative medical contraindications.
3. Identify individuals who should be referred for further medical testing.
4. Determine the appropriate test mode (eg, treadmill versus bicycle, isotonic versus isokinetic) and test protocol (eg, Bruce treadmill test).
5. Standardize all testing procedures.
6. Obtain all necessary pre-test data (eg, the resting levels of heart rate and blood pressure).
7. Know the specific test procedure.
8. Determine the order of testing.
9. Determine what measures will be obtained pre-test (eg, heart rate, blood pressure, ECG monitoring).
10. Plan safety and emergency procedures.
11. Prepare and organize equipment and tools.
12. Calibrate equipment, if necessary.
13. Include a warm-up period before the test.

14. Obtain an informed consent from the client. An informed consent implies that the client is aware of any potential risks and benefits of the test procedure and consents to being tested.

TEST RESPONSIBILITIES

1. Explain the test procedures.
2. Demonstrate the test procedures, if necessary.
3. Utilize test trials, if necessary.
4. Determine what measures will be obtained during the test (eg, heart rate, blood pressure, $\dot{V}O_2$, ECG monitoring, rating of perceived exertion).
5. Provide the same degree of motivation and encouragement to all the clients.

POST-TEST RESPONSIBILITIES

1. Determine the client's body posture (eg, standing, sitting, supine) for obtaining post-test data.
2. Determine what measures will be obtained post-test (eg, heart rate, blood pressure, ECG monitoring, rating of perceived exertion) and how long each measure will be monitored before releasing the client.
3. Include a cool-down period after the test.
4. Remove equipment (eg, ECG electrodes, heart rate monitoring system) from the client, if applicable.
5. Inform the client regarding his or her next step (eg, referral back to physician, further testing, scheduling an appointment for beginning the rehabilitation or conditioning program).
6. Organize and interpret the test results.

Characteristics of Effective Testing

The following represents characteristics of effective testing and may be used by the clinician to design or adapt various testing protocols[13,14,16,18]:

1. The testing protocol should have the following administrative characteristics:
   a. Test should be cost-effective.
   b. Test should not be time-consuming.
   c. Test should be relatively easy to administer.
   d. Test scoring and calculations should provide accurate results.
   e. Norms should be population specific.
2. The testing protocol should be reliable, valid, and objective.
3. The testing protocol should be specific to the following factors:
   a. Muscle group (eg, upper versus lower body)
   b. Type of muscular contraction (ie, static, dynamic, isokinetic)
   c. Energy utilization (ie, aerobic versus anaerobic)
   d. Body position (eg, upright, seated, recumbent)
   e. Speed of movement (eg, rpm, mph, degrees per second)
   f. Limb position (eg, internal or external rotation, flexed or extended)
   g. Joint angle (eg, trunk flexion and extension in degrees)
   h. Work-related task
   i. Sport-related skill
4. The testing protocol and testing conditions should be standardized and reproducible (eg, verbal cues, stabilization techniques, positioning, environmental conditions such as temperature and humidity).
5. The testing protocol must be safe.
6. The test results should be interpreted by an appropriate professional (eg, physician, physical therapist, exercise physiologist).
7. Test administration should be rigidly controlled.
8. Testing should generally be performed on the uninvolved extremity first.

9. Testing should be repeated at designated intervals in order to determine the efficacy of specific interventions.
10. The testing equipment should be in safe operating order and appropriate emergency precautions should be taken.
11. The testing equipment should be calibrated according to standardized guidelines.
12. The client should warm up and cool down before and after each test procedure.
13. The client's rights must be respected (ie, the test purpose, procedures, and risks should be explained thoroughly).

GENERAL GUIDELINES AND CONTRAINDICATIONS TO EXERCISE TESTING

Table 1–3 outlines pre-test guidelines and instructions, and Table 1–4 describes various guidelines and contraindications to exercise testing.

GUIDELINES AND STANDARDS FOR TESTING SAFETY

Procedural Safety Guidelines

Every facility should have a written plan for handling emergencies that might occur during testing, conditioning, and rehabilitation. The medical director or on-site physician should determine specific policies and procedures for handling emergency situations. The following are general procedural safety guidelines to consider[2,10,17]:

1. All clinical personnel should be certified in cardiopulmonary resuscitation (CPR).
2. All clinical personnel should either be certified in first aid or have a good understanding of first aid procedures.
3. It is recommended that personnel performing exercise testing (especially maximal treadmill testing) be trained in Advanced Cardiac Life Support (ACLS).
4. Each clinician should be assigned specific responsibilities during any test procedure.
5. Appropriate cardiac emergency equipment and supplies should be available.
6. Several first aid kits should be visible and easily accessible throughout the clinic.
7. Telephone numbers for emergency assistance should be clearly posted on all telephones in the clinic.
8. Telephone numbers of the client's referring and family physician should be indicated in his or her chart.
9. Evacuation plans should be established and posted in the clinic.
10. All safety rules and regulations should be clearly posted in the clinic.
11. A policy regarding emergency transportation to the nearest emergency room should be established.

TABLE 1–3. PRE-TEST GUIDELINES AND INSTRUCTIONS FOR EXERCISE TESTING[1,5,7,9,11]

1. The testing area should be approximately 22°C (72°F) or less and the humidity 60% or less, if possible.
2. Instruct and encourage the client to:
   a. Not smoke or use tobacco products for a minimum of 2 hours before testing
   b. Not use products containing caffeine for a minimum of 2 hours before testing
   c. Not wear unnecessary jewelry on testing day
   d. Remain as calm and relaxed as possible on testing day

TABLE 1–4. GUIDELINES AND CONTRAINDICATIONS FOR EXERCISE TESTING[1,5-9,11]

1. The clinician should observe all pre-established testing standards, guidelines, absolute contraindications, relative contraindications, and indications for stopping exercise testing (eg, see Chapter 5).
2. Reschedule test procedures if the following conditions exist:
   a. Testing equipment is not functioning properly.
   b. The client is suspected to be under the influence of alcohol or other nonprescription drugs (eg, cocaine, marijuana).
   c. The client appears to be or states having an adverse reaction to any prescribed medications.
3. Consider rescheduling test procedures if the following conditions exist:
   a. The client varied his or her prescribed medications (eg, high blood pressure medication) before testing procedures without the clearance of a physician.
   b. The client did not wear the appropriate shoes or clothing (eg, soft-soled shoes, socks, shirt, shorts, and sweat jacket and pants, as appropriate).
   c. The client did not fast for at least 2 hours before the test.
   d. The client donated blood within 24 hours of the test.
   e. The client engaged in excessive physical activity on testing day.
   f. The client is having a severe allergic response (eg, pollens).
   g. The client is ill.
   h. The client appears to be or states having extreme emotional distress.

12. All medications taken by the client, as well as other pertinent medical history, should be indicated in his or her chart.
13. Conditioning and rehabilitation equipment should be inspected on a regular basis.
14. The client should be supervised at all times.
15. The client should not be taxed beyond his or her physical limits.
16. All emergency procedures should be practiced periodically.

Equipment Safety Guidelines

The following are general equipment safety guidelines to consider:

1. Properly calibrate all equipment.
2. Periodically check the equipment's supporting structures (eg, treadmill handrails, cables on strength equipment).
3. Periodically, lubricate all equipment.
4. Avoid using cheater plugs and extension cords, which adapt three-blade power plugs to two-blade receptacles (thus defeating grounding).[15]
5. Have equipment inspected on a regular basis by biomedical instrumentation specialists for verifying its electrical safety and performance.
6. Floors should generally have a nonslip surface.
7. Safety instructions should be mounted in a visible area on each piece of equipment.
8. A review of safety checklists that have been established by other clinicians is recommended.[3,12]

REFERENCES

1. American College of Sports Medicine. *Guidelines for Exercise Testing and Prescription.* 4th ed. Philadelphia, Pa: Lea & Febiger; 1991.
2. Armitage-Johnson S. Emergency procedures. *Nat Strength Condit Assoc J.* 1990;12(4): 39–43.
3. Armitage-Johnson S. Maintaining strength facility areas. *Nat Strength Condit Assoc J.* 1990;12(1):24–25.
4. Blum RW. Preparticipation evaluation of the adolescent athlete: Timing and content of the examination. *Postgrad Med.* 1985;78(2):52–69.

5. Brannon FJ, Geyer MJ, Foley MW. *Cardiac Rehabilitation*. Philadelphia, Pa: FA Davis Co; 1988.
6. Chung EK, ed. *Exercise Electrocardiography: Practical Approach*. 2nd ed. Baltimore, Md: Williams & Wilkins; 1983.
7. Fletcher GF. *Exercise in the Practice of Medicine*. 2nd ed. Mount Kisco, NY: Futura Publishing; 1988.
8. Franklin BA, Gordon S, Timmis GC. *Exercise in Modern Medicine*. Baltimore, Md: Williams & Wilkins; 1989.
9. Froelicher VF, Marcondes GD. *Manual of Exercise Testing*. Chicago, Ill: Year Book Medical Publishers, Inc; 1989.
10. Halling DH. Facility rules and regulations. *Nat Strength Condit Assoc J*. 1990;12(6):58–61.
11. Hellerstein HK, Franklin BA. Exercise testing and prescription. In: Wenger NK, Hellerstein HK, eds. *Rehabilitation of the Coronary Patient*. 2nd ed. New York, NY: John Wiley & Sons, Inc; 1984.
12. Kroll B. Evaluating strength training equipment. *Nat Strength Condit Assoc J*. 1990;12(3):56–65.
13. MacDougall JD, Wenger HA. The purpose of physiological testing. In: MacDougall JD, Wenger HA, Green HJ, eds. *Physiological Testing of the High-Performance Athlete*. 2nd ed. Champaign, Ill: Human Kinetics Publishers, Inc; 1991.
14. Miller DK. *Measurement by the Physical Educator: Why and How*. Carmel, Ind: Benchmark Press; 1988.
15. Ritter HTM. Instrumentation considerations: Operating principles, purchase, management and safety. In: Michlovitz SL, ed. *Thermal Agents in Rehabilitation*. Philadelphia, Pa: FA Davis Co; 1986.
16. Sharkey BJ. Specificity of testing. In: Grana WA, Lomardo JA, Sharkey BJ, et al, eds. *Advances in Sports Medicine and Fitness*. Chicago, Ill: Year Book Medical Publishers, Inc; 1988;1.
17. Strauss WE, Scaramuzzi MS, Panton-Lapsley D, et al. Emergency plans and procedures for an exercise facility. In: Blair SN, Painter P, Pate RR, et al, eds. *Resource Manual for Guidelines for Exercise Testing and Prescription (American College of Sports Medicine)*. Philadelphia, Pa: Lea & Febiger; 1988.
18. Wilk K. Dynamic muscle strength testing. In: Amundsen LR. *Muscle Strength Testing. Instrumented and Non Instrumented Systems*. New York, NY: Churchill Livingstone; 1990.
19. Zito M. Musculoskeletal injuries of young athletes: The new trends. In: Gould JA, ed. *Orthopaedic and Sports Physical Therapy*. 2nd ed. St Louis, Mo: CV Mosby Co; 1990.

2

Principles of Exercise Prescription and Rehabilitation

CONCEPTS OF EXERCISE PRESCRIPTION AND REHABILITATION

Components of Exercise Prescription

Throughout this book, the parameters for individual exercise prescription (ie, mode, intensity, frequency, and duration of exercise) have generally been referenced from the original source. This format allows the clinician the option of adapting the exercise prescription parameters to meet personal and clinical standards.

The following list outlines the components of an ideal exercise prescription:

1. Pre-exercise warm-up session
2. Pre-exercise stretching session
3. Conditioning/training or rehabilitation session:
   a. Mode of exercise—indicates the type of exercise to be performed
   b. Intensity of exercise—indicates how hard the exercise should be performed
   c. Frequency of exercise—indicates how many times the individual exercise should be performed or the number of exercise sessions per day or per week
   d. Duration of exercise—indicates how long the individual exercise should be performed or the total duration of the exercise session or both
4. Post-exercise cool-down session
5. Post-exercise stretching session

The term *warm-up* refers to preliminary exercise procedures rather than the use of hot showers, counterirritants, massage, diathermy, or other forms of passive warm-up. The purpose of a warm-up session is as follows[2,7,12-14]:

1. To raise the general body temperature
2. To raise the deep muscle temperature
3. To stretch collagenous tissues
4. To reduce muscle viscosity, thus producing an improvement in mechanical efficiency
5. To increase the speed of nerve impulses and augment the sensitivity of nerve receptors
6. To improve cardiovascular response to sudden exercise

The purpose of a stretching session is to permit unrestricted full range of joint motion, which in turn prevents injury. Finally, the purpose of a cool-down session is to prevent the blood from pooling in the extremities and to gradually bring the cardiovascular system to near resting levels in a safe manner.[3]

The client should perform a pre-exercise warm-up and stretching session in order to prepare the body both physiologically and psychologically for physical activity, while the post-exercise session allows the body to taper off from intense physical activity.

Factors Affecting the Exercise Prescription

There are various factors that may affect human performance in a positive or negative manner. For this reason, clinicians should be aware of the following factors when designing conditioning and rehabilitation programs for their clients[4,5,15,16]:

1. Medical factors
   a. Congenital abnormalities (eg, coronary anomalies, aortic stenosis)
   b. Medical history (eg, hypertension, diabetes)
   c. Disease history (eg, rheumatoid arthritis)
2. Assistive factors
   a. Orthotics
   b. Cane, crutches, or walker
   c. Wheelchair
   d. Braces (eg, knee, back)
3. Personal factors
   a. Client's age, weight, and height
   b. Client's goals (eg, weight loss, injury rehabilitation, athletic competition)
   c. Client's budget
   d. Client's activity interests
   e. Client's activity skills
4. Structural factors
   a. Equipment availability (eg, type of shoe, types of strength training and cardiovascular equipment)
   b. Facility availability (eg, rehabilitation clinic, health club, home program)
   c. Types of terrain (eg, track, sand, gravel, grass)
5. Environmental factors
   a. Air pollution (eg, ozone, sulfur dioxide, carbon monoxide, lead)
   b. Climate (eg, temperature, humidity, barometric pressure, precipitation, sunshine, cloudiness, wind)
   c. Geographic location (eg, mountains, plains, desert, ocean)
   d. Altitude
   e. Allergens (eg, pollens)
6. Ergogenic factors
   a. Mechanical aids (eg, sport-specific specialty clothing, sport-specific specialty equipment, weight lifting belt)
   b. Nutritional aids (eg, protein supplements, carbohydrate loading)
   c. Pharmacological aids (eg, anabolic steroids, amphetamines)

      d. Physiological aids (eg, blood doping, oxygen rebreathing, alkaline salts)

      e. Psychological aids (eg, visualization, hypnosis)

      f. Restorational aids (eg, whirlpool therapy)

  7. Ergolytic factors
   - a. Alcohol
   - b. Tobacco
   - c. Marijuana
   - d. Cocaine

  8. Nutritional factors
   - a. Nutrient deficiencies (ie, vitamin, mineral, protein, carbohydrate, fat, water)
   - b. Food poisoning

  9. Anatomical factors
   - a. Body type (eg, ectomorph, mesomorph, endomorph)
   - b. Body frame size (eg, large, medium, small)
   - c. Unique body characteristics (eg, deformities, limb length inequality)

 10. Physiological factors
   - a. Current fitness level (eg, strength, cardiovascular, flexibility, range of motion, etc)
   - b. Current and previous injuries
   - c. Training system utilized
   - d. Length of sleep
   - e. Muscular soreness (ie, acute onset and delayed onset soreness, muscle stiffness, muscle cramps)

 11. Psychological factors
   - a. Work-related stress
   - b. Family-related stress
   - c. Sports competition–related stress
   - d. Client's motivational levels

Components of Conditioning and Training

The following lists components of conditioning and training programs:

1. General components
   - a. Flexibility
   - b. General muscular strength
   - c. General muscular endurance
   - d. General cardiovascular endurance
2. Specific components
   - a. Skill- or task-specific muscular strength
   - b. Skill- or task-specific muscular endurance
   - c. Skill- or task-specific cardiovascular endurance
   - d. Power
   - e. Speed
   - f. Agility
   - g. Balance
   - h. Sport-specific skill
   - i. Work-specific task

Components of Rehabilitation

The following lists the components of physical rehabilitation programs:

MEDICAL INTERVENTIONS

1. Medical evaluation and consultation
2. Medications
3. Surgery

THERAPEUTIC INTERVENTIONS[11]

1. Exercise therapy
   a. Passive exercise
   b. Active-assistive exercise
   c. Active exercise
   d. Resistive exercise
      (1) Manual
      (2) Isometric
      (3) Isotonic
      (4) Isokinetic
2. Manual therapy
   a. Joint mobilization
   b. Joint manipulation
   c. Stretching
   d. Range of motion
   e. Muscle energy technique
3. Modality therapy
   a. Cold
      (1) Ice packs
      (2) Gel packs
      (3) Ice massage
      (4) Ethyl chloride spray
   b. Heat
      (1) Moist heat packs
      (2) Infrared
      (3) Hydrotherapy
      (4) Shortwave diathermy
      (5) Microwave diathermy
      (6) Ultrasound
   c. Electrotherapeutic
      (1) Electrical stimulation (alternating or direct current)
      (2) TENS (transcutaneous electrical nerve stimulation)
      (3) MENS (microcurrent electrical neural stimulation)
   d. Traction
      (1) Manual
      (2) Motorized
   e. Massage (eg, effleurage, pétrissage, friction)
4. Stress therapy
   a. EMG biofeedback
   b. Relaxation techniques
   c. Stress management
   d. Visualization
5. Educational therapy
   a. Back school

Principles of Conditioning and Rehabilitation

The following outlines the principles of conditioning and rehabilitation:

1. Overload principle
2. Specificity principle
   a. Energy source specificity
   b. Contraction specificity
   c. Muscle group specificity
   d. Speed specificity
3. Reversibility principle
4. Individual differences principle

TABLE 2–1. PRE-EXERCISE GUIDELINES AND INSTRUCTIONS FOR EXERCISE PRESCRIPTION AND REHABILITATION[1,6,8,10]

1. The exercise area should be between 4 to 24°C (40 to 70°F) and below 65% relative humidity.
2. Encourage the client to:
   a. Eat approximately 2 hours before and after an exercise session.
   b. Not smoke or use tobacco products for a minimum of 2 hours before an exercise session. If possible, encourage the client to quit smoking and using tobacco products altogether.
   c. Report any unusual signs or symptoms experienced before, during, or after exercise.
   d. Not withhold any pertinent medical history from the clinical staff.
   e. Eat a variety of nutritious foods (eg, meats, fruits, vegetables, dairy products, whole grains, nuts, water).
   f. Obtain ample sleep (ie, 7 to 9 hours nightly) for optimal training effects.

GENERAL GUIDELINES AND CONTRAINDICATIONS TO EXERCISE PRESCRIPTION AND REHABILITATION

Table 2–1 outlines pre-exercise guidelines and instructions, and Table 2–2 describes various guidelines and contraindications for exercise prescription and rehabilitation.

GUIDELINES AND STANDARDS FOR EXERCISE SAFETY

For specific procedural and equipment safety guidelines during exercise, the clinician may utilize many of the principles in the Guidelines and Standards for Testing Safety section of Chapter 1.

Training Safety Guidelines
The following are general training safety guidelines to consider:

1. The client should be instructed to lift and exercise recognizing sound biomechanical principles.
2. The client should be instructed to avoid uncontrolled and rapid movement patterns during exercise (unless it is inherent to a sport-related skill or work-related task).
3. The client should be "spotted" when performing exercises near his or her maximal lifting capacity.[9]

TABLE 2–2. GUIDELINES AND CONTRAINDICATIONS FOR EXERCISE PRESCRIPTION AND REHABILITATION[1,8,10]

1. The clinician should observe all pre-established exercise prescription and rehabilitation standards, guidelines, absolute contraindications, relative contraindications, and indications for stopping exercise and rehabilitation programs (eg, see Chapter 5).
2. Reschedule or modify the exercise session if the following conditions exist:
   a. The equipment is not functioning properly.
   b. The client is suspected to be under the influence of alcohol or other nonprescription drugs (eg, cocaine, marijuana).
   c. The client appears to be or states having an adverse reaction to any prescribed medications.
3. Consider rescheduling or modifying the exercise session if the following conditions exist:
   a. The client varied his or her prescribed medications (eg, high blood pressure medication) before testing procedures without the clearance of a physician.
   b. The client did not wear the appropriate shoes or clothing (eg, soft-soled shoes, socks, shirt, shorts, and sweat jacket and pants, as appropriate). Encourage the client to wear and utilize appropriate clothing and equipment for exercising in various environmental conditions (eg, heat, cold, rain, hilly terrain).
   c. The client did not fast for at least 2 hours before the test.
   d. The client donated blood within 24 hours of the test.
   e. The client engaged in excessive physical activity on testing day.
   f. The client is having a severe allergic response (eg, pollens).
   g. The client is ill.
   h. The client appears to be or states having extreme emotional distress.

4. Conditioning and rehabilitation equipment should be spaced far enough apart to prevent restricted movement patterns.
5. The conditioning and rehabilitation area should be kept free of unnecessary equipment and objects that may cause obstructions.
6. The client should consult with the clinical staff before attempting to perform new or additional exercises, modify the exercise program, or go beyond the exercise prescription parameters (ie, intensity, frequency, duration).
7. The client should warm up and stretch for approximately 5 to 10 minutes before starting an exercise session.
8. The client should cool down and stretch for approximately 5 to 10 minutes after completing an exercise session.
9. The client should avoid holding his or her breath during lifting (ie, Valsalva's maneuver).
10. The client should exercise in a slow, smooth, and controlled manner, thus avoiding quick, and "jerky" motions.
11. The client should not use a sauna, steam bath, or whirlpool and should not take an extremely hot shower immediately (ie, within 5 to 10 minutes) after an exercise session.
12. The client should not exercise when feeling excessively fatigued or sore.
13. The client should not exercise when feeling ill.
14. The client should train with a partner for safety and motivation, if appropriate.
15. The clinical staff should monitor each client for signs of overtraining (eg, nausea after exercise, chronic fatigue, sleeplessness, joint pain, fainting, inability to finish the exercise program).

REFERENCES

1. American College of Sports Medicine. *Guidelines for Exercise Testing and Prescription*. 4th ed. Philadelphia, Pa: Lea & Febiger; 1991.
2. Barnard RJ, Gardner GW, Diaco NV, et al. Cardiovascular responses to sudden strenuous exercise—heart rate, blood pressure and ECG. *J Appl Physiol*. 1973;34:833–837.
3. Dimsdale JE, Hartley LH, Guiney T, et al. Postexercise peril: Plasma catecholamines and exercise. *JAMA*. 1984;251:630–632.
4. Eichner ER. Ergolytic drugs. *Sports Sci Exchange* (Chicago, Ill: Gatorade Sports Science Institute). 1989;2(15):1–5.
5. Eichner ER. Ergolytic drugs. *Int Med Specialist*. 1990;11(1):74–80.
6. Fardy PS, Yanowitz FG, Wilson PK. *Cardiac Rehabilitation, Adult Fitness and Exercise Testing*. 2nd ed. Philadelphia, Pa: Lea & Febiger; 1988.
7. Foster C, Dymond DS, Carpenter J, et al. Effect of warm-up on left ventricular response to sudden strenuous exercise. *J Appl Physiol*. 1982;53:380.
8. Franklin BA, Gordon S, Timmis GC. *Exercise in Modern Medicine*. Baltimore, Md: Williams & Wilkins; 1989.
9. Halling D. Safety considerations: Spotting. *Nat Strength Condit Assoc J*. 1991;13(2):54–55.
10. Hellerstein HK, Franklin BA. Exercise testing and prescription. In: Wenger NK, Hellerstein HK, eds. *Rehabilitation of the Coronary Patient*. 2nd ed. New York, NY: John Wiley & Sons, Inc; 1984.
11. Kaplan PE, Tanner ED. *Musculoskeletal Pain and Disability*. Norwalk, Conn: Appleton & Lange; 1989.
12. Shellock FG. Physiological benefits of warm-up. *Physician Sportsmed*. 1983;11(10): 134–139.
13. Shellock FG. Physiological, psychological, and injury prevention aspects of warm-up. *Nat Strength Condit Assoc J*. 1986;8(5):24–27.
14. Shellock FG, Prentice WE. Warming-up and stretching for improved physical performance and prevention of sports-related injuries. *Sports Med*. 1985;2:267–278.
15. Torg JS, Welsh RP, Shephard RJ. *Current Therapy in Sports Medicine*. Philadelphia, Pa: BC Decker, Inc; 1990;2.
16. Williams MH. *Beyond Training: How Athletes Enhance Performance Legally and Illegally*. Champaign, Ill: Human Kinetics Publishers, Inc; 1989.

Section Two 2

Clinical Guidelines for Exercise Testing

Chapter Three 3

Flexibility and Range of Motion Testing

METHODS OF TESTING

Goniometric Measurement Principles

Introduction

1. Measurements may be taken passively or actively.
2. A goniometer is ideal for measuring extremity range of motion but may also be used for measuring hip and trunk range of motion.

Equipment

1. Universal goniometers (plastic or metal), which may be either a full-circle (0 to 360 degrees) or half-circle (0 to 180 degrees) protractor with two arms. The one arm is called a stationary arm and is fixed during the measurement; the other arm is called a moving arm and is adjustable during the measurement.

Test Administration

1. For specific techniques of joint range-of-motion measurement, the clinician should refer to established guidelines.[2,5,8-11,32,34]
2. Record range of motion in degrees.

Special Considerations

1. To obtain accurate range-of-motion measurements, proper positioning of the client and goniometer is essential.
2. Describe or demonstrate the test procedure to the client to increase the accuracy of the measurement.[32]
3. The client should be instructed to remove clothing that restricts full range of motion. The clinician should properly drape the client for modesty and comfort, if necessary.[32]

19

4. Measurement procedures should be planned in advance to reduce unnecessary patient positioning. A proper sequencing may be as follows:

$$supine \rightarrow prone \rightarrow sitting \rightarrow standing$$

5. Extremities should be measured bilaterally to utilize the noninvolved extremity as a baseline measure for the client.

Fluid-filled Inclinometer Measurement Principles

Introduction

1. Measurements may be taken passively or actively.
2. The fluid-filled inclinometer is ideal for measuring spinal range of motion but may also be used for measuring extremity range of motion.

Equipment

1. Hand-held, fluid-filled inclinometer

Test Administration

1. For specific techniques of joint range-of-motion measurement, the clinician should refer to established guidelines.[9,22,29,30]
2. Record range of motion in degrees.

Special Considerations

1. To obtain accurate range of motion measurements, proper positioning of the client and inclinometer is essential.
2. Describe or demonstrate the test procedure to the client to increase the accuracy of the measurement.[32]
3. The client should be instructed to remove clothing that restricts full range of motion. The clinician should properly drape the client for modesty and comfort, if necessary.[32]
4. Measurement procedures should be planned in advance to reduce unnecessary patient positioning. A proper sequencing may be as follows:

$$supine \rightarrow prone \rightarrow sitting \rightarrow standing$$

5. Extremities should be measured bilaterally to utilize the noninvolved extremity as a baseline measure for the client.

Tape or Ruler Measurement Principles

Introduction

1. Measurements are most often taken actively.
2. A tape or ruler may be used for measuring spinal range of motion.

Equipment

1. Tape measure, constructed out of a nonstretchable material
2. Ruler

Test Administration

1. For specific techniques of joint range-of-motion measurement, the clinician should refer to established guidelines.[5,30,32]
2. Record range of motion in inches or centimeters.

Special Considerations

1. To obtain accurate range-of-motion measurements, proper positioning of the client and tape measure or ruler is essential.
2. Describe or demonstrate the test procedure to the client to increase the accuracy of the measurement.[32]

3. The client should be instructed to remove clothing that restricts full range of motion. The clinician should properly drape the client for modesty and comfort, if necessary.[32]

4. Measurement procedures should be planned in advance to reduce unnecessary patient positioning. A proper sequencing may be as follows:

$$supine \rightarrow prone \rightarrow sitting \rightarrow standing$$

Leighton Flexometer Measurement Principles

Introduction

1. Measurements may be taken passively or actively.
2. The Leighton flexometer may be used for measuring extremity range of motion but may also be used for measuring hip and trunk range of motion.

Equipment

1. Leighton flexometer (a gravity-type goniometer, that consists of a weighted, 360-degree dial and a weighted pointer mounted in a case) [27,33]

Test Administration

1. For specific techniques of joint range-of-motion measurement, the clinician should refer to established guidelines.[16,25-27,38]
2. Record range of motion in degrees.

Special Considerations

1. To obtain accurate range-of-motion measurements, proper positioning of the client and flexometer is essential.
2. Describe or demonstrate the test procedure to the client to increase the accuracy of the measurement.[32]
3. The client should be instructed to remove clothing that restricts full range of motion. The clinician should properly drape the client for modesty and comfort, if necessary.[32]
4. Measurement procedures should be planned in advance to reduce unnecessary patient positioning. A proper sequencing may be as follows:

$$supine \rightarrow prone \rightarrow sitting \rightarrow standing$$

5. Extremities should be measured bilaterally to utilize the noninvolved extremity as a baseline measure for the client.

Electrogoniometric Measurement Principles

Introduction

1. The electrogoniometer has a potentiometer (a device that provides an electrical signal proportional to the angle of the joint) that can give continuous recordings of the degrees of rotation of a joint being tested.[1,12,20,21]
2. The electrogoniometer may provide accurate and realistic measurements of functional flexibility during physical activity.[12]

Flexomeasure, Ruler, or Sliding Caliper Measurement Principles

Introduction

1. Measurements are most often taken actively.
2. The flexomeasure, ruler, or sliding caliper may be used for measuring hip and trunk range of motion but may also be used for extremity range of motion.

Equipment

1. Flexomeasure, ruler, or sliding caliper

Test Administration

1. Field tests, such as trunk flexion (ie, sit and reach), trunk extension, shoulder elevation, shoulder rotation, ankle extension, and ankle flexion, may be used to measure joint range of motion and flexibility. The clinician should refer to established guidelines for specific techniques of measurement.[6,12,14,17,18,24,31,35,40]
2. Record range of motion in inches or centimeters.

Special Considerations

1. To obtain accurate range-of-motion measurements, proper positioning of the client and flexomeasure, ruler, or sliding caliper is essential.
2. Describe or demonstrate the test procedure to the client to increase the accuracy of the measurement.[32]
3. The client should be instructed to remove clothing that restricts full range of motion. The clinician should properly drape the client for modesty and comfort, if necessary.[32]
4. Measurement procedures should be planned in advance to reduce unnecessary patient positioning. A proper sequencing may be as follows:

$$supine \rightarrow prone \rightarrow sitting \rightarrow standing$$

5. Measurement techniques with the flexomeasure, ruler, or sliding caliper have been criticized because the results may be influenced by the lengths and widths of body segments.[33,39]

Manual Clinical Test Principles

Introduction

1. Manual clinical tests, such as Ely's test (measuring rectus femoris tightness), Ober's test (measuring tensor fasciae latae tightness), Thomas test (measuring iliopsoas tightness), piriformis tightness test, hamstring tightness test, gastrocnemius/soleus tightness test, pectoralis minor tightness test, latissimus dorsi tightness test, and straight leg raise test, may be used to measure muscle tightness, flexibility, and range of motion. For specific techniques of measurement, the clinician should refer to established guidelines.[15,23,28]
2. Manual clinical tests, such as cervical anterior and posterior glide and medial and lateral displacement of the patella, may be used to measure joint play movements. For specific techniques of measurement, the clinician should refer to established guidelines.[7,19,28]
3. This test is ideal for measuring specific muscle tightness.

Additional Measurement Methods

1. Flexicurve[3,4,30]
2. Hand-held computerized device[30]
3. Optical methods[30,37]
4. Spondylometer[30]
5. Stereoradiography[30,36]
6. Three-dimensional digitizer[30]
7. Vector stereography[13,30]

CLASSIFYING AND REPORTING

Table 3–1 presents one type of classification system for identifying normal joint range of motion; others are also available for clinical use.[2,5,10,11,15,16,23,28,32,34] Figure 3–1 may be used for recording joint range of motion, muscle tightness, and flexibility status during testing procedures.

TABLE 3–1. JOINT RANGE-OF-MOTION CLASSIFICATIONS

Joint	Motion	Normal Ranges (degrees)
Cervical[a]	Flexion	0–60
	Extension	0–75
	Lateral flexion	0–45
	Rotation[b]	0–80
Shoulder	Flexion	0–180
	Extension	0–50
	Abduction	0–180
	Adduction	0–50
	Internal rotation[c]	0–90
	External rotation[c]	0–90
Elbow	Flexion	0–140
Radioulnar	Supination	0–80
	Pronation	0–80
Wrist	Flexion	0–60
	Extension	0–60
	Ulnar deviation	0–30
	Radial deviation	0–20
Thoracic[a]	Flexion	0–50
	Rotation	0–30
Lumbar[a]	Flexion	0–60+
	Extension	0–25
	Lateral flexion	0–25
Hip	Flexion	0–100
	Extension	0–30
	Abduction	0–40
	Adduction	0–20
	Internal rotation[d]	0–40
	External rotation[d]	0–50
Knee	Flexion	0–150
Ankle	Dorsiflexion	0–20
	Plantar flexion	0–40
Subtalar	Inversion	0–30
	Eversion	0–20
Metatarsophalangeal	Great toe dorsiflexion	0–50
	Great toe plantar flexion	0–30

[a]Measurements obtained with an inclinometer (sometimes called a gravity inclinometer, pendulum goniometer, or bubble goniometer).
[b]Measurements obtained with the client in a supine position and the head in a neutral position. Consider the client's nose pointing to the ceiling as the neutral position (0 degrees).
[c]Measurements obtained with the shoulder in 90 degrees of abduction.
[d]Measurements obtained with the client in a supine position and the foot in a neutral position. Consider the client's foot pointing to the ceiling as the neutral position (0 degrees).
Adapted from Engelberg AL, ed. Guides to the Evaluation of Permanent Impairment. 3rd ed (revised). Chicago, Ill: American Medical Association; 1990.

NAME: _____ DATE: _____

AGE: _____ SEX: M F HEIGHT: _____ in _____ cm WEIGHT: _____ lb _____ kg

RANGE OF MOTION

	Right	Left			Right	Left
CERVICAL SPINE			**KNEE**			
Flexion	____		Flexion		____	____
Extension	____		**ANKLE**			
Lateral flexion	____	____	Dorsiflexion		____	____
Rotation	____	____	Plantarflexion		____	____
LUMBAR SPINE			Inversion		____	____
Flexion	____		Eversion		____	
Extension	____		**ADDITIONAL**			
Lateral flexion	____	____	Straight leg raise		____	____
Rotation	____	____				

SHOULDER

	Right	Left
Flexion	____	____
Extension	____	____
Abduction	____	____
Internal rotation	____	____
External rotation	____	____

ELBOW

	Right	Left
Flexion	____	____

FOREARM

	Right	Left
Supination	____	____
Pronation	____	____

WRIST

	Right	Left
Flexion	____	____
Extension	____	____
Ulnar deviation	____	____
Radial deviation	____	____

HIP

	Right	Left
Flexion	____	____
Extension	____	____
Abduction	____	____
Internal rotation	____	____
External rotation	____	____

FLEXIBILITY

CLINICAL TESTS

	Right	Left
Thomas test (iliopsoas)	____	____
Ely's test (rectus femoris)	____	____
Ober's test (iliotibial band)	____	____
Hamstring tightness test	____	____
Piriformis tightness test	____	____
Gastrocnemius/soleus tightness test	____	____
Pectoralis minor tightness test	____	____
Latissimus dorsi tightness test	____	____

FIELD TESTS

Sit and reach test	____
Shoulder elevation test	____
Shoulder rotation test	____
Trunk extension test	____
Ankle flexion test	____
Ankle extension test	____

COMMENTS:

_____

_____

24 **Figure 3–1.** Sample data sheet for range of motion, muscle tightness, and flexibility measures.

REFERENCES

1. Adrian MJ. An introduction to electrogoniometry. In: O'Connell AL, ed. *Kinesiology Review*. Washington, DC: American Alliance for Health, Physical Education, Recreation and Dance; 1968.
2. American Academy of Orthopaedic Surgeons. *Joint Motion: Method of Measuring and Recording*. Park Ridge, Ill: American Academy of Orthopaedic Surgeons; 1965.
3. Anderson J, Sweetman B. A combined flexi-rule/hydrogoniometer for measurement of lumbar spine and its sagittal movement. *Rheumatol Rehab*. 1975;14:173–179.
4. Burton A. Regional lumbar sagittal mobility: Measurement of flexicurves. *Clin Biomech*. 1986;1:20–26.
5. Clarkson HM, Gilewich GB. *Musculoskeletal Assessment: Joint Range of Motion and Manual Muscle Strength*. Baltimore, Md: Williams & Wilkins; 1989.
6. Cureton TK. Flexibility as an aspect of fitness. *Res Q*. 1941;12:381–391.
7. Donatelli R, Wooden MJ, eds. *Orthopaedic Physical Therapy*. New York, NY: Churchill Livingstone; 1989.
8. Ekstrand J, Wiktorsson M, Oberg B, et al. Lower extremity goniometric measurements: A study to determine their reliability. *Arch Phys Med Rehabil*. 1982;63.171–175.
9. Engelberg AL, ed. *Guides to the Evaluation of Permanent Impairment*. 3rd ed (revised). Chicago, Ill: American Medical Association; 1990.
10. Esch D, Lepley M. *Evaluation of Joint Motion: Methods of Measuring and Recording*. Minneapolis, Minn: University of Minnesota Press; 1974.
11. Gerhardt J, Russe O. *International SFTR Method of Measuring and Recording Joint Motion*. Bern, Switzerland: Hans Huber Publishers; 1975.
12. Gettman LR. Fitness testing. In: Blair SN, Painter P, Pate RR, et al, eds. *Resource Manual for Guidelines for Exercise Testing and Prescription (American College of Sports Medicine)*. Philadelphia, Pa: Lea & Febiger; 1988.
13. Grew N, Harris J. A method of measuring human body shape and movement—The "vector stereograph." *Engineering Med*. 1979;8:115–118.
14. Heyward VH. *Advanced Fitness Assessment and Exercise Prescription*. 2nd ed. Champaign, Ill: Human Kinetics Publishers, Inc; 1991.
15. Hoppenfeld S. *Physical Examination of the Spine and Extremities*. Norwalk, Conn: Appleton-Century-Crofts; 1976.
16. Hubley-Kozey CL. Testing flexibility. In: MacDougall JD, Wenger HA, Green HJ, eds. *Physiological Testing of the High-Performance Athlete*. 2nd ed. Champaign, Ill: Human Kinetics Publishers, Inc; 1991.
17. Johnson BL. *Practical Flexibility Measurements with the Flexomeasure*. Portland, Tex: Brown and Littleman Co; 1977.
18. Johnson BL, Nelson JK. *Practical Measurements for Evaluation in Physical Education*. 4th ed. New York, NY: Macmillan Publishing Co; 1986.
19. Kaltenborn FM. *Mobilization of the Extremity Joints: Examination and Basic Treatment Techniques*. Oslo, Norway: Olaf Norlis Bokhandel; 1980.
20. Karpovich PV, Karpovich GP. Electrogoniometer: A new device for study of joints in action. *Fed Proc*. 1959;18:79.
21. Karpovich PV, Sinning WE. *Physiology of Muscular Activity*. Philadelphia, Pa: WB Saunders Co; 1971.
22. Keeley J, Mayer T, Cox R, et al. Quantification of lumbar function—Part 5: Reliability of range of motion measures in the sagittal plane and in in vivo torso rotation measurement technique. *Spine*. 1986;11:31–35.
23. Kendall FP, McCreary EK. *Muscles: Testing and Function*. 3rd ed. Baltimore, Md: Williams & Wilkins; 1983.
24. Leger L, Cantin F. Equivalences between the Wells and Dillon and the Cureton hip flexion tests. *Can Assoc Health, Physical Education, Recreation J*. 1983;50:10–12.
25. Leighton JR. An instrument and technique for the measurement of range of joint motion. *Arch Phys Med Rehabil*. 1955;36:571–578.
26. Leighton JR. The Leighton flexometer and flexibility test. *J Assoc Phys Ment Rehabil*. 1966;20:86–93.
27. Leighton JR. *Manual of Instruction for Leighton Flexometer*. Spokane, Wash: Jack R Leighton; 1987.
28. Magee DJ. *Orthopedic Physical Assessment*. 2nd ed. Philadelphia, Pa: WB Saunders Co; 1992.

29. Mayer T, Tencer A, Kristofferson S, et al. Use of noninvasive techniques for quantification of spinal range of motion in normal subjects and chronic low-back dysfunction patients. *Spine*. 1984;9:588–595.
30. Mayer TG, Gatchel RJ. *Functional Restoration for Spinal Disorders: The Sports Medicine Approach*. Philadelphia, Pa: Lea & Febiger; 1988.
31. Miller DK. *Measurement by the Physical Educator: Why and How*. Carmel, Ind: Benchmark Press; 1988.
32. Minor MAD, Minor SD. *Patient Evaluation Methods for the Health Professional*. Reston, Va: Reston Publishing Company, Inc (A Prentice-Hall Company); 1985.
33. Moffatt RJ. Strength and flexibility considerations for exercise prescription. In: Blair SN, Painter P, Pate RR, et al, eds. *Resource Manual for Guidelines for Exercise Testing and Prescription* (American College of Sports Medicine). Philadelphia, Pa: Lea & Febiger; 1988.
34. Norkin CC, White DJ. *Measurement of Joint Motion: A Guide to Goniometry*. Philadelphia, Pa: FA Davis Co; 1985.
35. Pollock ML, Wilmore JH. *Exercise in Health and Disease: Evaluation and Prescription for Prevention and Rehabilitation*. 2nd ed. Philadelphia, Pa: WB Saunders Co; 1990.
36. Seligman J, Gertzbein S, Tile M, et al. Computer analysis of spinal segment motion in degenerative disk disease with and without axial loading. *Spine*. 1984;9:566–573.
37. Thurston A, Harris G. Normal kinematics of the lumbar spine and pelvis. *Spine*. 1983;8:199–205.
38. Verducci FM. *Measurement Concepts in Physical Education*. St Louis, Mo: CV Mosby Co; 1980.
39. Wear CL. Relationship of flexibility measurements to length of body segments. *Res Q*. 1963;34:234–238.
40. Wells KF, Dillon EK. The sit and reach: A test of back and leg flexibility. *Res Q*. 1952;23:115–118.

Muscular Strength and Endurance Testing

METHODS OF TESTING

ACTIVITIES OF DAILY LIVING ASSESSMENT

Activities of Daily Living (ADL) Assessment Principles

Introduction

1. An activities of daily living (ADL) assessment is not specifically classified as strength testing. However, ADLs do represent important strength components and therefore may be used for assessing functional activities of daily living such as maneuvering from supine to sitting or from sitting to standing, climbing stairs, propelling a wheelchair, dressing, feeding, and personal hygiene.[4]
2. ADL questionnaires and rating forms have been established by clinicians for ease of assessment.[4,26,38,39,42,47,48,60,68]

LOW-LEVEL FUNCTIONAL TESTING

Low-level Functional Test Principles

Introduction

1. When specific patterns of difficulty are demonstrated during an ADL assessment (eg, stair climbing), a specific functional test (eg, step test) may be used to quantify strength and weakness relationships in specific muscles.[4]
2. Specific functional testing parameters (eg, step test, wheelchair push-ups) have been established by various clinicians.[4,22,58]

HIGH-LEVEL FUNCTIONAL TESTING

Isoinertial Test Procedures[44,51]

Name of Test
Progressive Isoinertial Lifting Evaluation (PILE)

Introduction

1. Isoinertial tests are ideal for assessing a worker's functional lifting ability.

Equipment

1. Sturdy plastic box
2. Free weights (in 5- and 10-lb increments)
3. Heart rate monitor
4. Stopwatch

Test Administration

Mayer and Gatchel[52] describe the test procedures for Progressive Isoinertial Lifting Evaluation (PILE) as follows:

1. The client should warm up the cardiovascular and muscular systems and perform specific trunk and leg stretches prior to testing.
2. Lifting is performed with a plastic box.
3. Women begin with a 5-lb load and increase in 5-lb increments whereas men begin with a 10-lb load and increase in 10-lb increments.
4. Weights are added every 20 seconds with a rate of four lifting movements during each 20-second interval.
5. A lifting movement involves the lifting of the weighted plastic box from one of the following heights:
   a. Floor to waist (0 to 30 in)
   b. Waist to shoulder (30 to 54 in)
6. For example, in the floor-to-waist–height lifting test, the client progressively lifts the box from floor to waist level for the previously identified test parameters (ie, four lifts during a 20-second interval) until one of the following end-points is reached:
   a. The client terminates the test secondary to complaints of fatigue or excessive pain (psychophysical end-point).
   b. The client attains a predetermined exercise end-point intensity, which is a specific intensity that can vary between 65% to 85% of age-predicted maximal heart rate (aerobic end-point).
   c. The client attains a predetermined "safe limit" of 45% to 55% of body weight (safety end-point).
7. Results of the test may be expressed as follows:
   a. Maximum weight lifted
   b. Total duration during each stage
   c. Total duration of the test
   d. Final heart rate attained at the completion of the test

ISOMETRIC (STATIC) TESTING

Manual Muscle Test Principles

Introduction

1. Several clinicians have presented techniques and procedures for measuring muscle strength with manual muscle testing.[19,20,24,33,37,43,45,49]
2. Manual muscle testing may be performed by utilizing make tests or break tests or by applying resistance throughout the range of motion.[11,24]

3. Advantages include the following[30]:
   a. Test is easy to perform after the requisite skill has been developed.
   b. Test provides ability to test small muscles or groups of muscles.
   c. Clinically, the muscles of almost any client may be tested manually.
4. Disadvantages include the following[30]:
   a. Subjectivity plays a role in data interpretation.
   b. Test assesses less than full range of motion.
   c. Test does not address variables such as velocity, power, and endurance.
5. Test is ideal for assessing muscle strength in a short period of time without equipment.

Hand-held Dynamometry Test Principles

Introduction

1. Hand-held dynamometers are held in the hand of the clinician during muscle strength testing and may be spring or strain-gauge based.[11]
2. Hand-held dynamometry may be performed by using either make tests or break tests.[11]
3. Specific test procedures have been established by various clinicians.[2,11-13,65,66]
4. These instruments are ideal for assessing and quantifying muscle strength with the use of minimal equipment.

Dynamometry Test Principles

Introduction

1. Dynamometry is ideal for assessing muscular strength and muscular endurance of the hand, back, and leg.

Equipment

1. Hand-grip or back-leg-lift dynamometer

Test Administration

1. Specific grip-, back-, and leg-strength norms have been established by various clinicians.[1,21,50]

Special Considerations

1. Advantages include the following[11]:
   a. Portable
   b. Relatively easy to use
   c. Relatively safe

Calisthenic-type Exercise Test Principles

Introduction

1. These exercises may be used for assessing the muscular endurance through the use of calisthenic activities.
2. Specific testing procedures (eg, timed flexed arm hang from a pull-up bar) have been established by various clinicians.[35,56,61]

Cable Tensiometry Test Principles

Introduction

1. Cable tensiometry may be used for assessing muscular strength at specific angles in the range of motion.

Equipment

1. Cable tensiometer

Test Administration

1. For specific techniques of assessing various muscle groups throughout the body, the clinician should refer to established guidelines.[15-17]
2. Specific norms for males and females, 9 years old through college age, have been established by various clinicians.[14,18]

Special Considerations

1. Advantages include the following[41]:
   a. Lightweight
   b. Portable
   c. Relatively easy to use
   d. Relatively safe
   e. May be used for measuring virtually all angles in the range of motion of a specific joint
2. A disadvantage of cable tensiometry is that it is not sensitive for measuring low forces.[3]

Machine Test Principles

Introduction

1. The machine test may be used for assessing isometric strength and fatigue through various computerized machines (eg, Ariel, Biodex, Cybex, Kin-Com, Lido, Merac) and others.[3]

Additional Isometric Test Methods

1. Rate of force development[64]
2. Rate of relaxation[64]
3. Strength[64]

Table 4-1 outlines various advantages and disadvantages of isometric testing.

ISOTONIC (DYNAMIC) TESTING

Maximum Muscle Strength Test Principles

Introduction

1. This test may be used for assessing muscular strength.

TABLE 4–1. ADVANTAGES AND DISADVANTAGES OF ISOMETRIC TESTING

Advantages
1. Involves minimal or no equipment
2. May be performed in the clinic or a field setting
3. Easier to accomplish good stabilization as compared with isotonic and isokinetic testing[3]
4. Produces less systemic fatigue as compared with isotonic and isokinetic testing[3]
5. Preferable when there is the presence of a joint contracture or painful arcs of joint motion[3]
6. Helpful in distinguishing between contractile and noncontractile tissue pathology[3]

Disadvantages
1. May not be specific enough to assess the strength changes from an isotonic or isokinetic program
2. May be difficult to determine an objective measurement of the client's physical effort
3. Cannot evaluate power since the velocity is zero[62]
4. Reflects angle-specific strength
5. Associated with Valsalva's maneuver

Equipment

1. Barbells, dumbbells, exercise machines, or free weights

Test Administration

ABSOLUTE ONE-REPETITION MAXIMUM (1-RM) METHOD[8,10,69]

1. A starting weight is selected below the client's currently known or estimated maximum lifting capacity.
2. If one repetition is completed with proper form, then 1- to 5-kg weight increments may be added until maximum lifting capacity is reached.
3. The client should rest approximately 2 to 3 minutes between each trial.[64]
4. The final weight reached with proper form is the client's new 1-RM for that particular exercise.

RELATIVE ONE-REPETITION MAXIMUM (1-RM) METHOD

1. Testing with barbells, dumbbells, or exercise machines:
   a. A starting weight is selected below the client's currently known or estimated maximum lifting capacity.
   b. If one repetition is completed with proper form, then 1- to 5-kg weight increments may be added until maximum lifting capacity is reached.[41]
   c. The client should rest approximately 2 to 3 minutes between each trial.[64]
   d. The final weight reached with proper form is the client's new 1-RM for that particular exercise and is divided by the client's body weight (for obtaining the strength-to-body-weight ratio). The results are compared to the following established norms:
      (1) College-age men and women (for the bench press, leg press, arm curl, lateral pull-down, leg extension, and leg curl)[32]
      2 Men and women ranging from 20 to 60+ years of age (for the bench press and leg press)[34,36]
2. Testing with calisthenic-type activities:
   a. Weight plates (range from 2½, 5, 10, and 25 lb) are attached to the client for each test (eg, pull-up, dip, sit-up, bench squat). The relative strength score is calculated by taking the additional weight added to the client and dividing this value by the client's body weight.[40]
   b. Specific test protocols and norms have been established by other clinicians.[40,56]

Special Considerations

1. Free-weight plates should be calibrated with an accurate scale and labeled accordingly.
2. Safety stops (ie, bars or pins used to prevent excessive range) should be strategically placed during testing (especially during the bench press and squat) to prevent injuries.[64]
3. Testing should be standardized through the use of positioning, specific joint angles, and lifting form.

Maximum Muscle Endurance Test Principles

Introduction

1. This test may be used for assessing muscular endurance.

Equipment

1. Barbells, dumbbells, exercise machines, or calisthenic-type equipment (eg, for pull-ups)

Test Administration

SET PERCENTAGE OF ONE-REPETITION MAXIMUM (1-RM) METHOD[59]

1. Select a percentage (eg, 70%) of 1-RM value for each exercise being tested.
2. Have the client complete as many repetitions as possible with good form. Specific norms for this method have not yet been established. However, the average individual should be able to complete 12 to 15 repetitions and the competitive athlete, 20 to 25 repetitions at 70% of 1-RM for each of the exercises tested.

SET PERCENTAGE OF BODY WEIGHT METHOD[32]

1. Select a percentage of body weight for each exercise being tested (refer to Table 4-2 for the specific percentages).
2. The client is instructed to complete 15 repetitions (if possible) for each exercise and the results are compared to established norms (for the bench press, leg press, arm curl, lateral pull-down, leg extension, and leg curl) for college-age men and women.[32]

TIMED MAXIMUM REPETITION METHOD

1. Select the appropriate testing parameter. For example, in a 1-minute sit-up test, the client is instructed to perform as many correct sit-ups as possible in a 1-minute period.
2. Results are compared to established norms for men and women ranging from 20 to 60+ years of age[59] and others.[28,56]

MAXIMUM REPETITION METHOD

1. Testing with a barbell:
   a. The YMCA bench press protocol utilizes an 80-lb barbell for men and a 35-lb barbell for women. Clients perform the bench press to a rhythm kept by a metronome (ie, 60 beats per minute). The client's score is the total number of successful repetitions.[28]
   b. Results for the bench press test are compared to established norms.[28]
2. Testing by means of calisthenic-type activities:
   a. Select the appropriate testing parameter. For example, in a push-up test, the client is instructed to perform as many consecutive push-ups as possible, without rest.
   b. Results are compared to established norms for men and women ranging from 20 to 60+ years of age.[59]
   c. Other norms are available for sit-ups, push-ups, modified push-ups, pull-ups, modified pull-ups, dips, and squat thrusts.[6,7,29,40,55,56]

TABLE 4–2. PERCENT BODY WEIGHT TO BE LIFTED FOR VARIOUS EXERCISES

Exercise	Men (%)	Women (%)
Arm curl	33	25
Bench press	66	50
Lateral pull-down	66	50
Triceps extension	33	33
Leg extension	50	50
Leg curl	33	33

From "Assessing Muscular Strength and Endurance" in Advanced Fitness Assessment and Exercise Prescription. 2nd edition. (Table 4.5, p. 109) by Vivian H. Heyward, 1991. Champaign, Ill: Human Kinetics Publishers, Inc. Copyright 1991 by Vivian H. Heyward. Adapted by permission.

Machine Test Principles[64]

Introduction

1. Isotonic testing may be performed on various computerized machines (eg, Ariel, Dynatrac, Kin-Com, Lido, Merac).
2. These machines may be used for testing muscle strength and muscle endurance.

Table 4-3 outlines various advantages and disadvantages of isotonic testing.

ISOKINETIC (ISODYNAMIC) TESTING

Isokinetic Test Procedures

Introduction

1. For specific types of measurements and terms used in reporting isokinetic data, refer to Rothstein, Lamb, and Mayhew.[63] Data generated from isokinetic testing generally provide the following information:
   a. Strength—maximum force generated by muscle contraction through an active range of motion.[27]
   b. Endurance—duration of repetitive exercise until peak force decreases 50%.[27]
   c. Power—force moved through an active range of motion in fixed time (usually tested at greater than 180 degrees per second).[27]
   d. Limb comparison—comparing the injured extremity to the uninjured extremity and reporting the results as a ratio or percentage of deficit.[31]
   e. Ratios—expressing results as ratios for agonist to antagonist muscles or comparing contraction types within the same muscle group (ie, eccentric to concentric torque patterns).[9,31,57]

Equipment

1. Isokinetic dynamometer (eg, Ariel, Biodex, Cybex, Kin-Com, Lido, Merac)[64]

Test Administration

1. For isokinetic testing procedures, interpretations, and norms, refer to specific isokinetic manufacturer manuals[20] and other clinical sources.[75,64]
2. For eccentric isokinetic testing procedures, refer to specific isokinetic manufacturer manuals (eg, Biodex, Kin-Com, Lido) and various clinical sources.[31]

Special Considerations

1. Isokinetic devices range in speeds from 0 to 300 degrees per second, with some devices offering velocities above 400 degrees per second. Since many functional activities and sports may range in speeds from 900 to 2000 degrees per second, the clinician should be cautious when making specific inferences to the function or performance of tested clients.[31,45,46,53,67]

Table 4-4 outlines various advantages and disadvantages of isokinetic testing.

TABLE 4–3. ADVANTAGES AND DISADVANTAGES OF ISOTONIC TESTING

Advantages
1. Provides an objective documentation of results.
2. Easy to perform in a clinical and physical education-type setting.

Disadvantages
1. May require the client to be skilled in a particular movement or activity (eg, bench press).
2. Use of momentum by client during testing may lead to injury and/or inaccurate results.

TABLE 4—4. ADVANTAGES AND DISADVANTAGES OF ISOKINETIC TESTING

Advantages
1. Test provides an objective documentation of results.
2. Shape of torque curves through the active range of motion at selected speeds may assist the clinician in determining if a client is providing consistent force and/or deliberate submaximum efforts.
3. Test assists the clinician in determining strength deficits and/or muscle imbalances.
4. Maximum force can be applied during all phases of the movement (ie, active range of motion) at a constant velocity.[54]
5. Test results are accurate and reproducible.

Disadvantages
1. Test may be time-consuming when testing more than one joint.
2. Test requires on-site calibration system, including weight and time checks.[27]
3. Test may produce significant increases in blood pressure and heart rate.[27]
4. Test depends on the motivational level of a client to exert a maximum effort.[5]
5. Test requires specialized personnel for collecting and interpreting data.[27]
6. Equipment is costly.
7. Learning by the client must take place.

REPORTING

Figure 4-1 may be used for reporting the results of strength testing.

NAME: _____ DATE: _____

AGE: _____ SEX: M   F

HEIGHT: _____ in _____ cm   WEIGHT: _____ lb _____ kg

	Max (lb)	5-RM (lb)	10-RM (lb)
Bench press	_____	_____	_____
Squat	_____	_____	_____
Military press	_____	_____	_____
Bicep curl	_____	_____	_____
Tricep extension	_____	_____	_____
Pull-ups	_____		
Sit-ups	_____		
Push-ups	_____		

GRIP STRENGTH

Hand Dominance: Right _____ Left _____ Bilateral _____

	1	2	3	4	5	
Right hand	_____	_____	_____	_____	_____	(lb)
Left hand	_____	_____	_____	_____	_____	(lb)

COMMENTS:

_____

_____

_____

34   **Figure 4—1.** Sample data sheet for muscular strength and endurance testing.

REFERENCES

1. Adams GM. *Exercise Physiology Laboratory Manual*. Dubuque, Iowa: Wm C Brown Publishers; 1990.
2. Agre JC, Magness JL, Hull SZ, et al. Strength testing with a portable dynamometer: Reliability for upper and lower extremities. *Arch Phys Med Rehabil*. 1987;68:454.
3. Amundsen LR. Isometric muscle strength testing with fixed-load cells. In: Amundsen LR, ed. *Muscle Strength Testing: Instrumented and Non-Instrumented Systems*. New York, NY: Churchill Livingstone; 1990.
4. Amundsen LR. Measurement of muscle strength: An overview of instrumented and non-instrumented systems. In: Amundsen LR, ed. *Muscle Strength Testing: Instrumented and Non-Instrumented Systems*. New York, NY: Churchill Livingstone; 1990.
5. Åstrand P-O, Rodahl K. *Textbook of Work Physiology: Physiological Bases of Exercise*. 3rd ed. New York, NY: McGraw-Hill Book Co; 1986.
6. Baumgartner TA. Modified pull-up test. *Res Q*. 1978;49:80–84.
7. Baumgartner TA, East WB, Frye PA, et al. Equipment improvements and additional norms for the modified pull-up test. *Res Q Exerc Sport*. 1984;55:64–68.
8. Baumgartner TA, Jackson AS. *Measurement for Evaluation in Physical Education and Exercise Science*. 4th ed. Dubuque, Iowa: Wm C Brown Publishers; 1991.
9. Bennett JG, Stauber WT. Evaluation and treatment of anterior knee pain using eccentric exercise. *Med Sci Sports Exerc*. 1986;18:526.
10. Berger RA. *Applied Exercise Physiology*. Philadelphia, Pa: Lea & Febiger; 1982.
11. Bohannon RW. Muscle strength testing with hand-held dynamometers. In: Amundsen LR, ed. *Muscle Strength Testing: Instrumented and Non-Instrumented Systems*. New York, NY: Churchill Livingstone; 1990.
12. Bohannon RW, Saunders N. Hand held dynamometry: A single trial may be adequate when measuring muscle strength in healthy individuals. *Physiotherapy Canada*. 1990;46:6.
13. Byl NN, Richards S, Asturias J. Intrarater and interrater reliability of strength measurements of the biceps and deltoid using a hand-held dynamometer. *J Orthop Sports Phys Ther*. 1988;9:399.
14. Clarke DH. *Exercise Physiology*. Englewood Cliffs, NJ: Prentice-Hall; 1975.
15. Clarke HH. *Cable Tension Strength Tests: A Manual*. Springfield, Mass: Stuart E Murphy; 1953.
16. Clarke HH. *Muscular Strength and Endurance in Man*. Englewood Cliffs, NJ: Prentice-Hall; 1966.
17. Clarke HH, Bailey TL, Shay CT. New objective strength tests of muscle groups by cable-tension methods. *Res Q*. 1952;23:136.
18. Clarke HH, Monroe RA. *Test Manual: Oregon Cable-Tension Strength Test Batteries for Boys and Girls from Fourth Grade to College*. Eugene, Ore: University of Oregon; 1970.
19. Clarkson HM, Gilewich GB. *Musculoskeletal Assessment: Joint Range of Motion and Manual Muscle Strength*. Baltimore, Md: Williams & Wilkins; 1989.
20. Cole JH, Furness AL, Twomey LT. *Muscles in Action: An Approach to Manual Muscle Testing*. New York, NY: Churchill Livingstone; 1988.
21. Corbin CB, Dowell LJ, Lindsey R, et al. *Concepts in Physical Education*. Dubuque, Iowa: Wm C Brown Publishers; 1978.
22. Csuka M, McCarthy DJ. Simple method for measurement of lower extremity muscle strength. *Am J Med*. 1985;78:77.
23. Cybex, A Division of Lumex Inc. *Isolated-Joint Testing and Exercise: A Handbook for Using Cybex II and U.B.X.T.* Ronkonkoma, NY: Cybex, A Division of Lumex Inc; 1983.
24. Daniels L, Worthingham C. *Muscle Testing: Techniques of Manual Examination*. 5th ed. Philadelphia, Pa: WB Saunders Co; 1986.
25. Davies GJ. *A Compendium of Isokinetics in Clinical Usage and Rehabilitation Techniques*. 3rd ed. LaCrosse, Wis: S & S Publishers; 1987.
26. DeSouza L, Hewer R, Lynn P, et al. Assessment of recovery of arms control in hemiplegic stroke patients. 1. Arm function tests. *Int Rehabil Med*. 1980;2:3.
27. Drez D, ed. *Therapeutic Modalities for Sports Injuries*. Chicago, Ill: Year Book Medical Publishers, Inc; 1989.
28. Golding LA, Myers CR, Sinning WE, eds. *Y's Way to Physical Fitness: The Complete Guide to Fitness Testing and Instruction*. 3rd ed. Champaign, Ill: Human Kinetics Publishers, Inc; 1989.
29. Government of Canada. *Fitness and Amateur Sports: Canadian Standardized Test of Fitness Operations Manual*. 3rd ed. Ottawa, Ontario: Minister of State, FAS 73-78; 1986.

30. Guffey JS, Burton BJ. A critical look at muscle testing. *Clin Management*. 1991;11(2):15–19.

31. Hageman PA, Sorensen TA. Eccentric isokinetics. In: Albert M. *Eccentric Muscle Training in Sports and Orthopaedics*. New York, NY: Churchill Livingstone; 1991.

32. Heyward VH. *Advanced Fitness Assessment and Exercise Prescription*. 2nd ed. Champaign, Ill: Human Kinetics Publishers, Inc; 1991.

33. Hoppenfeld S. *Physical Examination of the Spine and Extremities*. Norwalk, Conn: Appleton-Century-Crofts; 1976.

34. Institute for Aerobics Research. *Physical Fitness Norms*. Dallas, Tex: Institute for Aerobics Research; 1985 (unpublished data).

35. Institute for Aerobics Research. *Fitnessgram User's Manual*. Dallas, Tex: Institute for Aerobics Research; 1987.

36. Jackson A, Watkins M, Patton R. A factor analysis of twelve selected maximal isotonic strength performances on the Universal Gym. *Med Sci Sports Exerc*. 1980;12:274–277.

37. Janda V. *Muscle Function Testing*. Boston, Mass: Butterworths; 1983.

38. Jebsen R, Taylor N, Trieschmann R, et al. An objective and standardized test of hand function. *Arch Phys Med Rehabil*. 1965;50:311.

39. Jette AM. State of the art in functional status assessment. In: Rothstein JM, ed. *Measurement in Physical Therapy*. New York, NY: Churchill Livingstone; 1985.

40. Johnson BL, Nelson JK. *Practical Measurement for Evaluation and Physical Education*. 4th ed. Minneapolis, Minn: Burgess Publishing Co; 1986.

41. Katch FI, Katch VL, McArdle WD. Physiologic fitness: The basis of sports medicine. In: Grana WA, Kalenak A, eds. *Clinical Sports Medicine*. Philadelphia, Pa: WB Saunders Co; 1991.

42. Katz S. Assessing self-maintenance: Activities of daily living, mobility and instrumental activities of daily living. *J Am Geriatr Soc*. 1983;31:721.

43. Kendall FP, McCreary EK. *Muscles: Testing and Function*. 3rd ed. Baltimore, Md: Williams & Wilkins; 1983.

44. Kroemer K. An isoinertial technique to assess individual lifting capability. *Hum Factors*. 1983;25:493–506.

45. Lamb RL. Manual muscle testing. In: Rothstein JM, ed. *Measurement in Physical Therapy*. New York, NY: Churchill Livingstone; 1985.

46. Lankhorst GJ, Van de Stadt RJ, Van der Korst JK. The relationships of functional capacity, pain and isometric and isokinetic torque in osteoarthrosis of the knee. *Scand J Rehabil Med*. 1985;17:167.

47. Law M, Letts L. A critical review of scales of activities of daily living. *Am J Occup Ther*. 1989;43:522.

48. Lawton EB. Activities of daily living test: Geriatric considerations. *Phys Occup Ther Geriatrics*. 1980;1:11.

49. Lynch L. Manual muscle strength testing of the distal muscles. In: Amundsen LR, ed. *Muscle Strength Testing: Instrumented and Non-Instrumented Systems*. New York, NY: Churchill Livingstone; 1990.

50. Mathiowetz V. Grip and pinch strength measurements. In: Amundsen LR, ed. *Muscle Strength Testing: Instrumented and Non-Instrumented Systems*. New York, NY: Churchill Livingstone; 1990.

51. Mayer TG, Barnes D, Nichols G, et al. Progressive isoinertial lifting evaluation, II: A comparison with isokinetic lifting in a disabled chronic low-back industrial population. *Spine*. 1988;13:998.

52. Mayer TG, Gatchel RJ. *Functional Restoration for Spinal Disorders: The Sports Medicine Approach*. Philadelphia, PA: Lea & Febiger; 1988.

53. Mayhew TP, Rothstein JM. Measurement of muscle performance with instruments. In: Rothstein JM, ed. *Measurement in Physical Therapy*. New York, NY: Churchill Livingstone; 1985.

54. McArdle WD, Katch FI, Katch VL. *Exercise Physiology: Energy, Nutrition and Human Performance*. 3rd ed. Philadelphia, Pa: Lea & Febiger; 1991.

55. McSwegan P, Pemberton C, Petray C, et al. *Physical Best: The AAHPERD Guide to Physical Fitness Education and Assessment*. Reston, Va: American Alliance for Health, Physical Education, Recreation and Dance; 1989.

56. Miller DK. *Measurement by the Physical Educator: Why and How*. Carmel, Ind: Benchmark Press; 1988.

57. Nosse LJ. Assessment of selected reports on the strength relationship of the knee musculature. *J Orthop Sports Phys Ther*. 1982;4:78.

58. Olaogun M, Abereoje O, Obajuluwa V. Forward upward leading step test for the clinical evaluation of locomotor ability. *Clin Rehabil.* 1989;3:41.
59. Pollock ML, Wilmore JH, Fox SM. *Health and Fitness through Physical Activity.* New York, NY: John Wiley & Sons, Inc; 1978.
60. Porter ML, Stockley I, Purves WK. Functional index: A new objective assessment applicable to wrist fractures. In: Whittle M, Harris D, eds. *Biomechanical Measurement in Orthopaedic Practice.* Oxford, England: Clarendon Press; 1985.
61. President's Council on Physical Fitness and Sports. *The Presidential Physical Fitness Award Program.* Washington, DC: President's Council on Physical Fitness and Sports; 1987.
62. Ross RM, Jackson AS. *Exercise Concepts, Calculations and Computer Applications.* Carmel, Ind: Benchmark Press; 1990.
63. Rothstein JM, Lamb RL, Mayhew TP. Clinical uses of isokinetic measurements: Critical issues. *Phys Ther.* 1988;67;1840.
64. Sale DG. Testing strength and power. In: MacDougall JD, Wenger HA, Green HJ, eds. *Physiological Testing of the High-Performance Athlete.* 2nd ed. Champaign, Ill: Human Kinetics Publishers, Inc; 1991.
65. Smidt GL. *Muscle Strength Testing: A System Based on Mechanics.* Iowa City, Iowa: Spark Instruments and Academics; 1984.
66. Sullivan SJ, Chesley A, Hebert G, et al. The validity and reliability of hand-held dynamometry in assessing isometric external rotator performance. *J Orthop Sports Phys Ther.* 1988;10:213.
67. Thorstensson A, Karlsson J. Fatigability and fibre composition of human skeletal muscle. *Acta Physiol Scand.* 1976;98:318.
68. Wade DT, Collin C. The Barthel ADL index: A standard measure of physical disability? *Int Disabil Stud.* 1988;10:64.
69. Wilk K. Dynamic muscle strength testing. In: Amundsen LR. *Muscle Strength Testing: Instrumented and Non-Instrumented Systems.* New York, NY: Churchill Livingstone; 1990.

Chapter Five

Cardiovascular Endurance Testing

GUIDELINES FOR TESTING

Testing Standards and Guidelines

Rehabilitation facilities need to be cognizant of legal policies and procedures related to exercise testing and prescription.[2,65-67] To reduce the risk of litigation related to negligence, rehabilitation facilities should adhere to standards and guidelines defined by the following professional associations:

1. Aerobics Fitness Association of America[38]
2. American Association of Cardiovascular and Pulmonary Rehabilitation (AACPR)[5]
3. American College of Cardiology (ACC)[6]
4. American College of Sports Medicine (ACSM)[7,29]
5. American Heart Association (AHA)[8-10,12,14,15]
6. American Medical Association (AMA)[16-18]
7. American Physical Therapy Association (APTA)[19]
8. National Council of YMCAs[60]

The following section presents examples of guidelines for exercise testing and participation from the American College of Physicians/American College of Cardiology/American Heart Association and the American College of Sports Medicine.

American College of Physicians/American College of Cardiology/American Heart Association Guidelines and Standards

The American College of Physicians (ACP), the American College of Cardiology (ACC), and the American Heart Association (AHA) identify the minimum education, training, experience, and cognitive and technical skills necessary for the competent performance of cardiovascular exercise testing.[14] The ACP/ACC/AHA guidelines identify the physician as the testing specialist but state that "in selected patients, exercise testing can be safely performed by properly trained nurses,

TABLE 5–1. COGNITIVE SKILLS NEEDED TO PERFORM EXERCISE TESTS COMPETENTLY

1. Knowledge of appropriate indications for exercise testing
2. Knowledge of appropriate contraindications and risks of testing
3. Knowledge to promptly recognize and treat complications of exercise testing
4. Competence in cardiopulmonary resuscitation and successful completion of an AHA-sponsored course in advanced cardiac life support
5. Knowledge of specificity, sensitivity, and diagnostic accuracy of exercise testing in different patient populations
6. Knowledge of how to apply Bayes' theorem to interpret test results
7. Knowledge of various exercise protocols (Bruce, Naughton, Balke-Ware, USAFSAM, etc) and indications for each
8. Knowledge of basic cardiovascular and exercise physiology, including blood pressure and heart rate response to exercise
9. Knowledge of electrocardiography and changes in the electrocardiogram that may result from exercise, hyperventilation, ischemia, hypertrophy, conduction disorders, electrolyte disturbances, and drugs
10. Knowledge of cardiac arrhythmias and treatment of serious arrhythmias
11. Knowledge of cardiovascular drugs and how they affect exercise performance, hemodynamics, and the electrocardiogram
12. Knowledge of conditions and circumstances that can cause false-positive, indeterminate, or false-negative test results
13. Knowledge of the effects of age and disease on hemodynamic and electrocardiographic responses to exercise
14. Knowledge of principles and details of exercise testing, including proper lead placement and skin preparation
15. Knowledge of prognostic value of exercise testing
16. Knowledge of alternative diagnostic procedures to exercise testing
17. Knowledge of end-points of exercise testing and indications to terminate exercise testing
18. Knowledge of the concept of metabolic equivalent (MET) and estimation of exercise intensity in different modes of exercise
19. Ability and commitment to communicate diagnostic accuracy, risks, and results of the test to the patient, the medical record, and other physicians so that appropriately informed patient consent can be obtained

Reprinted with permission from the American Heart Association (AHA). Position Statement: Clinical Competence in Exercise Testing—A Statement for Physicians from the American College of Physicians (ACP)/American College of Cardiology (ACC)/American Heart Association (AHA) Task Force on Clinical Privileges in Cardiology. Circulation. Copyright 1990;82(5):1884–1888. Dallas, Tex: American Heart Association.

exercise physiologists, physical therapists, or medical technicians working directly under the supervision of the physician, who should be in the immediate vicinity and available for emergencies. However, the physician should be present to observe the patient continuously when the test is performed on a patient with severe angina pectoris, possible unstable angina pectoris, or exertional left ventricular dysfunction or arrhythmia."

The ACP/ACC/AHA identifies cognitive skills needed to perform cardiovascular exercise tests competently (see Table 5–1).

American College of Sports Medicine Guidelines

Tables 5–2 to 5–4 identify the American College of Sports Medicine's (ACSM) guidelines for exercise testing and participation.

Test Contraindications

Tables 5–5 and 5–6 outline contraindications to cardiovascular exercise testing.

Test Termination Criteria

Tables 5–7 to 5–9 identify indications for stopping a cardiovascular exercise test.

Test Selection Criteria

Tables 5–10 to 5–12 are not intended to serve as definitive standards for selecting cardiovascular exercise tests. These tables provide general test selection criteria to

TABLE 5–2. GUIDELINES FOR EXERCISE TESTING AND PARTICIPATION

	Apparently Healthy		Higher Risk[a]		With Disease[b]
	Younger ≤ 40 years (men) ≤ 50 years (women)	Older	No symptoms	Symptoms	
Medical exam and diagnostic exercise test recommended prior to:					
Moderate exercise[c]	No[e]	No	No	Yes	Yes
Vigorous exercise[d]	No	Yes[f]	Yes	Yes	Yes
Physician supervision recommended during exercise test:					
Submaximal testing	No	No	No	Yes	Yes
Maximal testing	No	Yes	Yes	Yes	Yes

[a] Persons with two or more risk factors (see Table 5–3) or symptoms (see Table 5–4).

[b] Persons with known cardiac, pulmonary, or metabolic disease.

[c] Moderate exercise (exercise intensity 40% to 60% $\dot{V}O_{2max}$). Exercise intensity well within the individual's current capacity and can be comfortably sustained for a prolonged period of time, ie, 60 minutes, slow progression, and generally noncompetitive.

[d] Vigorous exercise (exercise intensity > 60% $\dot{V}O_{2max}$). Exercise intense enough to represent a substantial challenge and which would ordinarily result in fatigue within 20 minutes.

[e] The "no" responses in this table mean that an item is "not necessary." The "no" response does not mean that the item should not be done.

[f] A "yes" response means that an item is recommended.

Reprinted with permission from the American College of Sports Medicine. Guidelines for Exercise Testing and Prescription. 4th ed. Philadelphia, Pa: Lea & Febiger; 1991:8.

TABLE 5–3. MAJOR CORONARY RISK FACTORS

1. Diagnosed hypertension or systolic blood pressure $\geq$ 160 or diastolic blood pressure $\geq$ 90 mm Hg on at least two separate occasions, or on antihypertensive medication
2. Serum cholesterol $\geq$ 6.20 mmol/L ($\geq$ 240 mg/dL)
3. Cigarette smoking
4. Diabetes mellitus[a]
5. Family history of coronary or other atherosclerotic disease in parents or siblings prior to age 55

[a]Persons with insulin-dependent diabetes mellitus (IDDM) who are over 30 years of age, or have had IDDM for more than 15 years, and persons with noninsulin-dependent diabetes mellitus who are over 35 years of age should be classified as patients with disease and treated according to the guidelines in Table 5–2.
Reprinted with permission from the American College of Sports Medicine. Guidelines for Exercise Testing and Prescription. 4th ed. Philadelphia, Pa: Lea & Febiger; 1991:6.

TABLE 5–4. MAJOR SYMPTOMS OR SIGNS SUGGESTIVE OF CARDIOPULMONARY OR METABOLIC DISEASE[a]

1. Pain or discomfort in the chest or surrounding areas that appears to be ischemic in nature
2. Unaccustomed shortness of breath or shortness of breath with mild exertion
3. Dizziness or syncope
4. Orthopnea/paroxysmal nocturnal dyspnea
5. Ankle edema
6. Palpitations or tachycardia
7. Claudication
8. Known heart murmur

[a]These symptoms must be interpreted in the clinical context in which they appear, since they are not all specific for cardiopulmonary or metabolic disease.
Reprinted with permission from the American College of Sports Medicine. Guidelines for Exercise Testing and Prescription. 4th ed. Philadelphia, Pa: Lea & Febiger; 1991:6.

TABLE 5–5. CONTRAINDICATIONS TO EXERCISE TESTING

Absolute Contraindications
1. A recent significant change in the resting ECG suggesting infarction or other acute cardiac events
2. Recent complicated myocardial infarction
3. Unstable angina
4. Uncontrolled ventricular dysrhythmia
5. Uncontrolled atrial dysrhythmia that compromises cardiac function
6. Third-degree A-V block
7. Acute congestive heart failure
8. Severe aortic stenosis
9. Suspected or known dissecting aneurysm
10. Active or suspected myocarditis or pericarditis
11. Thrombophlebitis or intracardiac thrombi
12. Recent systemic or pulmonary embolus
13. Acute infection
14. Significant emotional distress (psychosis)

Relative Contraindications
1. Resting diastolic blood pressure > 120 mm Hg or resting systolic blood pressure > 200 mm Hg
2. Moderate valvular heart disease
3. Known electrolyte abnormalities (hypokalemia, hypomagnesemia)
4. Fixed-rate pacemaker (rarely used)
5. Frequent or complex ventricular ectopy
6. Ventricular aneurysm
7. Cardiomyopathy, including hypertrophic cardiomyopathy
8. Uncontrolled metabolic disease (eg, diabetes, thyrotoxicosis, or myxedema)
9. Chronic infectious disease (eg, mononucleosis, hepatitis, AIDS)
10. Neuromuscular, musculoskeletal, or rheumatoid disorders that are exacerbated by exercise
11. Advanced or complicated pregnancy

Reprinted with permission from the American College of Sports Medicine. Guidelines for Exercise Testing and Prescription. 4th ed. Philadelphia, Pa: Lea & Febiger; 1991:59.

TABLE 5—6. ADDITIONAL CONTRAINDICATIONS TO EXERCISE TESTING[17,53,64,117,118]

1. The client does not wish to be tested
2. Unwillingness of the client to give informed consent
3. Suspected intoxication and/or drug abuse by the client
4. Any acute general illness
5. Locomotion problem
6. Uncontrolled hypertension
7. Severe anemia
8. Severe electrolyte imbalance
9. Morbid obesity
10. Severe physical handicap

TABLE 5—7. INDICATIONS FOR STOPPING AN EXERCISE TEST

1. Progressive angina (stop at 3+ level or earlier on a scale of 1+ to 4+) (see Table 5–8)
2. Ventricular tachycardia
3. Any significant drop (20 mm Hg) of systolic blood pressure or a failure of the systolic blood pressure to rise with an increase in exercise load
4. Lightheadedness, confusion, ataxia, pallor, cyanosis, nausea, or signs of severe peripheral circulatory insufficiency
5. > 4 mm horizontal or down-sloping ST depression or elevation (in the absence of other indicators of ischemia)
6. Onset of second- or third-degree A-V block
7. Increasing ventricular ectopy, multiform PVCs, or R on T PVCs
8. Excessive rise in blood pressure: systolic pressure > 250 mm Hg; diastolic pressure > 120 mm Hg
9. Chronotropic impairment
10. Sustained supraventricular tachycardia
11. Exercise-induced left bundle branch block
12. Subject requests to stop
13. Failure of the monitoring system

Reprinted with permission from the American College of Sports Medicine. Guidelines for Exercise Testing and Prescription. 4th ed. Philadelphia, Pa: Lea & Febiger, 1991:72.

TABLE 5—8. ANGINA AND DYSPNEA SCALES

Angina Scale

1+	Light, barely noticeable
2+	Moderate, bothersome
3+	Severe, very uncomfortable
4+	Most severe pain ever experienced

Dyspnea Scale

+1	Mild, noticeable to patient but not observer
+2	Mild, some difficulty, noticeable to observer
+3	Moderate difficulty, but can continue
+4	Severe difficulty, patient cannot continue

Reprinted with permission from the American College of Sports Medicine. Guidelines for Exercise Testing and Prescription. 4th ed. Philadelphia, Pa: Lea & Febiger; 1991:73.

TABLE 5—9. ADDITIONAL INDICATIONS FOR STOPPING AN EXERCISE TEST[7,17,118]

1. The testing clinician stops the test at his or her own discretion.
2. The client is unable to keep pace with the treadmill without attempting to hold onto the handrail.
3. The client attains a predetermined exercise end-point intensity for submaximal testing (ie, a specific intensity that can vary between 65% to 85% of age-predicted maximal heart rate) determined before testing by the clinician.
4. The client completes designated time of protocol.
5. The client responds to general questions in a confused state.
6. The client exhibits central nervous system symptoms (eg, vertigo or visual disturbances).
7. The client has leg cramps or intermittent claudication.
8. The client shows marked fatigue or shortness of breath.
9. The client is wheezing.
10. The client has radiating pain.

TABLE 5–10. CRITERIA FOR SELECTING CARDIOVASCULAR EXERCISE TESTS

Client's Limitations or Tasks	Treadmill Tests	Leg Cycle Ergometer Tests	Arm Cycle Ergometer Tests	Step Tests	Field Tests	Task/Skill Specific Tests
Limited sitting tolerance	Suggested test	Not advisable	Not advisable	Clinician discretion	Optional test	Clinician discretion
Limited standing tolerance	Not advisable	Suggested test	Optional test	Not advisable	Not advisable	Clinician discretion
Limited walking tolerance	Not advisable	Suggested test	Optional test	Not advisable	Not advisable	Clinician discretion
Limited lumbar flexion	Suggested test	Not advisable	Not advisable	Not advisable	Optional test	Clinician discretion
Limited lumbar extension	Clinician discretion	Clinician discretion	Clinician discretion	Not advisable	Clinician discretion	Clinician discretion
Sacroiliac dysfunction	Not advisable	Clinician discretion	Clinician discretion	Not advisable	Not advisable	Clinician discretion
Lower extremity pathology	Not advisable	Clinician discretion	Suggested test	Not advisable	Not advisable	Clinician discretion
Upper extremity pathology	Optional test	Suggested test	Not advisable	Clinician discretion	Optional test	Clinician discretion
Lower extremity sport- or work-related tasks	Suggested test	Suggested test	Optional test	Optional test	Optional test	Optional test
Upper extremity sport- or work-related tasks	Optional test	Optional test	Suggested test	Optional test	Optional test	Optional test

TABLE 5–11. MAXIMAL VERSUS SUBMAXIMAL EXERCISE TESTING[7,52,56,57]

Maximal Exercise Testing
1. Subjective maximal exercise testing may generally be defined as when a client is unable to continue the specified protocol due to intolerable fatigue, dyspnea, or pain.[117]
2. It is attained when a client appears to give a true maximal effort (point of bodily exhaustion) or when other clinical points are reached (see Tables 5–7 to 5–9).[15]
3. It is attained when, during a maximal test, the measured oxygen consumption reaches a value that will not increase despite an increase in the workload.[57]
4. It is more sensitive than a submaximal test in detecting underlying cardiovascular abnormalities.
5. It provides a more reliable and objective measure of cardiovascular fitness.
6. It is used as a diagnostic tool for detecting underlying cardiovascular abnormalities.

Submaximal Exercise Testing
1. Maximal testing protocols may be adapted for submaximal testing by terminating the test when the client attains a predetermined exercise end-point intensity (ie, a specific intensity that can vary between 65% and 85% of age-predicted maximal heart rate).
2. It is useful for determining a client's fitness level when a diagnostic test is not required.
3. It is useful in monitoring changes in cardiovascular fitness levels.
4. The most vulnerable clients are stressed to a relatively greater extent during an age-predicted heart rate-targeted submaximal test, whereas less impaired clients are limited by the submaximal target heart rate.[15,57]

TABLE 5–11. (Continued)

5. The max $\dot{V}O_2$ predicted from submaximal heart rate is generally within 10 to 20% of a person's actual value and is limited by the following:[92]
  a. Assumes a near linear relationship between heart rate, oxygen uptake, and work intensity for light to moderate workloads. However, the relationship between oxygen uptake and work intensity becomes curvilinear at heavier workloads.[23,46,69,92]
  b. Assumes a constant economy or mechanical efficiency. The max $\dot{V}O_2$ will be underestimated in a client with poor mechanical efficiency because the heart rate will be elevated due to the added oxygen cost of the inefficient exercise.[92]
  c. Assumes that the maximal heart rate for subjects of a given age is similar. Maximal heart rate has been shown to vary as much as plus or minus 10 beats per minute for individuals of the same age.[69,92]
  d. Variations in day-to-day heart rate.[92]

TABLE 5–12. CONTINUOUS VERSUS INTERMITTENT EXERCISE TESTING[44,93]

Continuous Tests
1. These are designed with no rest periods between the work increments.[92]
2. An advantage is that it takes less time to administer the test and, therefore, a larger number of individuals may be tested.[92]
3. A disadvantage may be that the client experiences localized muscle discomfort (eg, thigh discomfort during a bicycling test and low back and gastrocnemius discomfort during a treadmill test) during the test.[92]

Discontinuous Tests
1. These are designed with a 5- to 10-minute rest interval between the workloads.[69]
2. An advantage may be that there is less localized muscle fatigue during testing.[124]
3. A disadvantage is the time involved in waiting out the rest periods (which may vary from several minutes to a day or more) between the exercise bouts.[124]

aid clinicians in choosing an appropriate test for their clients. Table 5–10 categorizes each test as follows:

1. Clinician discretion implies that clinicians must choose the test based on their own clinical expertise and the client's specific medical limitations. However, it should be noted that all the tests are ultimately under the direct discretion of the clinician.
2. Suggested test—implies that this test is the most preferred for this category.
3. Optional test—implies that this test may also be considered by the clinician.
4. Not advisable—implies that this test may have contraindications for this category.

Predicting and Measuring Maximal Oxygen Consumption

Indirect Methods of Predicting or Estimating $\dot{V}O_2$ Max

SUBMAXIMAL TESTING
Predicted maximal MET level and $\dot{V}O_2$ may be attained from the following methods:[46]

1. Graphs (see Figure 5–1)[60]
2. Tables[64,106]
3. Nomograms[35,69]
4. Formulas and calculations[7,69,106]

MAXIMAL TESTING
Predicted maximal MET level and $\dot{V}O_2$ may be attained from maximal exercise time or peak-attained workloads through the use of the following methods:[46,52]

1. Graphs (see Figure 5–2)[7]
2. Tables[64,69]
3. Nomograms[35]
4. Formulas and calculations[7,69,106]

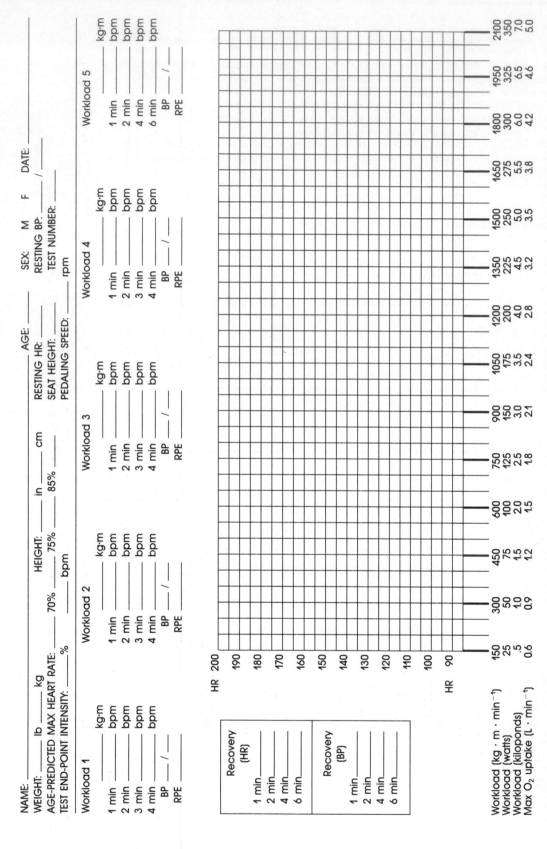

NAME: _____
WEIGHT: _____ lb _____ kg
AGE-PREDICTED MAX HEART RATE: _____%
TEST END-POINT INTENSITY: _____%

HEIGHT: _____ in _____ cm
70%   75%   85%   _____ bpm

AGE: _____   SEX: M   F   DATE: _____
RESTING HR: _____   RESTING BP: _____ / _____
SEAT HEIGHT: _____   TEST NUMBER: _____
PEDALING SPEED: _____ rpm

Workload 1

	kg·m
1 min	_____ bpm
2 min	_____ bpm
3 min	_____ bpm
4 min	_____ bpm
BP	___/___
RPE	_____

Workload 2

	kg·m
1 min	_____ bpm
2 min	_____ bpm
3 min	_____ bpm
4 min	_____ bpm
BP	___/___
RPE	_____

Workload 3

	kg·m
1 min	_____ bpm
2 min	_____ bpm
3 min	_____ bpm
4 min	_____ bpm
BP	___/___
RPE	_____

Workload 4

	kg·m
1 min	_____ bpm
2 min	_____ bpm
3 min	_____ bpm
4 min	_____ bpm
BP	___/___
RPE	_____

Workload 5

	kg·m
1 min	_____ bpm
2 min	_____ bpm
4 min	_____ bpm
6 min	_____ bpm
BP	___/___
RPE	_____

Recovery (HR)

1 min	_____
2 min	_____
4 min	_____
6 min	_____

Recovery (BP)

1 min	_____
2 min	_____
4 min	_____
6 min	_____

HR 200
190
180
170
160
150
140
130
120
110
100
HR 90

Workload (kg · m · min⁻¹)	150	300	450	600	750	900	1050	1200	1350	1500	1650	1800	1950	2100
Workload (watts)	25	50	75	100	125	150	175	200	225	250	275	300	325	350
Workload (kiloponds)	.5	1.0	1.5	2.0	2.5	3.0	3.5	4.0	4.5	5.0	5.5	6.0	6.5	7.0
Max O₂ uptake (L · min⁻¹)	0.6	0.9	1.2	1.5	1.8	2.1	2.4	2.8	3.2	3.5	3.8	4.2	4.6	5.0

Figure 5–1. Graph for plotting predicted maximal aerobic capacity. $\dot{V}O_2$ can be estimated from a formula that gives reasonable estimates of the $\dot{V}O_2$ up to work rates of about 1200 kg · m · min⁻¹ (ACSM[7]: $\dot{V}O_2$ (mL · min⁻¹) = 2 mL · kg⁻¹ · m⁻¹ × kg · m · min⁻¹ + 300 mL · min⁻¹. *Adapted with permission from Golding LA, Myers CR, Sinning WE, eds. Y's Ways to Physical Fitness. 3rd ed. Champaign, Ill: Human Kinetics Publishers, Inc; 1989:100, YMCA of the USA, 101 N Wacker Dr, Chicago, Ill 60606.*

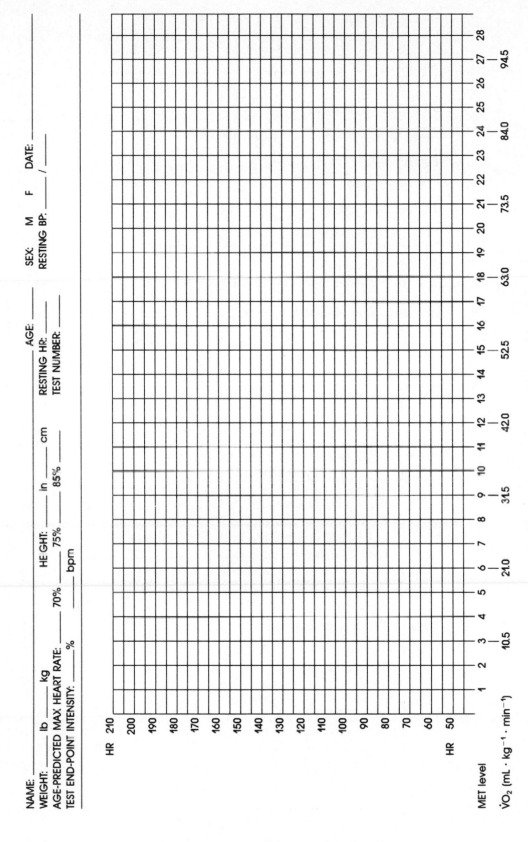

NAME: _____ AGE: _____

WEIGHT: _____ lb _____ kg   HE GHT: _____ in _____ cm   SEX: M   F

AGE-PREDICTED MAX HEART RATE: _____ 70% _____ 75% _____ 85% _____   RESTING HR: _____   DATE: _____ / _____

TEST END-POINT INTENSITY: _____ %   _____ bpm   RESTING BP: _____

TEST NUMBER: _____

HR 210
200
190
180
170
160
150
140
130
120
110
100
90
80
70
60
50
HR

MET level   1   2   3   4   5   6   7   8   9   10   11   12   13   14   15   16   17   18   19   20   21   22   23   24   25   26   27   28

V̇O₂ (mL · kg⁻¹ · min⁻¹)   10.5   21.0   31.5   42.0   52.5   63.0   73.5   84.0   94.5

Figure 5–2. Graph for plotting predicted maximal aerobic capacity.

47

Direct Methods of Measuring V̇O₂ Max

One can also directly measure $\dot{V}O_2$ max through open-circuit spirometry (ie, a Douglas bag or portable spirometer); however, this text will not describe this procedure.

METHODS OF TESTING

Heart Rate Measurement Procedures[69,73,74,103,106]

Equipment

1. Stopwatch

Test Administration

1. Auscultation method
   a. The stethoscope bell is placed over the 3rd intercostal space to the left of the sternum.
   b. For determining heart rate per minute, count for 10, 15, 30, or 60 seconds and multiply by 6, 4, 2, or 1, respectively.
2. Palpation method
   a. The pulse may be palpated at the brachial, carotid, or radial arteries.
   b. For determining resting heart rate per minute, one may count for 10, 15, 30, or 60 seconds and multiply by 6, 4, 2, or 1, respectively (see Special Considerations section for measuring post-exercise heart rate).
3. ECG method
   a. For regular rhythms: Find a specific R wave that falls on a heavy black line. Then count off 300, 150, 100, 75, 60, 50 for each heavy black line that follows. Where the next R wave falls determines the rate (assuming a constant paper speed of 25 mm/s).[43,111]
   b. For irregular rhythms: Count the number of QRS complexes in a 6-second interval (included within two time markers at the top border of the ECG paper). Find the complex that coincides with the time marker at the top of the ECG paper. Then count the number of QRS complexes in a span of 30 boxes (two groups of 15 boxes distinguished by a time marker at the top of the ECG paper) and multiply by 10 to determine the heart rate per 60 seconds (assuming a constant paper speed of 25 mm/s). Note that each large box equals 0.2 second and thus, 30 large boxes equal $30 \times 0.2 = 6$ seconds.[111]

Special Considerations

1. Post-exercise heart rate measurement:
   a. One should attempt to complete the measurement of heart rate within 15 seconds after the cessation of exercise. Since it takes a few seconds to position the hand for palpating the heartbeat, it is recommended to use a 10-second pulse count (multiplying by 6 to obtain heart rate per minute) to avoid errors resulting from the deceleration of the heartbeat.[105,106]
   b. One may also use a 15-second pulse count (multiplying by 4 to obtain heart rate per minute) for measuring post-exercise heart rate; however, a 5% to 10% error may result from this method.[40,95,106]
2. Disadvantages of using the palpation method may include:[46]
   a. Taking too much time to locate a pulse
   b. Inaccuracies in counting beats
   c. Inaccuracies associated with timing device
   d. Recovery pulse rates not reflecting exercise rates
3. Ideally, the client should be either supine or sitting quietly for 5 to 10 minutes before the resting heart rate is taken.

4. Resting heart rate may fluctuate secondary to the following: going from a lying to a standing position, eating, smoking, emotional stress, consumption of caffeine, time of day, medications, and temperature.
5. Avoid using the thumb (while using the palpation method) since it has a pulse of its own.[69]
6. A reflex slowing of the heart rate may occur if excessive pressure is placed on the carotid artery.
7. Resting heart rate should be evaluated periodically since it decreases secondary to exercise training.
8. In order to avoid inaccuracies associated with the variability of resting heart rate, one should obtain multiple readings of resting heart rate on different days under standardized conditions.[106]

Blood Pressure Measurement Procedures[1,11,13,24,68,69,73,74,83,103,106]

Equipment

1. Stethoscope
2. Mercury sphygmomanometer, calibrated aneroid manometer, or a validated electronic device

Test Administration

1. The client should be seated with the arm bare and supported by either the clinician's hand or a table. The elbow may be slightly bent and the palm facing upward (ie, supinated).
2. Wrap the cuff firmly around the upper arm and position the arm at heart level (horizontal level of the fourth intercostal space at the sternum during measurement in the seated and upright positions). Raising the arm above this position lowers blood pressure and lowering the arm increases blood pressure. The aneroid manometer may be at any height, and the mercury manometer should be level with the clinician's eyes.
3. Align the arrows of the cuff with the brachial artery and make sure the lower margin of the cuff is about 2.5 cm above the antecubital fossa.
4. Place the stethoscope about 1 cm below the antecubital space over the brachial artery.
5. Quickly inflate the cuff to one of the following levels[1]:
   a. 160 to 200 mm Hg
   b. 20 mm Hg above the expected or known systolic pressure
   c. 30 mm Hg above the disappearance of the radial pulse
6. Slowly release the pressure at a rate of 2 to 3 mm Hg per heartbeat or 2 to 5 mm Hg per second.[1] Note when you hear the first Korotkoffs sound, which is a sudden rush of blood as the artery opens. The reading at this point corresponds to the systolic pressure.
7. Continue reducing the pressure until the sound disappears (fifth phase). This point provides the most accurate index of diastolic pressure.
8. Open the valve completely to exhaust all the air from the cuff.
9. Take blood pressure on the left and right arms because there may be arterial obstructions. In follow-up evaluations, the arm that was found to have the higher pressure should be used.[106]

Special Considerations

1. Take blood pressure in a quiet room. Ideally, the client should be sitting quietly for at least 5 minutes before blood pressure is taken.
2. The testing area should be approximately 72°F or less and the humidity 60% or less, if possible.[7]
3. The client's upper arm should be bare for best results.

TABLE 5–13. CLASSIFICATION OF BLOOD PRESSURE IN ADULTS AGED 18 YEARS OR OLDER[a]

	Blood Pressure Range (mm Hg)	Category
Diastolic	< 85	Normal blood pressure
	85–89	High-normal blood pressure
	90–104	Mild hypertension
	105–114	Moderate hypertension
	≥ 115	Severe hypertension
Systolic[b]	< 140	Normal blood pressure
	140–159	Borderline isolated systolic hypertension
	≥ 160	Isolated systolic hypertension

[a]Classification based on the average of two or more readings on two or more occasions.
[b]When diastolic blood pressure is less than 90 mm Hg.
Adapted from the National Heart, Lung and Blood Institute (National High Blood Pressure Education Program). The 1988 report of the Joint National Committee on Detection, Evaluation and Treatment of High Blood Pressure. Arch Intern Med. 1988;148:1023–1038. Chicago, Ill: American Medical Association.

4. Use the proper size cuff for a child (13 to 20 cm), an adult (17 to 26 cm), or a large adult (32 to 42 cm). The measurement in the parentheses refers to the arm circumference at midpoint.[13,106]

5. Two or more blood pressure readings should be averaged. If the first two readings differ by more than 5 mm Hg, then the clinician should obtain additional readings.[100]

6. Allow at least 30 seconds between blood pressure measurements, thus allowing normal circulation to return.[106]

7. Ideally, the client should not consume any stimulants (eg, caffeine) or depressants (eg, alcohol) on testing day.

8. For the classification of blood pressure of adults 18 years or older, refer to Table 5–13.

9. Blood pressure may be taken in a lying, sitting, or standing position to assess any variances.

10. Blood pressure may also be taken at the following areas:
    a. Upper leg—with the client in a prone position, the cuff (generally, a large or thigh cuff) is applied over the posterior aspect of the midthigh. The stethoscope is placed over the artery in the popliteal fossa.
    b. Lower leg—with the client in a supine position, the cuff (generally, a normal or large cuff) is applied to the lower leg with the distal border of the cuff being at the malleoli level. The stethoscope is placed over the posterior tibial or dorsalis pedis arteries.
    c. Forearm—with the client in a sitting position, the cuff (generally, a small or normal cuff) is applied to the forearm 13 cm from the elbow. The stethoscope is placed over the radial artery at the wrist.

11. Extraneous factors that may alter blood pressure:[78]
    a. Recent smoking or eating
    b. Anxiety
    c. Talking
    d. Physical exertion
    e. Cold
    f. Medications (eg, estrogens, adrenal steroids, adrenergic drugs)
    g. Bladder distension

12. Sources of potential error in measuring blood pressure:[78]
    a. Improper cuff size
    b. Equipment not calibrated
    c. Arm not positioned at heart level
    d. Arm held without support
    e. Too slow bladder inflation

f. Too rapid bladder deflation

g. Clinician bias owing to digit preference

13. The following are ways to improve the loudness and sharpness of the Korotkoffs sounds[78]:

   a. Rapid inflation of the bladder

   b. Raising the arm above heart level for a few seconds prior to inflating the bladder

   c. Having the client open and close his or her hand 10 times before the bladder is inflated

14. Clinicians interested in cardiovascular responses to strength training should refer to Fleck.[47]

15. The sphygmomanometer should be calibrated periodically using the manufacturer's manual for specific guidelines and other sources.[13,72,83] In general, the pointer should rest within the zero (0) when the cuff is completely deflated. If not, the sphygmomanometer should be checked for accuracy.

Rating of Perceived Exertion (RPE) Measurement Procedures[7,30–32,53,64,88,106,132]

Equipment

1. RPE scale chart (see Table 5–14)

Test Administration

1. Tell the client a 6 on the 15-point scale represents the easiest exercise that he or she has ever experienced and may be imagined as walking at a comfortable pace without any noticeable strain.[88]

2. Tell the client a 20 on the 15-point scale represents the most difficult exercise that he or she has ever experienced and may be imagined as exercise in which he or she cannot take another step without stopping.[88]

3. The client may provide differentiated ratings as follows[99]:

   a. Central rating arising from the heart and lungs

   b. Local rating from the muscles under stress (eg, legs)

   c. Overall rating, which considers all stimuli from every source

4. The client is told that there is no right or wrong answer and that he or she is free to choose any rating.

TABLE 5–14. RATING OF PERCEIVED EXERTION SCALES[a,b]

6		0	Nothing at all
7	Very, very light	0.5	Very, very weak
8		1	Very weak
9	Very light	2	Weak
10		3	Moderate
11	Fairly light	4	Somewhat strong
12		5	Strong
13	Somewhat hard	6	
14		7	Very strong
15	Hard	8	
16		9	
17	Very hard	10	Very, very strong
18		●	Maximal
19	Very, very hard		
20			

[a]The Borg scale can assist a clinician in judging the degree of fatigue reached by the client from one test to another or to correlate the level of fatigue during testing with that experienced during activities of daily living.[15]
[b]For Borg's latest terminology, refer to Borg.[32]
Reprinted with permission from Borg G. Psychophysical bases of perceived exertion. Med Sci Sports Exerc. Copyright 1982;14(5):377–381. Indianapolis, Ind: American College of Sports Medicine.

Special Considerations

1. The rating of perceived exertion (RPE) scale was first introduced by Borg[31] and can be defined as a method to determine the subjective experience during exercise and as a means to quantify the participant's sensations to the exercise intensity.
2. Studies have shown RPE to be highly correlated with several physiologic determinants, such as work intensity, oxygen uptake, and heart rate, particularly when expressed as percentages of their respective maximums.
3. The RPE scale may assist the clinician in further quantifying levels of exertion in response to testing and training.

ECG Monitoring Principles[1,58,61,112,126]

Introduction

1. It is not the purpose of this section to give details on how to place electrodes on a client, record an ECG, or interpret a basic ECG pattern.
2. The electrocardiogram (ECG) represents a visible record of the heart's electrical activity. A stylus traces the activity on a moving strip of special heat-sensitive paper.
3. The ECG gives important information concerning the spread of excitation to the different parts of the heart and is of value in the diagnosis of cases of abnormal cardiac rhythm and myocardial damage.

Equipment

1. Electrocardiograph
2. Treadmill or cycle ergometer, if performing exercise testing
3. Stethoscope and sphygmomanometer, if performing exercise testing

Special Considerations

1. Resting ECG strips may be obtained while the client is in the supine, sitting, or standing positions.
2. Resting ECG strips may be obtained during hyperventilation and breath-holding maneuvers.
3. Exercise ECG strips may be obtained for 10 seconds during each minute of the cardiovascular exercise test.
4. Minute-by-minute exercise ECG recordings may be obtained for approximately 7 minutes post-exercise or until the pre-test resting heart rate and blood pressure values are obtained. Monitoring may also be continued if there is persistent ST-segment depression or elevation, persistent angina, unstable dysrhythmias, or unusual signs and symptoms.
5. The ECG should be calibrated periodically using the manufacturer's manual for specific guidelines and other sources.[10,72]

TABLE 5–15. BRUCE PROTOCOL[a,b,34,35,46,69]

Stage	Grade (%)	Speed (mph)	Duration (min)	METs
*	0	1.5 or 1.7	3	—
**	5	1.5 or 1.7	3	3
1	10	1.7	3	4
2	12	2.5	3	7
3	14	3.4	3	10
4	16	4.2	3	13
5	18	5.0	3	16

[a]Continuous test.
[b]The Bruce Protocol is often modified with preliminary stages consisting of 0% or 5% grades or both at either 1.5 or 1.7 mph.

TREADMILL TESTING

Maximal Treadmill Test Protocols
Tables 5–15 to 5–19 outline and list various maximal treadmill test protocols.

Submaximal Treadmill Test Protocols
Tables 5–20 and 5–21 outline various submaximal treadmill test protocols.

TABLE 5–16. MODIFIED NAUGHTON PROTOCOL[a,46,101]

Stage	Grade (%)	Speed (mph)	Duration (min)	METs
1	0	2.0	3	2
2	3.5	2.0	3	3
3	7.0	2.0	3	4
4	10.5	2.0	3	5
5	14.0	2.0	3	6
6	17.5	2.0	3	7
7	12.5	3.0	3	8
8	15.0	3.0	3	9
9	17.5	3.0	3	10

[a]Continuous test.

TABLE 5–17. MODIFIED BALKE PROTOCOL[a,7,26]

Stage	Grade (%)	Speed (mph)	Duration (min)	METs
1	0	2.0	3	2.5
2	3.5	2.0	3	3.5
3	7.0	2.0	3	4.5
4	10.5	2.0	3	5.4
5	14.0	2.0	3	6.4
6	17.5	2.0	3	7.4
7	12.5	3.0	3	8.5
8	15.0	3.0	3	9.5
9	17.5	3.0	3	10.5
10	20.0	3.0	3	11.6
11	22.5	3.0	3	12.6

[a]Continuous test.

TABLE 5–18. LOW LEVEL PROTOCOL[a,122]

Stage	Grade (%)	Speed (mph)	Duration (min)	METs
1	0	1.2	3	2.1
2	3.0	1.2	3	2.4
3	6.0	1.2	3	2.7
4	3.5	2.0	3	3.5
5	7.0	2.0	3	4.5
6	10.5	2.0	3	5.4
7	12.0	2.5	3	6.4

[a]Continuous test.

TABLE 5–19. ADDITIONAL MAXIMAL TREADMILL TEST PROTOCOLS[a]

1. Branching protocol[7]
2. Ellestad protocol[44,46]
3. Kattus protocol[69,82]
4. Treadmill time tests[1,3,49,55]
5. US Air Force School of Aerospace Medicine (USAFSAM) protocol[46,136]
6. Wilson protocol[134]

[a]Continuous tests.

TABLE 5–20. SUBMAXIMAL TREADMILL TEST PROTOCOLS AND THE ESTIMATED STEADY-STATE ENERGY COST FOR THE LAST MINUTE OF EACH STAGE[a,b,c]

Stage	Grade (%)	Speed (mph)	Duration (min)	Energy Cost[d] $\dot{V}O_2$ $(mL \cdot kg^{-1} \cdot min^{-1})$	METs
Bruce Protocol					
1	10	1.7	3	13.4	3.82
2	12	2.5	3	21.4	6.12
3	14	3.4	3	31.5	9.01
Ross Protocol—Female					
1	0	3.4[e]	3	14.9	4.25
2	3	3.4	3	18.4	5.27
3	6	3.4	3	22.0	6.29
4	9	3.4	3	25.6	7.31
5	12	3.4	3	29.2	8.33
Ross Protocol—Male					
1	0	3.4[e]	3	14.9	4.25
2	4	3.4	3	19.6	5.61
3	8	3.4	3	24.4	6.97
4	12	3.4	3	29.2	8.33
5	16	3.4	3	33.9	9.09

[a]Continuous test.
[b]Either the Bruce or Ross protocol may be used for single or multi-stage equations in the predicting of $\dot{V}O_2$ max.
[c]Specific formulas are provided by Pollock and Wilmore[106] and Ross and Jackson[110] for calculating $\dot{V}O_2$ max for both the Bruce and Ross protocols.
[d]$\dot{V}O_2$ $(mL \cdot kg^{-1} \cdot min^{-1}) = \{[75 + (6 \times \%)] \times (mph/60)\} \times 3.5.$[109]
[e]A speed of 3.0 mph can be used and is especially useful for someone not accustomed to treadmill walking. The energy cost for the first stage would then be 3.75 METs.[108]
Adapted from Ted A. Baumgartner and Andrew S. Jackson. Measurement for Evaluation in Physical Education and Exercise Science. 4th ed. Copyright 1991, Dubuque, Iowa: Wm C Brown Publishers; p. 310. All rights reserved. Adapted by permission.

TABLE 5–21. ADDITIONAL SUBMAXIMAL TREADMILL TEST PROTOCOLS[a]

1. Prediction equation[23]
2. Prediction equations[127,87]

[a]Continuous tests.

Treadmill Test Procedures[7,27,52,53,69,77,92,106,110,117,118,130]

Introduction

All the treadmill tests listed as protocols may be adapted for performing submaximal and maximal testing. This section specifically describes methods and calculations for graphing the results obtained from testing. As previously mentioned, clinicians may also utilize nomograms, tables, and formulas for predicting $\dot{V}O_2$ max.

Equipment

1. Motorized treadmill with adjustable grade and speed (eg, Quinton):
   a. Clinical use recommendations—grade from 0% to 14% and speed from 1 to 10 mph[77]
   b. Research use recommendations—grade from 0% to 25% and speed from 1 to 25 mph[77]
2. Stethoscope and sphygmomanometer
3. Heart rate monitor
4. Electrocardiograph, if applicable

Test Administration

PRE-TEST DUTIES

1. Make sure all equipment is properly calibrated.
2. Complete health screening questionnaire (see Appendix, Figure D–1).
3. Screen for potential contraindications prior to cardiovascular exercise testing (see Tables 5–5 and 5–6).
4. Performing a physical evaluation (see Appendix, Figure D–2) prior to cardiovascular assessment is recommended to rule out any orthopedic-related contraindications.
5. Record resting heart rate, resting blood pressure, age-predicted maximal heart rate, and predetermined exercise end-point intensity (see Figure 5–3).
6. Determine whether the test will be:
   a. Submaximal or maximal.
   b. Continuous or discontinuous.
   c. Multi-stage or single-stage.
7. Select the test protocol that will be utilized.
8. Obtain informed consent in writing prior to testing (see Appendix, Table D–1).
9. Prepare the client for testing (ie, attach a heart rate monitor or ECG leads).
10. Discuss the following testing procedures with the client:
    a. Describe the purpose of the test.
    b. Explain stage changes in the protocol.
    c. Instruct the client to give a 10- to 15-second warning, if possible, before self-terminating the test.
    d. Describe the use of the RPE scale (see Table 5–14).
    e. The test will be stopped when the client self-terminates the test or when pre-established criteria are met (see Table 5–7 to 5–9).

PRE-TEST PROCEDURES

1. Have the client straddle the treadmill belt and hold onto the handrail for support. Turn on the treadmill power and have the client stroke the belt with one foot. Once the client is comfortable, have him or her practice by stepping onto the treadmill belt and walking in a normal heel-toe gait pattern.
2. Instruct the client to remove his or her hands from the handrails and walk normally. Holding the handrail should be highly discouraged during the test since this can reduce the oxygen cost of exercise by as much as 30%.[9]
3. Instruct the client to avoid looking down at the treadmill belt.

TEST PROCEDURES

1. Start the treadmill test and record the following (see Figure 5–4):
   a. Heart rate during the last 15 seconds of each minute.
   b. Blood pressure at the beginning and end of each stage. The blood pressure cuff may be taped to the client or slightly inflated in order to keep it in place.
   c. RPE at the beginning and end of each stage and at any time that the client offers a rating.
   d. Appearance of the client (eg, gait abnormalities, facial grimacing), as appropriate.
   e. The exact time the client experiences symptom(s) (eg, radiating low back pain) during the test.
   f. ECG strip (if applicable) during any abnormal monitor readings or physical signs or symptoms.
2. Continue the test until one or more criteria in Tables 5–7 to 5–9 are met.

NAME: _____ DATE: _____

A. TEST INFORMATION:

Test mode: Leg Cycle _____   Treadmill _____   Arm Cycle _____

Step _____   Field _____

Test Protocol: _____

Intensity of test: Submaximal _____   Maximal _____

B. TEST RESULTS:

Predicted max METs: _____

Predicted max $\dot{V}O_2$: _____ $mL \cdot kg^{-1} \cdot min^{-1}$

Predicted functional MET range: _____

Predicted fitness classification: _____

C. CALCULATIONS:

D. COMMENTS:

_____

_____

_____

_____

_____

_____

_____

_____

_____

_____

_____

Figure 5–3. Sample data sheet for cardiovascular exercise testing.

STAGE (#)	ELEVATION (% grade)	SPEED (mph)	DURATION (min)	METs	TIME (min)	HR (bpm)	BP (mm Hg)	PE
							/	
							/	
							/	
							/	
							/	
							/	
							/	
							/	
							/	
							/	
							/	
							/	
							/	
Max Data							/	
Walk			1 Minute post-exercise				/	
			2 Minute post-exercise				/	
Sit			4 Minute post-exercise				/	
			6 Minute post-exercise				/	

Figure 5–4. Sample protocol and data sheet for treadmill testing.

POST-TEST PROCEDURES

1. Once the test is terminated, proceed with a brief cool-down period with the client on the treadmill and holding onto the handrail.[46] Monitor the heart rate until it is within 15 to 25 beats per minute of the resting heart rate and the systolic blood pressure is within 20 mm Hg.
2. Monitor ECG changes, if applicable, for the test procedure. If the client is symptomatic, continue monitoring until arrhythmias have stabilized and the client is asymptomatic.[74]
3. Record the total duration and the reason(s) for terminating the test (see Figure 5–3).
4. Explain to the client that the test data will be analyzed in order to develop an appropriate cardiovascular training program.

Calculations

1. Determine the client's estimated maximal heart rate by either referring to Table 11–3 or subtracting the client's age from 220.
2. Refer to Figure 5–2 for plotting the following points on the graph:
   a. Draw a horizontal line corresponding to the client's maximal heart rate.
   b. Plot the highest heart rate versus MET level per treadmill stage.
   c. Draw a straight line through the points plotted and extend to the maximal heart rate line.
   d. Drop a perpendicular line from this intersection to the baseline of the graph (ie, METs).
   e. Record the predicted maximal MET level. Convert into predicted $\dot{V}O_2$ max by multiplying by 3.5.

Special Considerations

1. The following are general guidelines for designing and modifying treadmill tests:
   a. Provide a warm-up for the first few minutes of the test.
   b. Intensity of each stage may range from ½ to 3 METs.
   c. Duration of each stage may range from 2 to 4 minutes.
   d. Heart rate should be measured every 1 to 2 minutes and blood pressure at least during the last minute of each stage.
   e. Record ECG (if applicable) at least at the beginning and end of the test and during points where the client expresses chest pain or discomfort.
   f. Provide a recovery period for up to 10 minutes or longer (if indicated) while monitoring the heart rate, blood pressure, signs or symptoms, and ECG (if applicable).
2. Spotters may be utilized at the discretion of the testing clinician for safety purposes.
3. The treadmill should be calibrated periodically using the manufacturer's manual for specific guidelines and other sources.[10,63,72]
4. Refer to Table 5–22 for advantages and disadvantages of treadmill testing.

LEG CYCLE ERGOMETER TESTING

Maximal Leg Cycle Ergometer Test Protocols
Tables 5–23 to 5–25 outline and list various maximal leg cycle ergometer test protocols.

Submaximal Leg Cycle Ergometer Test Protocols
Figure 5–5 and Table 5–26 outline and list various submaximal leg cycle ergometer test protocols.

Leg Cycle Ergometer Test Procedures[7,52,53,60,69,77,92,102,106,110,117,118,130]

Name of Test
YMCA Bicycle Protocol

Introduction
This test is based on the fact that heart rate and oxygen uptake are linear functions of the rate of work. However, this linearity exists only at certain heart rates. For instance, at low heart rates external stimuli such as laughter, talking, and stress may affect the heart rate. Linearity is stated to begin at approximately 110 beats per minute. The basis of this YMCA test is to obtain two heart rates between 110 and 150 beats per minute at two different workloads. However, a steady-state heart rate (a heart rate that is within 5 beats) must be attained at each workload. Steady-state heart rate is said usually to occur within 3 minutes; however, it may take longer.[60]

TABLE 5–22. ADVANTAGES AND DISADVANTAGES OF TREADMILL TESTING[46,69,119,125,129]

Advantages

1. Walking is an activity that is familiar to everyone.
2. Treadmill allows the clinician to vary both speed and grade over a wide range of exercise intensities.
3. The treadmill provides a more precise control of work than the bicycle ergometer because cycling is controlled by the client and not by the ergometer (this holds true for ergometers with rate-dependent exercise intensity).
4. Walking is an activity that generally does not overload one specific muscle group in an unnatural pattern (eg, bicycle ergometry overloads the quadriceps in a nonweight-bearing manner; therefore, clients who are not accustomed to cycling will often be unable to reach maximal heart rates due to leg fatigue).
5. Maximal $\dot{V}O_2$ is generally 5% to 11% higher with treadmill testing, as compared to cycle ergometer testing.[129]

Disadvantages

1. May be frightening to some clients.
2. May be noisy.
3. May be too bulky.
4. May be expensive.
5. Handrails, arm boards, mouthpieces (if measuring oxygen uptake), and blood-pressure measuring devices used during testing may reduce the client's actual work rate.
6. May require the use of spotters in case a client loses his or her balance on the motorized belt.
7. May be difficult to spot a client at high speeds and increased grades.
8. Difficult to quantify metabolic workload.
9. Requires some coordination by the client.
10. Movement artifacts may be noted on the ECG monitor due to arm and torso movement.
11. The client must be able to bear weight on his or her lower extremities.
12. May be difficult to obtain exercise heart rates and blood pressure.
13. MET values for treadmill protocols are applicable only if the client is in a steady state and not holding onto the handrails during exercise.

TABLE 5–23. ÅSTRAND PROTOCOL[a,21,69]

| | Workload kg · m · min^{-1} (watts) | | Speed | Duration |
Stage	Men	Women	(rpm)[b]	(min)
1	600 (100)	300 (50)	50	2–3
2	900 (150)	450 (75)	50	2–3
3	1200 (200)	600 (100)	50	2–3
4	1500 (250)	750 (125)	50	2–3
5	1800 (300)	900 (150)	50	2–3

[a]Continuous test.
[b]rpm = revolutions per minute.

TABLE 5–24. MCARDLE, KATCH, AND PECHAR PROTOCOL[a,69,93]

Stage	Workload kg · m · min^{-1} (watts)	Speed (rpm)	Duration (min)
1	900 (150)	60	2
2	1080	60	2
3	1260 (230)	60	2
4	1440	60	2
5	1620 (270)	60	2
6	1800	60	2
7	1980 (360)	60	2

[a]Continuous test.

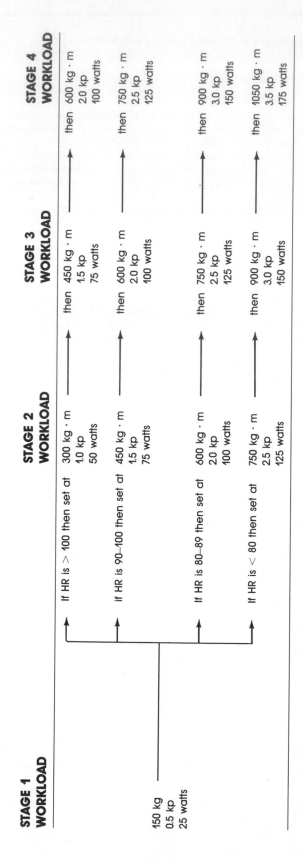

Figure 5–5. YMCA bicycle protocol for both males and females (continuous test). The duration of each stage is 3 to 4 minutes. If the heart rate differs by more than 5 bpm in the last 30 seconds of minutes 1 and 2, then the workload is extended 1 additional minute until a steady state is attained. The pedaling speed is set at 50 rpm for all testing workloads. The client should warm up for about 1 to 5 minutes prior to testing. The test is started by setting the initial workload at 150 kg · m · min⁻¹ (0.5 kp). The symbols (<) equal less than and (>) equal greater than.
Adapted with permission from Golding LA, Myers CR, Sinning WE, eds. Y's Way to Physical Fitness. 3rd ed. Champaign, Ill: Human Kinetics Publishers, Inc; 1989:91, YMCA of the USA, 101 N Wacker Dr, Chicago, IL 60606.

60

TABLE 5–25. ADDITIONAL MAXIMAL LEG CYCLE ERGOMETER TEST PROTOCOLS[a]

1. Åstrand protocol[22]
2. Fox protocol[50]

[a]Discontinuous tests.

TABLE 5–26. ADDITIONAL SUBMAXIMAL LEG CYCLE ERGOMETER TEST PROTOCOLS[a]

1. American College of Sports Medicine protocol[7]
2. Åstrand-Ryhming nomogram[123,69]
3. Fox protocol[50,69]
4. Physical Working Capacity (PWC$_{170}$) protocol[169,123]

[a]Continuous tests.

Equipment

1. Leg cycle ergometer (eg, Monark), which is a constant torque ergometer with a range of 0 to 2100 kg · m · min^{-1}. Each major gradation should be at 300 kg · m with intermediate marks at 150 kg · m[60]
2. Metronome (not needed if the cycle has an rpm counter)
3. Stethoscope and sphygmomanometer
4. Heart rate monitor
5. Stopwatch
6. Electrocardiograph, if applicable

Test Administration

PRE-TEST DUTIES

1. Make sure all equipment is properly calibrated.
2. Complete health screening questionnaire (see Appendix, Figure D–1).
3. Screen for potential contraindications prior to cardiovascular exercise testing (see Tables 5–5 and 5–6).
4. Performing a physical evaluation (see Appendix, Figure D–2) prior to cardiovascular assessment is recommended to rule out any orthopedic-related contraindications.
5. Record resting heart rate, resting blood pressure, age-predicted maximal heart rate and predetermined exercise end-point intensity (see Figure 5–3).
6. Obtain informed consent in writing prior to test (see Appendix, Table D–1).
7. Prepare the client for testing (ie, attach a heart rate monitor).
8. Discuss the following testing procedures with the client:
   a. Describe the purpose of the test.
   b. Explain stage changes in the protocol.
   c. Instruct the client to give a 10- to 15-second warning, if possible, before self-terminating the test.
   d. The test will be stopped when the client self-terminates the test or when pre-established criteria are met (see Table 5–7 to 5–9).

PRE-TEST PROCEDURES

1. The seat height should be adjusted so that there is no more than 5 to 10 degrees of flexion in the knee at the lowest pedal position.[74]
2. Select the appropriate pedaling rate (50 revolutions per minute for the YMCA protocol) and instruct the client to maintain this rate throughout the test.
3. Instruct the client to look straight ahead and maintain good sitting posture throughout the test.
4. Instruct the client to hold the bicycle handlebars but not to grip them too tightly or to tense the upper trunk muscles unnecessarily.

TEST PROCEDURES

1. Have a warm-up period for 1 to 3 minutes to allow the client to adjust to the pedaling rate.
2. Adjust the first workload according to the protocol utilized and all subsequent workloads according to the client's heart rate response.
3. Client should cycle for a minimum of 3 minutes at each workload; however, an additional minute may be required to reach steady state.
4. Record the following during the test:
   a. Heart rate during the last 15 seconds of each minute.
   b. Workload according to the client's heart rate response based on the selected test protocol (see Figure 5–5).
   c. Blood pressure at the beginning and end of each stage. The blood pressure cuff may be taped to the client or slightly inflated in order to keep it in place.
   d. Appearance of client (eg, gait abnormalities, facial grimacing), as appropriate.
   e. The exact time the client experiences symptom(s) (eg, radiating low back pain) during the test.
5. Continue the test until one or more criteria in Tables 5–7 to 5–9 are met.

POST-TEST PROCEDURES

1. Once the test is terminated, proceed with a brief cool-down period with the client sitting on the bicycle.[46] Monitor the heart rate until it is within 15 to 25 beats per minute of the resting heart rate and the systolic blood pressure is within 20 mm Hg.
2. Monitor ECG changes, if applicable, for the test procedure. If the client is symptomatic, continue monitoring until arrhythmias have stabilized and the client is asymptomatic.[74]
3. Record the total duration and the reason(s) for terminating the test (see Figure 5–3).
4. Explain to the client that the test data will be analyzed to develop an appropriate cardiovascular training program.

Calculations

1. Determine the client's estimated maximal heart rate by either referring to Table 11–3 or subtracting the client's age from 220.
2. Refer to Figure 5–1 for plotting the following points on the graph:
   a. Draw a horizontal line corresponding to the client's maximal heart rate.
   b. Plot the steady-state heart rate of the last two workloads.
   c. Draw a straight line through the points plotted and extend to the maximal heart rate line.
   d. Drop a perpendicular line from this intersection to the baseline of the graph (ie, workload).
   e. Record the maximal oxygen uptake ($L \cdot min^{-1}$) according to the predicted maximal workload. Convert $L \cdot min^{-1}$ to $mL \cdot min^{-1}$ by multiplying by 1000. Then calculate $\dot{V}O_2$ ($mL \cdot kg^{-1} \cdot min^{-1}$) by dividing $mL \cdot min^{-1}$ by the client's body weight in kilograms. Finally, calculate the METs by dividing $\dot{V}O_2$ ($mL \cdot kg^{-1} \cdot min^{-1}$) by 3.5.

Special Considerations

1. The following are general guidelines for designing and modifying leg cycle ergometer tests:
   a. Provide a warm-up for the first few minutes of the test at the lowest resistance.
   b. Maintain a constant pedal speed of 50 to 60 revolutions per minute

throughout the test. The client may need encouragement to maintain the designated pedal speed.

   c. Increase the external work by 25 to 50 watts per stage.

   d. Intensity of each stage may range from ½ to 3 METs.

   e. Duration of each stage may range from 2 to 4 minutes.

   f. Heart rate should be measured every 1 to 2 minutes and blood pressure at least during the last minute of each stage.

   g. Record ECG (if applicable) at least at the beginning and end of the test and during points where the client expresses chest pain or discomfort.

   h. Provide a recovery period for up to 10 minutes or longer (if indicated) while monitoring the heart rate, blood pressure, signs or symptoms, and ECG (if applicable).

2. Competitive cyclists generally pedal between 90 and 120 revolutions per minute. Therefore, clinicians may find it difficult to test elite cyclists on standard leg cycle ergometers.[106]

3. The leg cycle ergometer should be calibrated periodically using the manufacturer's manual for specific guidelines and other sources.[10,21,63,72]

4. It should also be noted that the magnitude of training changes may vary considerably depending on the mode of testing (ie, individuals trained on a leg cycle ergometer show greater improvements when tested on a bicycle than on a treadmill).[92]

5. Refer to Table 5–27 for advantages and disadvantages of leg cycle ergometer testing.

TABLE 5–27. ADVANTAGES AND DISADVANTAGES OF LEG CYCLE ERGOMETER TESTING[42,57,69,119,125,129]

Advantages

1. Inexpensive as compared to a quality treadmill.
2. Portable.
3. Occupies less space as compared to a treadmill.
4. Less noisy as compared to a treadmill.
5. Safer because it requires less coordination since the client is supported.
6. Easier to spot the client.
7. Fewer movement artifacts are noted on the ECG monitor due to less arm and torso movement.
8. Relatively easy to obtain exercise heart rates and blood pressure.
9. Accurately quantifies external work (the work rate–$\dot{V}O_2$ relationship).
10. The client does not have to bear weight on his or her lower extremities.
11. Easily calibrated.

Disadvantages

1. Most individuals have a lower maximal $\dot{V}O_2$ and anaerobic threshold on the leg cycle ergometer than on the treadmill, even though maximal heart rate, maximal minute ventilation (ie, the volume of air taken into or exhaled from the body in one minute), and maximal lactate are similar on both ergometers.[129]
2. Some clients are unable to cycle at a prescribed rate. Mechanically braked cycles, using an adjustable brake to provide resistance to pedaling, require exact pedaling frequencies for work quantification. Electrically braked cycles, using a magnetic field to produce a resistance to pedaling, maintain a given work rate despite minor fluctuations in pedaling frequency.
3. Some clients experience "seat pain" due to friction.
4. Bike requires frequent calibration.
5. Bike places a greater stress on the cardiovascular system in terms of the double product (ie, heart rate multiplied by systolic blood pressure) at any given oxygen uptake than does treadmill exercise. Isometric tension developed by the arms and hands holding onto the cycle handlebars also contribute to the increased stress levels.
6. Localized muscular fatigue may prevent some individuals from reaching a true cardiovascular functional limit.
7. In friction bikes, successive testing and time may decrease the accuracy to quantify work output secondary to belt tension variations.

TABLE 5–28. FIELD TEST PROTOCOLS

1. Montana bicycle test[1,115]
2. 12-Minute cycling test[37,97]
3. 1-Mile and 1.5-mile run test[14,37]
4. 9- and 12-minute run test[4,37]
5. 600-Yard run-walk test[48]
6. 12-Minute swimming test[37,97]
7. 1-Mile walk test[84]
8. Post-50 walk test[128]
9. 3-Mile walking test[37,97]
10. 12-Minute walking test[96]
11. Rockport fitness walking test[69,107]

FIELD TESTING

Field Test Protocols
Table 5–28 lists various field test protocols.

Field Test Procedures[7,69,84,106,107]

Name of Test
Rockport Fitness Walking Test

Equipment

1. Comfortable walking shoes
2. Loose fitting clothing
3. Stethoscope and sphygmomanometer
4. Stopwatch

Test Administration

PRE-TEST DUTIES

1. Make sure that the course is 1 mile in distance, flat, and clear of obstacles (a ¼-mile track is preferable).
2. Complete health screening questionnaire (see Appendix, Figure D–1).
3. Screen for potential contraindications prior to cardiovascular exercise testing (see Tables 5–5 and 5–6).
4. Performing a physical evaluation (see Appendix, Figure D–2) prior to cardiovascular assessment is recommended to rule out any orthopedic-related contraindications.
5. Record resting heart rate, resting blood pressure, age-predicted maximal heart rate, and predetermined exercise end-point intensity (see Tables 5–7 to 5–9).
6. Obtain informed consent in writing prior to test (see Appendix, Table D–1).
7. Explain to the client:
   a. Purpose of the test.
   b. That the test will be stopped when the client self-terminates the test or when pre-established criteria are met (see Tables 5–7 to 5–9).

TEST PROCEDURES

1. The client should stretch 5 to 10 minutes before the test.
2. Instruct the client to walk 1 mile as quickly as possible.
3. Take a 15-second pulse immediately after completing the test.

POST-TEST PROCEDURES

1. Once the test is terminated, proceed with a brief cool-down period. Monitor the heart rate until it is within 15 to 25 beats per minute of the resting heart rate and the systolic blood pressure is within 20 mm Hg.

TABLE 5–29. ADVANTAGES AND DISADVANTAGES OF FIELD TESTING

Advantages
1. Versatile
2. Inexpensive
3. May be used to test groups of individuals
4. May be repeated frequently since they are easy to administer

Disadvantages
1. Limited ability to assess exercise heart rate, blood pressure, ECG, and signs or symptoms

2. Record the total duration and the reason(s) for terminating the test (see Figure 5–3).
3. Explain to the client that the test data will be analyzed to develop an appropriate cardiovascular training program.

Calculations

1. The following generalized equation for men and women may be used to estimate $\dot{V}O_2$ in mL $\cdot$ kg^{-1} $\cdot$ min^{-1}:

$$\dot{V}O_2 \text{ max} = 132.853 - (0.0769 \times BW) - (0.3877 \times age) + (6.3150 \times sex) - (3.2649 \times time) - (0.1565 \times HR)$$

where BW = weight in pounds
age = rounded to the nearest year
sex = 0 for female and 1 for male
time = walk time to the nearest hundredth of a minute
HR = heart rate in beats per minute during the last lap of the test.

Special Considerations

1. Refer to Table 5–29 for advantages and disadvantages of field testing.

STEP TESTING

Step Test Protocols
Tables 5–30 and 5–31 outline and list various step test protocols.

Step Test Principles[69,106]

Equipment

1. Platform with adjustable heights and nonslip surface (a handrail for safety may be attached)
2. Metronome
3. Stethoscope and sphygmomanometer
4. Heart rate monitor
5. Stopwatch
6. Electrocardiograph, if applicable

Special Considerations

1. Refer to Table 5–32 for advantages and disadvantages of step testing.

ARM CYCLE ERGOMETER TESTING

Arm Cycle Ergometer Test Protocols
Tables 5–33 and 5–34 outline and list various arm cycle ergometer test protocols.

Arm Cycle Ergometry Test Principles[7,52,53,60,69,77,92,102,106,110,117,118]

TABLE 5–30. STEP TEST PROTOCOLS

Test Name (Reference)	Stepping Rate (steps · min⁻¹)	Bench Height (in)	Duration of Exercise (min)
Canadian Aerobic Fitness Test (CAFT)[62,76,120,121]	—[a]	8	—[b]
Harvard Step Test[33]	30	20	5
Three-Minute Step Test[70]	24	18	3
Queens College Step Test[94]	22	16.25	3
YMCA Three-Minute Step Test[60,79]	24	12	3
Ohio State University (OSU) Step Test[85]	24–30	15 and 20	18 innings[c] 50 seconds each Phase I: 6 innings, 24 steps · min⁻¹, 15-in bench Phase II: 6 innings, 30 steps · min⁻¹, 15-in bench Phase III: 6 innings, 30 steps · min⁻¹, 20-in bench
Cotten Revision of OSU Step Test[39]	24–36	17	18 innings[c] 50 seconds each Phase I: 6 innings, 24 steps · min⁻¹, 17-in bench Phase II: 6 innings, 30 steps · min⁻¹, 17-in bench Phase III: 6 innings, 36 steps · min⁻¹, 17-in bench
Eastern Michigan University Step Test[135]	24–30	14–20	20 innings[c] 50 seconds each Phase I: 5 innings, 24 steps · min⁻¹, 14-in bench Phase II: 5 innings, 30 steps · min⁻¹, 14-in bench Phase III: 5 innings, 30 steps · min⁻¹, 17-in bench Phase IV: 5 innings, 30 steps · min⁻¹, 20-in bench

[a] Steps per minute is based on age and identified in the test.
[b] The duration of exercise is based on the individual's fitness level.
[c] Each inning consists of 30 seconds of stepping and 20 seconds of rest.

Adapted from Heyward VH. Advanced Fitness Assessment and Exercise Prescription. 2nd ed. Champaign, Ill: Human Kinetics Publishers, Inc.; 1991; and Pollock ML, Wilmore JH. Exercise in Health and Disease: Evaluation and Prescription for Prevention and Rehabilitation. 2nd ed. Philadelphia, Pa: WB Saunders Co; 1990.

TABLE 5–31. ADDITIONAL STEP TEST PROTOCOLS[a]

1. California State University, Long Beach (CSULB) Step Test[191]
2. Forestry step test[1,114]
3. Graded step test[99]
4. Kasch step test[180]
5. Katch and McArdle step test[81,106]
6. Maritz, Morrison, Peter et al. step test[89]
7. Master step test[190]
8. Post-50 step test[128]
9. Stairmaster step-treadmill test[71,106]
10. Techumseh step test[181,98]

[a]Refer to the American College of Sports Medicine[7] and Heyward[69] for further step test calculations.

TABLE 5–32. ADVANTAGES AND DISADVANTAGES OF STEP TESTING[119]

Advantages
1. Portable
2. Inexpensive
3. May be used to test groups of individuals
4. Useful for individuals whose occupational activities require sustained climbing

Disadvantages
1. Requires coordination by the client
2. The client must be able to bear weight on his or her lower extremities
3. Places individuals with knee or ankle problems at risk

TABLE 5–33. ARM CYCLE ERGOMETER TEST PROTOCOLS

Reference	Initial Workload (kg · m · min⁻¹)	Workload per stage (kg · m · min⁻¹)	Stage Duration (min)	Cranking Rate (rev · min⁻¹)
___a,e	200	100	3	40
___b,f	Zero resistance	150	3	50
___c,f	150	150	4	60
___d,e	100	___g	3	60

[a]Shaw, Crawford, Karliner, et al.[116]
[b]Schwade, Blomqvist, Shapiro.[113]
[c]Fardy, Webb, Hellerstein.[45]
[d]Lazarus, Cullinane, Thompson.[86]
[e]Continuous test.
[f]Discontinuous test.
[g]Stage 1 = 150; 100 increments thereafter.
Adapted with permission from Franklin BA, Gordon S, Timmis GC, eds. Exercise in Modern Medicine. Copyright 1989, Baltimore, Md: Williams & Wilkins; p. 50.

TABLE 5–34. ADDITIONAL ARM CYCLE ERGOMETER TEST PROTOCOLS[52]

1. Balady, Weiner, McCabe et al. protocol[25]
2. DeBusk, Valdez, Houston et al. protocol[41]
3. Golding, Horvat, Horvat-Beutal et al. protocol (wheelchair ergometry)[59]
4. Pitetti, Snell, Gundersen-Stray protocol (wheelchair ergometry)[104]
5. Wahren, Bygdeman protocol[128]
6. Williams, Cottrell, Powers et al. protocol[131]

Equipment

1. Mounted bicycle ergometer (eg, Monark)
2. Metronome (not needed if cycle has rpm counter)
3. Stethoscope and sphygmomanometer
4. Heart rate monitor
5. Stopwatch
6. Electrocardiograph, if applicable

Special Considerations

1. The following are general guidelines for designing and modifying arm cycle ergometer tests:
   a. Provide a warm-up for the first few minutes of the test at the lowest resistance.
   b. Cranking rate may range from 40 to 60 revolutions per minute. The client may need encouragement to maintain the designated rate.
   c. May be performed seated or standing (which permits greater use of torso and postural muscle groups).
   d. If performing a seated test, mount the cycle ergometer on a table at a height of 68 to 70 cm. Have the client in an upright position with feet flat on the floor. During cranking, the arms should be alternately extended at right angles to the body, allowing for a slight bend at the elbow at maximal reach.
   e. Protocols may be continuous, increasing by 25-watt increments per stage every 2 to 4 minutes. Protocols may also be discontinuous, increasing by 25-watt increments per stage every 2 to 4 minutes separated by 1 to 2 minutes of rest. Discontinuous protocols may be better tolerated by some clients and permit a more frequent measure of blood pressure. It should be noted that leg cycle ergometer tests may be adapted for arm cycle ergometry provided the power output increments are lower for arm cycle ergometry.
   f. Intensity of each stage may range from ½ to 3 METs.
   g. Heart rate should be measured every 1 to 2 minutes and blood pressure at least during the last minute of each stage.
   h. Record ECG (if applicable) at least at the beginning and end of the test and during points where the client complains of chest pain or discomfort.
   i. Provide a recovery period of 10 minutes or longer (if indicated) while monitoring the heart rate, blood pressure, signs or symptoms, and ECG (if applicable). Blood pressure measurements may be taken on one arm while cranking at submaximal intensities or immediately after the completion of a stage.
2. Heart rate response to arm cycle ergometry exceeds that seen at the same submaximal work rate in leg cycle ergometry. However, the peak heart rate is less in arm cycle ergometry than in leg cycle ergometry by usually 10 to 15 beats per minute.[92]
3. McArdle, Katch, and Katch[92] note that the correlation between max $\dot{V}O_2$ for arm and leg exercise is low. Therefore, it is not possible to accurately predict one's capacity for arm exercise from a test using the legs.
4. Refer to Table 5–35 for advantages and disadvantages of arm cycle ergometer testing.

CLASSIFYING AND REPORTING

Tables 5–36 and 5–37 contain several types of classification systems for identifying cardiorespiratory fitness, and Figure 5–3 may be used for recording cardiovascular status during testing procedures. For further aerobic fitness classifications, refer to Adams,[1] Åstrand,[20] Cooper,[36] Government of Canada,[62] Jackson and Ross,[75] and Sharkey[115] and for sport-specific values of maximal oxygen uptake, refer to Wilmore and Costill.[133]

TABLE 5–35. ADVANTAGES AND DISADVANTAGES OF ARM CYCLE ERGOMETER TESTING[7,25,51-54,57,69,92,106,124,127,129]

Advantages

1. Useful for individuals who have lower extremity orthopedic, vascular, or neurologic impairments.
2. Useful for individuals with a lower extremity deformity or handicap.
3. Useful for individuals whose occupational or leisure activities require sustained upper body effort.
4. May be considered an acceptable mode of testing pregnant women.

Disadvantages

1. $\dot{V}O_2$ max determined by arm cycle ergometry is lower than $\dot{V}O_2$ max in leg ergometry (ie, treadmill or leg cycle ergometry) by 20% to 30%.[106]
2. Blood pressure is difficult to assess.
3. $\dot{V}O_2$ max for arm cycling approximates 50% to 70% of that for leg cycling, assuming the client is in normal health and has not undergone specific upper extremity training.[129]

TABLE 5–36. NORMAL VALUES OF MAXIMUM OXYGEN UPTAKE AT DIFFERENT AGES[a]

Age (yrs)	Men	Women
20–29	43 (± 22)	36 (± 21)
	[12 METs[b]]	[10 METs]
30–39	42 (± 22)	34 (± 21)
	[12 METs]	[10 METs]
40–49	40 (± 22)	32 (± 21)
	[11 METs]	[9 METs]
50–59	36 (± 22)	29 (± 22)
	[10 METs]	[8 METs]
60–69	33 (± 22)	27 (± 22)
	[9 METs]	[8 METs]
70–79	29 (± 22)	27 (± 22)
	[8 METs]	[8 METs]

[a] $(mL \cdot kg^{-1} \cdot min^{-1})$
[b] MET, metabolic equivalent; 1 MET = 3.5 mL $\cdot$ kg^{-1} $\cdot$ min^{-1} oxygen uptake.
Reprinted with permission from the American Heart Association (AHA). AHA Medical/Scientific Statement: Exercise Standards—A Statement for Health Professionals from the American Heart Association. Circulation. 1990;82(6): 2286-2322. Dallas, Tex: Copyright 1991, American Heart Association.

TABLE 5–37. CLINICALLY SIGNIFICANT KEY METABOLIC EQUIVALENTS FOR MAXIMUM EXERCISE[a]

1 MET = resting

2 METs = level walking at 2 mph

4 METs = level walking at 4 mph

< 5 METs = poor prognosis; usual limit immediately after myocardial infarction; peak cost of basic activities of daily living

10 METs = prognosis with medical therapy as good as coronary artery bypass surgery

13 METs = excellent prognosis regardless of other exercise responses

18 METs = elite endurance athletes

20 METs = world class athletes

[a] MET, metabolic equivalent or a unit of sitting, resting oxygen uptake. 1 MET = 3.5 mL $\cdot$ kg^{-1} $\cdot$ min^{-1} oxygen uptake.
Reprinted with permission from the American Heart Association (AHA). AHA Medical/Scientific Statement: Exercise Standards—A Statement for Health Professionals from the American Heart Association. Circulation. 1990;82(6):2286-2322. Dallas, Tex: Copyright 1991, American Heart Association.

REFERENCES

1. Adams GM. *Exercise Physiology Laboratory Manual.* Dubuque, Iowa: Wm C Brown Publishers; 1990.
2. Alexander J, Holder AR, Wolfson S. Legal implications of exercise testing. *J Cardiovas Med.* 1978;3:1137.
3. Alexander JF, Liang MTC, Stull GA, et al. A comparison of the Bruce and Liang equations for predicting VO₂ max in young adult males. *Res Q Exerc Sport.* 1984;55(4):383–387.
4. American Alliance for Health, Physical Education, Recreation and Dance. *AAHPERD Health Related Physical Fitness Test Manual.* Reston, Va: American Alliance for Health, Physical Education, Recreation and Dance; 1980.
5. American Association of Cardiovascular and Pulmonary Rehabilitation. *Guidelines for Cardiac Rehabilitation Programs.* Champaign, Ill: Human Kinetics Publishers, Inc; 1991.
6. American College of Cardiology (ACC)/American Heart Association (AHA) (Subcommittee on Exercise Testing). Guidelines for exercise testing: A Report of the ACC/AHA Task Force on Assessment of Cardiovascular Procedures. *J Am Coll Cardiol.* 1986;8(3):725–738.
7. American College of Sports Medicine. *Guidelines for Exercise Testing and Prescription.* 4th ed. Philadelphia, Pa: Lea & Febiger; 1991.
8. American Heart Association. *Exercise Testing and Training of Apparently Healthy Individuals: A Handbook for Physicians.* Dallas, Tex: American Heart Association; 1972.
9. American Heart Association. *Exercise Testing and Training of Individuals with Heart Disease or at a High Risk for Its Development: A Handbook for Physicians.* Dallas, Tex: American Heart Association; 1975.
10. American Heart Association. *The Exercise Standards Book* (reprinted from *Circulation.* 1979;59:421A; *Circulation.* 1979;59:849A; *Circulation.* 1979;59:1084A; *Circulation.* 1980; 62:699A). Dallas, Tex: American Heart Association; 1980.
11. American Heart Association. *Recommendations for Human Blood Pressure Determination by Sphygmomanometers.* Dallas, Tex: American Heart Association; 1980.
12. American Heart Association. Guidelines for exercise testing. *Circulation.* 1986;75: 653A–667A.
13. American Heart Association. *Recommendations for Human Blood Pressure Determination by Sphygmomanometers.* Dallas, Tex: American Heart Association; 1987.
14. American Heart Association. Position Statement: Clinical competence in exercise testing—A Statement for Physicians from the American College of Physicians (ACP)/ American College of Cardiology (ACC)/American Heart Association (AHA) Task Force on Clinical Privileges in Cardiology. *Circulation.* 1990;82(5):1884–1888.
15. American Heart Association. AHA Medical/Scientific Statement: Exercise standards— A Statement for Health Professionals from the American Heart Association. *Circulation.* 1990;82(6):2286–2322.
16. American Medical Association (Committee on Exercise and Physical Fitness). Evaluation for exercise participation: The apparently healthy individual. *JAMA.* 1972;219: 900–901.
17. American Medical Association (Council on Scientific Affairs). Indications and contraindications for exercise testing. *JAMA.* 1981;246:1015–1018.
18. American Medical Association. Standards and Guidelines for Cardiopulmonary Resuscitation (CPR) and Emergency Cardiac Care (ECC). *JAMA.* 1986;255(21):2905–2984.
19. American Physical Therapy Association. Cardiopulmonary Specialty Council handout. Alexandria, Va: American Physical Therapy Association; 1991.
20. Åstrand I. Aerobic work capacity in men and women with special reference to age. *Acta Physiol Scand.* 1960;49(Suppl 169).
21. Åstrand P-O. *Work Tests with the Bicycle Ergometer.* Varberg, Sweden: Monark-Crescent AB; (undated).
22. Åstrand P-O. Human physical fitness with special reference to age and sex. *Physiol Rev.* 1956;36:307–335.
23. Åstrand P-O, Rhyming IA. A nomogram for calculation of aerobic capacity (physical fitness) from pulse rate during submaximal work. *J Appl Physiol.* 1954;7:218–221.
24. Atwood JA, Nielson D. Scope of cardiac rehabilitation. *Phys Ther.* 1985;65:22–29.

25. Balady GJ, Weiner DA, McCabe CH, et al. Value of arm exercise testing in detecting coronary artery disease. *Am J Cardiol.* 1985;55:37–39.
26. Balke B, Ware R. An experimental study of physical fitness of Air Force personnel. *US Armed Forces Med J.* 1959;10:675–688.
27. Baumgartner TA, Jackson AS. *Measurement for Evaluation in Physical Education and Exercise Science.* 4th ed. Dubuque, Iowa: Wm C Brown Publishers; 1991.
28. Bell RD, Collis ML, Hoshizaki TB. *The Post 50 "3-S" Physical Performance Test.* Victoria, BC: Durkin and Assoc, Ltd; 1984.
29. Blair SN, Painter P, Pate RR, et al, eds. *Resource Manual for Guidelines for Exercise Testing and Prescription* (American College of Sports Medicine). Philadelphia, Pa: Lea & Febiger; 1988.
30. Borg G. *Physical Performance and Perceived Exertion.* Lund, Sweden: Gleerup; 1962.
31. Borg G. Psychophysical bases of perceived exertion. *Med Sci Sports Exerc.* 1982;14: 377–387.
32. Borg G. An *Introduction to Borg's RPE-Scale.* Ithaca, NY: Mouvement Publications, Inc; 1985.
33. Brouha L. The step test: A simple method of measuring physical fitness for muscular work in young men. *Res Q.* 1943;14:31–36.
34. Bruce RA. Exercise testing of patients with coronary artery disease. *Ann Clin Res.* 1971;3:323–332.
35. Bruce RA, Kusumi F, Hosmer D. Maximal oxygen intake and nomographic assessment of functional aerobic impairment in cardiovascular disease. *Am Heart J.* 1973;85: 546–562.
36. Cooper KH. *The Aerobics Way.* New York, NY: Bantam Books, Inc; 1977.
37. Cooper KH. *The Aerobics Program for Total Well-Being.* New York, NY: M Evans and Company, Inc; 1982.
38. Cooper PG. *Aerobics Theory and Practice.* Sherman Oaks, Calif: Aerobics and Fitness Association of America; 1985.
39. Cotton DJ. A modified step test for group cardiovascular testing. *Res Q.* 1971;42:91–95.
40. Cotton FS, Dill DB. On the relationship between the heart rate during exercise and that of immediate post-exercise period. *Am J Physiol.* 1983;111:554–558.
41. DeBusk RF, Valdez R, Houston N, et al. Cardiovascular responses to dynamic and static effort soon after myocardial infarction: Application to occupational work assessment. *Circulation.* 1978;58:368–375.
42. DiNubile NA, ed. *The Exercise Prescription (Clinics in Sports Medicine).* Philadelphia, Pa: WB Saunders Co; 1991;10(1).
43. Dubin D. *Rapid Interpretation of EKG's.* 3rd ed. Tampa, Fla: Cover Publishing; 1974.
44. Ellestad MH. *Stress Testing: Principles and Practice.* 3rd ed. Philadelphia, Pa: FA Davis Co; 1986.
45. Fardy PS, Webb D, Hellerstein HK. Benefits of arm exercise in cardiac rehabilitation. *Physician Sportsmed.* 1977;5:30–41.
46. Fardy PS, Yanowitz FG, Wilson PK. *Cardiac Rehabilitation, Adult Fitness and Exercise Testing.* 2nd ed. Philadelphia, Pa: Lea & Febiger; 1988.
47. Fleck SJ. Cardiovascular response to strength training. In: Komi PV, ed. *Strength and Power in Sport (The Encyclopedia of Sports Medicine).* Boston, Mass: Blackwell Scientific Publications; 1992.
48. Fleishman EA. *The Structure and Measurement of Physical Fitness.* Englewood Cliffs, NJ: Prentice-Hall; 1964.
49. Foster C, Jackson AS, Pollock ML, et al. Generalized equations for predicting functional capacity from treadmill performance. *Am Heart J.* 1984;107:1229–1234.
50. Fox EL. A simple, accurate technique for predicting maximal aerobic power. *J Appl Physiol.* 1973;35:914–916.
51. Franklin BA. Exercise testing, training and arm ergometry. *Sports Med.* 1985;2:100–119.
52. Franklin BA, Gordon S, Timmis GC. *Exercise in Modern Medicine.* Baltimore, Md: Williams & Wilkins; 1989.
53. Franklin BA, Rubenfire M. *Cardiac Rehabilitation (Clinics in Sports Medicine).* Philadelphia, Pa: WB Saunders Co; 1984;3.
54. Franklin BA, Vander L, Wrisley D, et al. Aerobic requirements of arm ergometry: Implications for exercise testing and training. *Physician Sportsmed.* 1983;11:81–90.

55. Frid DJ, Ellefsen K, Porcari J, et al. Estimating VO_2 max from a modified Balke treadmill protocol: Validation in a young healthy population. *Med Sci Sports Exerc.* 1988;20 (Suppl, Abstract #3):S1.

56. Froelicher VF. *Exercise and the Heart: Clinical Concepts.* 2nd ed. Chicago, Ill: Year Book Medical Publishers, Inc; 1987.

57. Froelicher VF, Marcondes GD. *Manual of Exercise Testing.* Chicago, Ill: Year Book Medical Publishers, Inc; 1989.

58. Goldberger AL, Goldberger E. *Clinical Electrocardiography: A Simplified Approach.* St. Louis, Mo: CV Mosby Co; 1986.

59. Golding LA, Horvat MA, Horvat-Beutal T, et al. A graded exercise test protocol for spinal cord injured individuals. *J Cardiopul Rehabil.* 1986;6:362–367.

60. Golding LA, Myers CR, Sinning WE. *Y's Way to Physical Fitness: The Complete Guide to Testing and Instruction.* 3rd ed. Champaign, Ill: Human Kinetics Publishers, Inc; 1989.

61. Goldman MJ. *Principles of Clinical Electrocardiography.* 11th ed. Los Altos, Calif: Lange Medical Publications; 1982.

62. Government of Canada. *Fitness and Amateur Sports: Canadian Standardized Test of Fitness (CSTF) Operations Manual.* 3rd ed. Ottawa, Ontario: Minister of State, FAS 73-78; 1986.

63. Hellerstein HK. Specifications for exercise testing equipment. *Circulation.* 1979;59: 849a–854a.

64. Hellerstein HK, Franklin BA. Exercise testing and prescription. In: Wenger NK, Hellerstein HK, eds. *Rehabilitation of the Coronary Patient.* 2nd ed. New York, NY: John Wiley & Sons, Inc; 1984.

65. Herbert DL. *Legal Aspects of Sports Medicine.* Canton, Ohio: Professional Reports Corporation; 1990.

66. Herbert DL, Herbert WG. *Legal Aspects of Preventive and Rehabilitative Exercise Programs.* 2nd ed. Canton, Ohio: Professional Reports Corporation; 1989.

67. Herbert WG, Herbert DL. Legal considerations. In: Blair SN, Painter P, Pate RR, et al, eds. *Resource Manual for Guidelines for Exercise Testing and Prescription* (American College of Sports Medicine). Philadelphia, Pa: Lea & Febiger; 1988.

68. Heyward VH. *Designs for Fitness: A Guide to Physical Fitness Appraisal and Exercise Prescription.* Minneapolis, Minn: Burgess Publishing Co; 1984.

69. Heyward VH. *Advanced Fitness Assessment and Exercise Prescription.* 2nd ed. Champaign, Ill: Human Kinetics Publishers, Inc; 1991.

70. Hodgkins J, Skubic V. Cardiovascular efficiency test scores for college women in the United States. *Res Q.* 1963;34:454–461.

71. Holland GJ, Weber F, Heng MK, et al. Maximal step-treadmill exercise and treadmill exercise by patients with coronary heart disease: A comparison. *J Cardiopul Rehabil.* 1988;8:58–68.

72. Howley ET. The exercise testing laboratory. In: Blair SN, Painter P, Pate RR, et al, eds. *Resource Manual for Guidelines for Exercise Testing and Prescription* (American College of Sports Medicine). Philadelphia, Pa: Lea & Febiger; 1988.

73. Irwin S. Clinical manifestations and assessment of ischemic heart disease. *Phys Ther.* 1985;65(12):16–21.

74. Irwin S, Tecklin JS. *Cardiopulmonary Physical Therapy.* 2nd ed. St. Louis, Mo: CV Mosby Co; 1990.

75. Jackson AS, Ross RM. *Understanding Exercise for Health and Fitness.* Houston, Tex: Mac J-R Publishing; 1986.

76. Jette M, Campbell J, Mongeon J, et al. The Canadian home fitness test as a predictor of aerobic capacity. *Can Med Assoc J.* 1976;114:680–682.

77. Jones NL, Campbell EJM. *Clinical Exercise Testing.* 3rd ed. Philadelphia, Pa: WB Saunders Co; 1988.

78. Kaplan NM. *Clinical Hypertension.* 4th ed. Baltimore, Md: Williams & Wilkins; 1986.

79. Kasch FW, Boyer JL. *Adult Fitness.* Greeley, Colo: All American Productions and Publications; 1968.

80. Kasch FW, Boyer JL. *Adult Fitness Principles and Practice.* San Diego, Calif: San Diego State College; 1968.

81. Katch FI, McArdle WD. *Nutrition, Weight Control and Exercise.* 3rd ed. Philadelphia, Pa: Lea & Febiger; 1988.

82. Kattus AA, Hanafee WN, Longmire WP, et al. Diagnosis, medical and surgical management of coronary insufficiency. *Ann Intern Med.* 1968;69:115–136.

83. Kirkendall WM, Feinlieb M, Freis ED, et al. Recommendations for human blood pressure determination by sphygmomanometers. *Circulation*. 1980;62:1146A–1155A.

84. Kline GM, Porcari JP, Hintermeister R, et al. Estimation of VO_2 max from a one-mile track walk, gender, age and body weight. *Med Sci Sports Exerc*. 1987;19(3):253–259.

85. Kurucz R, Fox EL, Mathews DK. Construction of a submaximal cardiovascular step test. *Res Q*. 1969;40:115–122.

86. Lazarus B, Cullinane E, Thompson PD. Comparison of the results and reproducibility of arm and leg exercise tests in men with angina pectoris. *Am J Cardiol*. 1981;47: 1075–1079.

87. Mahar M, Jackson AS, Ross RM, et al. Predictive accuracy of single and double stage sub max treadmill work for estimating aerobic capacity. *Med Sci Sports Exerc*. 1985;17(2, Suppl, Abstract #4):206–207.

88. Maresh CM, Noble BJ. Utilization of perceived exertion ratings during exercise testing and training. In: Hall LK, Meyer GC, Hellerstein HK. *Cardiac Rehabilitation: Exercise Testing and Prescription*. New York, NY: Spectrum Publications, Inc; 1984.

89. Maritz JS, Morrison JF, Peter J, et al. A practical method of estimating an individual's maximal oxygen intake. *Ergonomics*. 1961;4:97.

90. Master AM, Oppenheimer ET. A simple exercise tolerance test for circulatory efficiency with standard tables for normal individuals. *Am J Med Sci*. 1929;177:223–243.

91. Mastropaolo J, Bigelow TW, Takei Y, et al. *Training Manual for the Practice of Exercise Physiology*. Huntington Beach, Calif: Ben Franklin Press; 1983.

92. McArdle WD, Katch FI, Katch VL. *Exercise Physiology: Energy, Nutrition and Human Performance*. 3rd ed. Philadelphia, Pa: Lea & Febiger; 1991.

93. McArdle WD, Katch FI, Pechar GS. Comparison of continuous and discontinuous treadmill and bicycle tests for VO_2 max. *Med Sci Sports*. 1973;5:156–160.

94. McArdle WD, Katch FI, Pechar GS, et al. Reliability and interrelationships between maximal oxygen intake, physical working capacity and step test scores in college women. *Med Sci Sports*. 1972;4:182–186.

95. McArdle WD, Swiren L, Magel JR. Validity of the post-exercise heart rate as a means of estimating heart rate during work for varying intensities. *Res Q*. 1969;40:523–528.

96. McGavin CR, Gupta SP, McHardy GJR. Twelve minute walking test for assessing disability in chronic bronchitis. *Br Med J*. 1976;1:822–823.

97. Miller DK. *Measurement by the Physical Educator: Why and How*. Carmel, Ind: Benchmark Press; 1988.

98. Montoye HJ, Willis PW, Cunningham DA, et al. Heart rate response to a modified Harvard step test: Males and females, 10–69. *Res Q*. 1969;40(1):153–162.

99. Nagle FS, Balke B, Naughton JP. Gradational step tests for assessing work capacity. *J Appl Physiol*. 1965;20:745–748.

100. National Heart, Lung and Blood Institute (National High Blood Pressure Education Program). The 1988 report of the Joint National Committee on Detection, Evaluation and Treatment of High Blood Pressure. *Arch Intern Med*. 1988;148:1023–1038.

101. Naughton J, Balke B, Nagle F. Refinement in methods of evaluation and physical conditioning before and after myocardial infarction. *Am J Cardiol*. 1964;14:837.

102. Nieman DC. *The Sports Medicine Fitness Course*. Palo Alto, Calif: Bull Publishing Co; 1986.

103. Perloff JK. *Physical Examination of the Heart and Circulation*. 2nd ed. Philadelphia, Pa: WB Saunders Co; 1990.

104. Pitetti KH, Snell PG, Gundersen-Stray J. Maximal response of wheelchair-confined subjects to four types of arm exercise. *Arch Phys Med Rehabil*. 1987;68:10–13.

105. Pollock ML, Broida J, Kendrick Z. Validity of palpation technique of heart rate determination and its estimation of training heart rate. *Res Q*. 1972;43:77–81.

106. Pollock ML, Wilmore JH. *Exercise in Health and Disease: Evaluation and Prescription for Prevention and Rehabilitation*. 2nd ed. Philadelphia, Pa: WB Saunders Co; 1990.

107. Rockport Walking Institute. *Rockport Fitness Walking Test*. Marlboro, Mass: Rockport Walking Institute; 1986.

108. Ross RM. *Understand Exercise*. Houston, Tex: Cardio-Stress; 1984.

109. Ross RM, Jackson AS. Development and validation of total work equations for estimating the energy cost of walking. *J Cardiopul Rehabil*. 1986;6:182–192.

110. Ross RM, Jackson AS. *Exercise Concepts, Calculations and Computer Applications*. Carmel, Ind: Benchmark Press; 1990.

111. Scheidt S. *Clinical Symposia: Basic Electrocardiography: Leads, Axes and Arrhythmias.* West Caldwell, NJ: CIBA Pharmaceutical Co; 1983;35(2).
112. Scheidt S. *Clinical Symposia: Basic Electrocardiography: Abnormalities of Electrographic Patterns.* West Caldwell, NJ: CIBA Pharmaceutical Co.; 1984;36(6).
113. Schwade J, Blomqvist CG, Shapiro W. A comparison of the response to arm and leg work in patients with ischemic heart disease. *Am Heart J.* 1977;94:203–208.
114. Sharkey BJ. *Fitness and Work Capacity* (Report FS-315). Washington, DC: US Department of Agriculture; 1977.
115. Sharkey BJ. *Physiology of Fitness.* 3rd ed. Champaign, Ill: Human Kinetics Publishers, Inc; 1990.
116. Shaw DJ, Crawford MH, Karliner JS, et al. Arm-crank ergometry: A new method for the evaluation of coronary artery disease. *Am J Cardiol.* 1974;33:801–805.
117. Sheffield LT. Exercise stress testing. In: Braunwald E, ed. *Heart Disease: A Textbook of Cardiovascular Medicine.* 3rd ed. Philadelphia, Pa: WB Saunders Co; 1988.
118. Sheffield LT. Exercise stress testing. In: Fletcher GF. *Exercise in the Practice of Medicine.* 2nd ed. Mount Kisco, NY: Futura Publishing; 1988.
119. Shephard RJ. *Exercise Physiology.* Philadelphia, Pa: BC Decker; 1987.
120. Shephard RJ, Bailey DA, Mirwald RL. Development of the Canadian home fitness test. *Can Med Assoc J.* 1976;114:675–679.
121. Shephard RJ, Thomas S, Weller I. The Canadian home fitness test: 1991 update. *Sports Med.* 1991;11(6):358–366.
122. Sivarajan ES, Lerman J, Mansfield LW, et al. Progressive ambulation and treadmill testing of patients with acute myocardial infarction during hospitalization: A feasibility study. *Arch Phys Med Rehabil.* 1977;58:241–247.
123. Sjostrand T. Changes in respiratory organs of workmen at an ore melting works. *Acta Med Scand.* 1947;128(Suppl 196): 687–699.
124. Skinner JS. *Exercise Testing and Exercise Prescription for Special Cases: Theoretical Basis and Clinical Application.* Philadelphia, Pa: Lea & Febiger; 1987.
125. Smodlaka VN. Treadmills versus bicycle ergometers. *Physician Sportsmed.* 1982;10(8): 75–80.
126. Thomas CL, ed. *Taber's Cyclopedic Medical Dictionary.* 15th ed. Philadelphia, Pa: FA Davis Co; 1985.
127. Vokac Z, Bell H, Bautz-Holter E, et al. Oxygen uptake/heart rate relationship in leg and arm exercise, sitting and standing. *J Appl Physiol.* 1975;39:54–59.
128. Wahren J, Bygdeman S. Onset of angina pectoris in relation to circulatory adaptation during arm and leg exercise. *Circulation.* 1971;44:432–441.
129. Wasserman K, Hansen JE, Sue DY, et al. *Principles of Exercise Testing and Interpretation.* Philadelphia, Pa: Lea & Febiger; 1987.
130. Weber KT, Janicki JS. *Cardiopulmonary Exercise Testing: Physiologic Principles and Clinical Applications.* Philadelphia, Pa: WB Saunders Co; 1986.
131. Williams J, Cottrell E, Powers SK, et al. Arm ergometry: A review of published protocols and the introduction of a new weight adjusted protocol. *J Sports Med Phys Fitness.* 1983;23:107–112.
132. Williams JG, Eston RG. Determination of the intensity dimension in vigorous exercise programmes with particular reference to the use of the rating of perceived exertion. *Sports Med.* 1989;8(3):177–189.
133. Wilmore JH, Costill DL. *Training for Sport and Activity: The Physiological Basis of the Conditioning Process.* 3rd ed. Dubuque, Iowa: Wm C Brown Publishers; 1988.
134. Wilson PK, Winga ER, Edgett JW, et al. *Policies and Procedures of a Cardiac Rehabilitation Program: Immediate to Long Term Care.* Philadelphia, Pa: Lea & Febiger; 1978.
135. Witten C. Construction of a submaximal cardiovascular step test for college females. *Res Q.* 1973;44:46–50.
136. Wolthuis RA, Froelicher VF, Fischer J, et al. New practical treadmill protocol for clinical use. *Am J Cardiol.* 1977;39:697–700.

Chapter Six

Kinanthropometric Testing

METHODS OF TESTING

Height Measurement Procedures[9,43,56]

Introduction

1. May be used in a clinical setting for:
   a. Use in formulas and equations
   b. Grouping of individuals for sports and activity participation
   c. Observing young individuals who significantly deviate from height norms for their age group and gender

Equipment

1. Platform scale with stadiometer or anthropometer

Test Administration

1. Socks and shoes should be removed prior to measurement.
2. The client should stand with his or her back to the measuring device, feet together, arms relaxed by the side, eyes directed straight ahead, and with an erect posture. The client is then instructed to stand as tall as possible and take a deep breath while the measurement is taken.
3. The stadiometer should be adjusted to rest lightly on top of the head (ie, as close as possible to the scalp) so that it forms a right angle.[1]
4. Record height to the nearest ¼ in or 0.5 cm.

Special Consideration

1. Ideally, height should be measured in the morning.

Weight Measurement Procedures[9,43,56]

Introduction

1. May be used in a clinical setting for:
   a. Use in formulas and equations

b. Grouping of individuals for sports and activity participation
c. Observing young individuals who significantly deviate from weight norms for their age group and gender

Equipment

1. Platform scale

Test Administration

1. All weighings should be performed using the same scale.
2. The zero position should be checked before each weighing.
3. A consistent method of measurement should be used. For example, the client should wear the same amount of clothing before and after measurements.
4. Record weight to the nearest ½ lb or 500 g.

Special Considerations

1. Ideally, weight should be measured before breakfast and after the bowel and bladder have been emptied.
2. A standard balance scale is preferred to a spring-balance or digital scale because it can be calibrated more easily.
3. A client's naked weight should be obtained when tests relate the fitness score to body weight, and exercise-clothed weight should be used for tests that require calculations of work or power.[1]
4. Scales should be calibrated periodically using known weights verified from a bureau of standards.

Height–Weight Table Classification Principles[4,43,51,52,54,55]

Introduction

1. The table projects "desirable weights" for men and women by determining height and frame size (ie, elbow breadth, ankle girth).
2. The 1959 and 1983 height–weight tables from the Metropolitan Life Insurance Company provide a crude categorization of body weights ("desirable weights") for men and women of various heights and frame sizes. However, it does not assess an individual's body composition (ie, there is no way to know if an individual is muscular or simply overfat).

GIRTH (CIRCUMFERENCE) MEASUREMENTS

Girth (Circumferential) Measurement Protocols
Table 6–1 outlines girth measurement protocols.

Girth (Circumference) Measurement Principles[19,27-31,49,74]

Introduction

1. Through the use of formulas, equations, and tables, an individual's percent fat may be predicted from girth measurements. Girth measures may also be used for assessing swelling and testing for patterns of weight loss and muscle gain.

TABLE 6–1. GIRTH (CIRCUMFERENTIAL) MEASUREMENT PROTOCOLS[28]

Men
1. College age[7]
2. Ages 18–22[38]

Women
1. College age[7]
2. Ages 20–70[73]

Equipment

1. Steel or heavy plastic measuring tape (one with a Gulick handle that has a spring attachment is preferred)

Test Administration

1. The client is instructed to stand in an erect and relaxed manner with the arms hanging loosely at the sides.
2. Tape should be wrapped around the body area smoothly and snugly without kinking or indenting the skin.
3. Two to three measures should be taken at each site for consistency.
4. For specific anatomic landmarks for measuring circumferences, refer to Callaway, Chumlea, Bouchard, et al.[13]
5. Record girth to the nearest ⅛ in or 0.5 cm.

Special Consideration

1. Ideally, girth should be measured in the morning and before heavy physical activity.

Limb Length Measurement Principles

Introduction

1. Limb length measurements may be used to determine if a discrepancy of length exists between paired body segments.[53]
2. Limb length measurements may be useful for comparing lengths of femurs following fracture, fitting assistive devices, monitoring growth of children, and determining if a limb length discrepancy may be contributing to a dysfunction in other body areas.[53]

Limb Volume Measurement Principles[6,53,71]

Introduction

1. Limb volume measurements are based on Archimedes' principle (ie, the law that a body immersed in a fluid is buoyed up by a force equal to the weight of the fluid displaced by the body) and may be used for monitoring edema.[70]

SKINFOLD MEASUREMENTS

Skinfold Measurement Protocols
Table 6–2 outlines skinfold measurement protocols.

Skinfold Measurement Procedures[17,18,24,28,48,58]

Introduction

1. Through the use of formulas, equations, and tables, an individual's percent body fat may be predicted from skinfold measurements. Skinfold measures may also provide patterns of regional fat loss or gain throughout the body.
2. Skinfold assessments are based on the principle that approximately 50% of stored body fat is located as subcutaneous fat, which is closely related to overall body fat. Also, it should be noted that stored body fat is distributed differently in men and women.
3. The skinfold equations were originally derived from underwater weighing techniques.[33]
4. Generally, skinfold measurements have an error factor of approximately 3% to 4%. However, the 3% to 4% error is with the assumption that the skinfold method is being measured accurately. Measurement inaccuracies may compound the percentage of error (see Special Considerations section for sources of error).[75]

TABLE 6–2. SKINFOLD MEASUREMENT PROTOCOLS

Men
1. Ages 6–11[8]
2. Ages 12–14[8]
3. Ages 15–17[8]
4. Ages 18–26[66]
5. Ages 18–61[32]
6. College athletes[21]
7. Nomogram for college age[69]
8. Nomogram for college age[5]
9. College age[23]

Women
1. Ages 6–10[8]
2. Ages 11–13[8]
3. Ages 14–15[8]
4. Ages 16–18[8]
5. Ages 17–25[67]
6. Ages 18–55[34]
7. College athletes[34]
8. Nomograms for college age[69]
9. Nomograms for college age[5]
10. College age[23]

Adapted from Heyward VH. *Advanced Fitness Assessment and Exercise Prescription. 2nd ed.* Champaign, Ill: Human Kinetics Publishers, Inc; 1991.

5. Skinfold thicknesses are soft-tissue measurements. Therefore, compressibility of both skin and adipose tissue varies with the state of hydration, age, size, and the individual.[43]
6. There are two types of skinfold prediction equations: population-specific and generalized. Population-specific equations are assumed to be valid only for individuals of the specific age group, sex, race, and fitness level for which the equation was developed. On the other hand, generalized equations, developed from a broader spectrum (ie, sex, age, and fitness level), make it possible to use one equation rather than several for estimating percent body fat.[33]

Equipment

1. Skinfold calipers (eg, Lange, Harpenden)

Test Administration

1. Use a Lange caliper for measurements[14,33] since the generalized equations of Jackson and Pollock[32] and Jackson, Pollock, and Ward[34] were developed using the Lange caliper. If a Harpenden caliper (or other caliper) is used, then adjustments should be made to allow for the differences between the calipers.[25]
2. Make all measurements on the right side of the body (unless otherwise indicated).[33]
3. The "bite" of the skinfold should cover two thicknesses of skin and subcutaneous fat, but not the muscle.[20]
4. Use Table 6–3 in identifying the skinfold sites for the Jackson and Pollock[32] and Jackson, Pollock, and Ward[34] generalized equations. For other skinfold equations, refer to Lohman, Roche, and Martorell[43] and Lohman, Roche, and Martorell.[44]
5. Select one of the appropriate sum of three skinfolds listed in Table 6–4.
6. Identify, measure, and mark each site appropriately with a felt tip pen.
7. Grasp the skinfold firmly by the thumb and index finger (grasped with the pads at the tip of the thumb and finger) and place the caliper perpendicular to the fold (proximally) at approximately 1 cm from the thumb and index finger.[33] Keep the skinfold elevated while taking the measurement.

TABLE 6-3. IDENTIFYING SKINFOLD SITES[32,34]

1. Chest—a diagonal fold taken half of the distance between the anterior axillary line and the nipple for men and one third of the distance from the anterior axillary line to the nipple for women.
2. Triceps—a vertical fold on the posterior midline of the upper arm (over the triceps muscle), halfway between the acromion and olecranon processes; the elbow should be extended and relaxed.
3. Subscapular—a fold taken on a diagonal line coming from the vertebral border to 1 to 2 cm from the inferior angle of the scapula.
4. Suprailium—a diagonal fold above the crest of the ilium at the spot where an imaginary line would come down from the anterior axillary line (many recommend that the measure be taken more laterally at the anterior axillary line).
5. Abdominal—a vertical fold taken at a lateral distance of approximately 2 cm from the umbilicus.
6. Thigh—a vertical fold on the anterior aspect of the thigh midway between hip and knee joints.

Adapted with permission from Jackson AS, Pollock ML. Practical assessment of body composition. Physician Sportsmed. Copyright 1985;13(5):76–90. New York, NY: McGraw-Hill Book Co.

8. Slowly release the caliper jaw pressure so that full tension is exerted on the skinfold. Read the dial on the caliper to the nearest 0.5 mm (ie, for Lange calipers; however, other caliper scales may be different) approximately 1 to 4 seconds after the caliper jaw pressure has been released.[33,43]
9. A minimum of two measurements should be taken at each site, and these measures should not differ by more than 1 mm.[33] Before taking a second measure, the clinician should pause briefly (approximately 15 seconds) to allow for body fluids to return to the area of the skinfold.[20] If repeated measures vary by more than 1 mm, then a third measure should be taken. Typically, the clinician should complete measurements at one site before moving to the next site.[33]
10. The three trials, which were measured to be within 1 mm of each other, are then averaged and recorded as the value for that particular site.[33]
11. Use Tables 6-5 to 6-8 for estimating the client's percent body fat.

Special Considerations

1. Possible sources of error:
   a. Wet or moist skin may result in the clinician grasping extra skin or fat and thus, obtaining larger values.[33] Therefore, the client's skin should be dry and lotion-free prior to measurement.
   b. Measurements taken immediately after exercise or when the client is overheated will increase skinfold size due to the shifting of body fluid to the skin.[33] For this reason, it is best to wait approximately 2 hours after exercise to obtain measurements.
   c. Dehydration may result in a decrease in skinfold as high as 15%.[10]
   d. Lack of experience of the measuring clinician.
   e. More than one tester (especially if both are not using the same technique).

TABLE 6-4. SELECTING SKINFOLD SITES[33]

Men[a]
1. Chest, abdomen, and thigh[b]
2. Chest, triceps, and subscapula[c]

Women[a]
1. Triceps, suprailium, and thigh[b]
2. Triceps, abdomen, and suprailium[c]

[a]The accuracy of the two sums of three skinfolds is similar.
[b]Provides a good representation of the total body and is highly correlated with the sum of seven skinfolds.
[c]May be more practical to use in a clinical setting.

TABLE 6–5. PERCENT FAT ESTIMATE FOR MEN: SUM OF CHEST, ABDOMEN, AND THIGH SKINFOLDS[a]

Sum of Skinfolds (mm)	Age to the Last Year								
	< 22	23–27	28–32	33–37	38–42	43–47	48–52	53–57	> 57
8–10	1.3	1.8	2.3	2.9	3.4	3.9	4.5	5.0	5.5
11–13	2.2	2.8	3.3	3.9	4.4	4.9	5.5	6.0	6.5
14–16	3.2	3.8	4.3	4.8	5.4	5.9	6.4	7.0	7.5
17–19	4.2	4.7	5.3	5.8	6.3	6.9	7.4	8.0	8.5
20–22	5.1	5.7	6.2	6.8	7.3	7.9	8.4	8.9	9.5
23–25	6.1	6.6	7.2	7.7	8.3	8.8	9.4	9.9	10.5
26–28	7.0	7.6	8.1	8.7	9.2	9.8	10.3	10.9	11.4
29–31	8.0	8.5	9.1	9.6	10.2	10.7	11.3	11.8	12.4
32–34	8.9	9.4	10.0	10.5	11.1	11.6	12.2	12.8	13.3
35–37	9.8	10.4	10.9	11.5	12.0	12.6	13.1	13.7	14.3
38–40	10.7	11.3	11.8	12.4	12.9	13.5	14.1	14.6	15.2
41–43	11.6	12.2	12.7	13.3	13.8	14.4	15.0	15.5	16.1
44–46	12.5	13.1	13.6	14.2	14.7	15.3	15.9	16.4	17.0
47–49	13.4	13.9	14.5	15.1	15.6	16.2	16.8	17.3	17.9
50–52	14.3	14.8	15.4	15.9	16.5	17.1	17.6	18.2	18.8
53–55	15.1	15.7	16.2	16.8	17.4	17.9	18.5	19.1	19.7
56–58	16.0	16.5	17.1	17.7	18.2	18.8	19.4	20.0	20.5
59–61	16.9	17.4	17.9	18.5	19.1	19.7	20.2	20.8	21.4
62–64	17.6	18.2	18.8	19.4	19.9	20.5	21.1	21.7	22.2
65–67	18.5	19.0	19.6	20.2	20.8	21.3	21.9	22.5	23.1
68–70	19.3	19.9	20.4	21.0	21.6	22.2	22.7	23.3	23.9
71–73	20.1	20.7	21.2	21.8	22.4	23.0	23.6	24.1	24.7
74–76	20.9	21.5	22.0	22.6	23.2	23.8	24.4	25.0	25.5
77–79	21.7	22.2	22.8	23.4	24.0	24.6	25.2	25.8	26.3
80–82	22.4	23.0	23.6	24.2	24.8	25.4	25.9	26.5	27.1
83–85	23.2	23.8	24.4	25.0	25.5	26.1	26.7	27.3	27.9
86–88	24.0	24.5	25.1	25.7	26.3	26.9	27.5	28.1	28.7
89–91	24.7	25.3	25.9	26.5	27.1	27.6	28.2	28.8	29.4
92–94	25.4	26.0	26.6	27.2	27.8	28.4	29.0	29.6	30.2
95–97	26.1	26.7	27.3	27.9	28.5	29.1	29.7	30.3	30.9
98–100	26.9	27.4	28.0	28.6	29.2	29.8	30.4	31.0	31.6
101–103	27.5	28.1	28.7	29.3	29.9	30.5	31.1	31.7	32.3
104–106	28.2	28.8	29.4	30.0	30.6	31.2	31.8	32.4	33.0
107–109	28.9	29.5	30.1	30.7	31.3	31.9	32.5	33.1	33.7
110–112	29.6	30.2	30.8	31.4	32.0	32.6	33.2	33.8	34.4
113–115	30.2	30.8	31.4	32.0	32.6	33.2	33.8	34.5	35.1
116–118	30.9	31.5	32.1	32.7	33.3	33.9	34.5	35.1	35.7
119–121	31.5	32.1	32.7	33.3	33.9	34.5	35.1	35.7	36.4
122–124	32.1	32.7	33.3	33.9	34.5	35.1	35.8	36.4	37.0
125–127	32.7	33.3	33.9	34.5	35.1	35.8	36.4	37.0	37.6

[a]This table was computer-generated using regression equations,[32,34] and body density was transformed to percent body fat using the Siri formula.[65]

Reprinted with permission from Jackson AS, Pollock ML. Practical assessment of body composition. Physician Sportsmed. Copyright 1985;13(5):76–90. New York, NY: McGraw-Hill Book Co.

    f. Nonstandardization of skinfold sites.

    g. Not using well-designed calipers that exert a constant pressure of 10 g · mm^{-2} throughout the full range of caliper opening.[55,57,68]

    h. Not using the same caliper as used in determining the original equation.

    i. Not using the appropriate equation for the population being tested.

    j. Difficulty in accurately measuring extremely obese or heavily muscled individuals.

2. Since there are many skinfold formulas and protocols, the clinician will have to choose one or several that are most appropriate for his or her client population.

3. For standardized skinfold sites and procedures, refer to the *Anthropometric Standardization Reference Manual.*[43,44]

4. Allow the skinfold to follow its natural cleavage lines (Langer's lines) when grasping the skin.[43]

TABLE 6–6. PERCENT FAT ESTIMATE FOR MEN: SUM OF CHEST, TRICEPS, AND SUBSCAPULA SKINFOLDS[a]

Sum of Skinfolds (mm)	Age to the Last Year								
	< 22	23–27	28–32	33–37	38–42	43–47	48–52	53–57	> 57
8–10	1.5	2.0	2.5	3.1	3.6	4.1	4.6	5.1	5.6
11–13	3.0	3.5	4.0	4.5	5.1	5.6	6.1	6.6	7.1
14–16	4.5	5.0	5.5	6.0	6.5	7.0	7.6	8.1	8.6
17–19	5.9	6.4	6.9	7.4	8.0	8.5	9.0	9.5	10.0
20–22	7.3	7.8	8.3	8.8	9.4	9.9	10.4	10.9	11.4
23–25	8.6	9.2	9.7	10.2	10.7	11.2	11.8	12.3	12.8
26–28	10.0	10.5	11.0	11.5	12.1	12.6	13.1	13.6	14.2
29–31	11.2	11.8	12.3	12.8	13.4	13.9	14.4	14.9	15.5
32–34	12.5	13.0	13.5	14.1	14.6	15.1	15.7	16.2	16.7
35–37	13.7	14.2	14.8	15.3	15.8	16.4	16.9	17.4	18.0
38–40	14.9	15.4	15.9	16.5	17.0	17.6	18.1	18.6	19.2
41–43	16.0	16.6	17.1	17.6	18.2	18.7	19.3	19.8	20.3
44–46	17.1	17.7	18.2	18.7	19.3	19.8	20.4	20.9	21.5
47–49	18.2	18.7	19.3	19.8	20.4	20.9	21.4	22.0	22.5
50–52	19.2	19.7	20.3	20.8	21.4	21.9	22.5	23.0	23.6
53–55	20.2	20.7	21.3	21.8	22.4	22.9	23.5	24.0	24.6
56–58	21.1	21.7	22.2	22.8	23.3	23.9	24.4	25.0	25.5
59–61	22.0	22.6	23.1	23.7	24.2	24.8	25.3	25.9	26.5
62–64	22.9	23.4	24.0	24.5	25.1	25.7	26.2	26.8	27.3
65–67	23.7	24.3	24.8	25.4	25.9	26.5	27.1	27.6	28.2
68–70	24.5	25.0	25.6	26.2	26.7	27.3	27.8	28.4	29.0
71–73	25.2	25.8	26.3	26.9	27.5	28.0	28.6	29.1	29.7
74–76	25.9	26.5	27.0	27.6	28.2	28.7	29.3	29.9	30.4
77–79	26.6	27.1	27.7	28.2	28.8	29.4	29.9	30.5	31.1
80–82	27.2	27.7	28.3	28.9	29.4	30.0	30.6	31.1	31.7
83–85	27.7	28.3	28.8	29.4	30.0	30.5	31.1	31.7	32.3
86–88	28.2	28.8	29.4	29.9	30.5	31.1	31.6	32.2	32.8
89–91	28.7	29.3	29.8	30.4	31.0	31.5	32.1	32.7	33.3
92–94	29.1	29.7	30.3	30.8	31.4	32.0	32.6	33.1	33.4
95–97	29.5	30.1	30.6	31.2	31.8	32.4	32.9	33.5	34.1
98–100	29.8	30.4	31.0	31.6	32.1	32.7	33.3	33.9	34.4
101–103	30.1	30.7	31.3	31.8	32.4	33.0	33.6	34.1	34.7
104–106	30.4	30.9	31.5	32.1	32.7	33.2	33.8	34.4	35.0
107–109	30.6	31.1	31.7	32.3	32.9	33.4	34.0	34.6	35.2
110–112	30.7	31.3	31.9	32.4	33.0	33.6	34.2	34.7	35.3
113–115	30.8	31.4	32.0	32.5	33.1	33.7	34.3	34.9	35.4
116–118	30.9	31.5	32.0	32.6	33.2	33.8	34.3	34.9	35.5

[a]This table was computer generated using regression equations,[23,31] and body density was transformed to percent body fat using the Siri formula.[65]

Reprinted with permission from Jackson AS, Pollock ML. Practical assessment of body composition. Physician Sportsmed. Copyright 1985;13(5):76–90. New York, NY: McGraw-Hill Book Co.

5. Some clinicians prefer taking skinfold measurements in a rotational order.[42,57]
6. It is advisable to train with skilled clinicians and compare the results in order to determine measurement accuracy.
7. Calipers should be calibrated periodically with a gauge block available from the manufacturer.
8. Refer to Table 6–9 for advantages and disadvantages of skinfold measurements.

Additional Measurement Methods

1. Bioelectrical impedance analysis[40,45,46,58,63]
2. Body mass index[1,41,61]
3. Chemical analysis of cadavers[39]
4. Computerized tomography (CT)[39,64,72]
5. Diameters[61,77]

TABLE 6–7. PERCENT FAT ESTIMATE FOR WOMEN: SUM OF TRICEPS, SUPRAILIUM, AND THIGH SKINFOLDS[a]

Sum of Skinfolds (mm)	Age to the Last Year								
	< 22	23–27	28–32	33–37	38–42	43–47	48–52	53–57	> 57
23–25	9.7	9.9	10.2	10.4	10.7	10.9	11.2	11.4	11.7
26–28	11.0	11.2	11.5	11.7	12.0	12.3	12.5	12.7	13.0
29–31	12.3	12.5	12.8	13.0	13.3	13.5	13.8	14.0	14.3
32–34	13.6	13.8	14.0	14.3	14.5	14.8	15.0	15.3	15.5
35–37	14.8	15.0	15.3	15.5	15.8	16.0	16.3	16.5	16.8
38–40	16.0	16.3	16.5	16.7	17.0	17.2	17.5	17.7	18.0
41–43	17.2	17.4	17.7	17.9	18.2	18.4	18.7	18.9	19.2
44–46	18.3	18.6	18.8	19.1	19.3	19.6	19.8	20.1	20.3
47–49	19.5	19.7	20.0	20.2	20.5	20.7	21.0	21.2	21.5
50–52	20.6	20.8	21.1	21.3	21.6	21.8	22.1	22.3	22.6
53–55	21.7	21.9	22.1	22.4	22.6	22.9	23.1	23.4	23.6
56–58	22.7	23.0	23.2	23.4	23.7	23.9	24.2	24.4	24.7
59–61	23.7	24.0	24.2	24.5	24.7	25.0	25.2	25.5	25.7
62–64	24.7	25.0	25.2	25.5	25.7	26.0	26.7	26.4	26.7
65–67	25.7	25.9	26.2	26.4	26.7	26.9	27.2	27.4	27.7
68–70	26.6	26.9	27.1	27.4	27.6	27.9	28.1	28.4	28.6
71–73	27.5	27.8	28.0	28.3	28.5	28.8	29.0	29.3	29.5
74–76	28.4	28.7	28.9	29.2	29.4	29.7	29.9	30.2	30.4
77–79	29.3	29.5	29.8	30.0	30.3	30.5	30.8	31.0	31.3
80–82	30.1	30.4	30.6	30.9	31.1	31.4	31.6	31.9	32.1
83–85	30.9	31.2	31.4	31.7	31.9	32.2	32.4	32.7	32.9
86–88	31.7	32.0	32.2	32.5	32.7	32.9	33.2	33.4	33.7
89–91	32.5	32.7	33.0	33.2	33.5	33.7	33.9	34.2	34.4
92–94	33.2	33.4	33.7	33.9	34.2	34.4	34.7	34.9	35.2
95–97	33.9	34.1	34.4	34.6	34.9	35.1	35.4	35.6	35.9
98–100	34.6	34.8	35.1	35.3	35.5	35.8	36.0	36.3	36.5
101–103	35.3	35.4	35.7	35.9	36.2	36.4	36.7	36.9	37.2
104–106	35.8	36.1	36.3	36.6	36.8	37.1	37.3	37.5	37.8
107–109	36.4	36.7	36.9	37.1	37.4	37.6	37.9	38.1	38.4
110–112	37.0	37.2	37.5	37.7	38.0	38.2	38.5	38.7	38.9
113–115	37.5	37.8	38.0	38.2	38.5	38.7	39.0	39.2	39.5
116–118	38.0	38.3	38.5	38.8	39.0	39.3	39.5	39.7	40.0
119–121	38.5	38.7	39.0	39.2	39.5	39.7	40.0	40.2	40.5
122–124	39.0	39.2	39.4	39.7	39.9	40.2	40.4	40.7	40.9
125–127	39.4	39.6	39.9	40.1	40.4	40.6	40.9	41.1	41.4
128–130	39.8	40.0	40.3	40.5	40.8	41.0	41.3	41.5	41.8

[a]This table was computer-generated using regression equations,[32,34] and body density was transformed to percent body fat using the Siri formula.[65]

Reprinted with permission from Jackson AS, Pollock ML. Practical assessment of body composition. Physician Sportsmed. Copyright 1985;13(5):76–90. New York, NY: McGraw-Hill Book Co.

6. Height-squared index[1,7]
7. Hydrostatic weighing (underwater weighing, densitometry)[1,7,11,28]
8. Isotope dilution[19,60]
9. Maturation[61]
10. Muscle metabolite excretion[12,50]
11. Near-infrared interactance[16,28]
12. Neutron activation[47]
13. O-Scale[61]
14. Photon absorptiometry[15]
15. Potassium-40[22]
16. Proportionality[61]
17. Somatotype classification[61]
18. Total body electrical conductivity[59,60,62]
19. Ultrasound[26,35,39]
20. X-ray[36,37,39]

TABLE 6–8. PERCENT FAT ESTIMATE FOR WOMEN: SUM OF TRICEPS, ABDOMEN, AND SUPRAILIUM SKINFOLDS[a]

Sum of Skinfolds (mm)	Age to the Last Year								
	18–22	*23–27*	*28–32*	*33–37*	*38–42*	*43–47*	*48–52*	*53–57*	*> 57*
8–12	8.8	9.0	9.2	9.4	9.5	9.7	9.9	10.1	10.3
13–17	10.8	10.9	11.1	11.3	11.5	11.7	11.8	12.0	12.2
18–22	12.6	12.8	13.0	13.2	13.4	13.5	13.7	13.9	14.1
23–27	14.5	14.6	14.8	15.0	15.2	15.4	15.6	15.7	15.9
28–32	16.2	16.4	16.6	16.8	17.0	17.1	17.3	17.5	17.7
33–37	17.9	18.1	18.3	18.5	18.7	18.9	19.0	19.2	19.4
38–42	19.6	19.8	20.0	20.2	20.3	20.5	20.7	20.9	21.1
43–47	21.2	21.4	21.6	21.8	21.9	22.1	22.3	22.5	22.7
48–52	22.8	22.9	23.1	23.3	23.5	23.7	23.8	24.0	24.2
53–57	24.2	24.4	24.6	24.8	25.0	25.2	25.3	25.5	25.7
58–62	25.7	25.9	26.0	26.2	26.4	26.6	26.8	27.0	27.1
63–67	27.1	27.2	27.4	27.6	27.8	28.0	28.2	28.3	28.5
68–72	28.4	28.6	28.7	28.9	29.1	29.3	29.5	29.7	29.8
73–77	29.6	29.8	30.0	30.2	30.4	30.6	30.7	30.9	31.1
78–82	30.9	31.0	31.2	31.4	31.6	31.8	31.9	32.1	32.3
83–87	32.0	32.2	32.4	32.6	32.7	32.9	33.1	33.3	33.5
88–92	33.1	33.3	33.5	33.7	33.8	34.0	34.2	34.4	34.6
93–97	34.1	34.3	34.5	34.7	34.9	35.1	35.2	35.4	35.6
98–102	35.1	35.3	35.5	35.7	35.9	36.0	36.2	36.4	36.6
103–107	36.1	36.2	36.4	36.6	36.8	37.0	37.2	37.3	37.5
108–112	36.9	37.1	37.3	37.5	37.7	37.9	38.0	38.2	38.4
113–117	37.8	37.9	38.1	38.3	39.2	39.4	39.6	39.8	39.2
118–122	38.5	38.7	38.9	39.1	39.4	39.6	39.8	40.0	40.0
123–127	39.2	39.4	39.6	39.8	40.0	40.1	40.3	40.5	40.7
128–132	39.9	40.1	40.2	40.4	40.6	40.8	41.0	41.2	41.3
133–137	40.5	40.7	40.8	41.0	41.2	41.4	41.6	41.7	41.9
138–142	41.0	41.2	41.4	41.6	41.7	41.9	42.1	42.3	42.5
143–147	41.5	41.7	41.9	42.0	42.2	42.4	42.6	42.8	43.0
148–152	41.9	42.1	42.3	42.8	42.6	42.8	43.0	43.2	43.4
153–157	42.3	42.5	42.6	42.8	43.0	43.2	43.4	43.6	43.7
158–162	42.6	42.8	43.0	43.1	43.3	43.5	43.7	43.9	44.1
163–167	42.9	43.0	43.2	43.4	43.6	43.8	44.0	44.1	44.3
168–172	43.1	43.2	43.4	43.6	43.8	44.0	44.2	44.3	44.5
173–177	43.2	43.4	43.6	43.8	43.9	44.1	44.3	44.5	44.7
178–182	43.3	43.5	43.7	43.8	44.0	44.2	44.4	44.6	44.8

[a]This table was computer-generated using regression equations,[32,34] and body density was transformed to percent body fat using the Siri formula.[66]
Reprinted with permission from Jackson AS, Pollock ML. Practical assessment of body composition. Physician Sportsmed. Copyright 1985;13(5):76–90. New York, NY: McGraw-Hill Book Co.

TABLE 6–9. ADVANTAGES AND DISADVANTAGES OF SKINFOLD MEASUREMENTS

Advantages
1. Relatively easy to perform
2. Relatively inexpensive
3. Relatively safe
4. Requires minimal client cooperation
5. Is not time-consuming
6. Relatively simple interpretation

Disadvantage
1. If sources of error are compounded, there may be a large prediction error.

CLASSIFYING AND REPORTING

Tables 6–10 and 6–11 provide the clinician with body fat classifications, and Table 6–12 will assist the clinician in determining ideal body weight. Figure 6–1 may be used for recording skinfolds, height, and weight during testing procedures.

TABLE 6–10. PERCENT BODY FAT CLASSIFICATIONS[a,b]

Age (yr)	Men				
	Poor	Fair	Average	Good	Excellent
20–29	>24	21–23	14–20	11–13	<10
30–39	>25	22–24	15–21	12–14	<11
40–49	>27	24–26	17–23	14–16	<13
50–59	>28	25–27	18–24	15–17	<14
60+	>29	26–28	17–25	16–18	<15

Age (yr)	Women				
	Poor	Fair	Average	Good	Excellent
20–29	>32	29–31	20–28	16–19	<15
30–39	>33	30–32	21–29	17–20	<16
40–49	>34	31–33	22–30	18–21	<17
50–59	>35	32–34	23–31	19–22	<18
60+	>36	33–35	24–32	20–23	<19

[a]Norms are based on the average fat percentage levels of 308 men between 18 and 61 years of age and 249 women between 18 and 55 years of age, who varied considerably in body structure, body composition, and exercise habits.
[b]For sport-specific values of relative percent fat, refer to Wilmore and Costill.[76]
Adapted from Gettman LR. Fitness testing. In: Blair SN, Painter P, Pate RR, et al, eds. Resource Manual for Guidelines for Exercise Testing and Prescription (American College of Sports Medicine). Philadelphia, Pa: Lea & Febiger; 1988. Data from Jackson and Pollock[32] and Jackson, Pollock, and Ward.[34]

TABLE 6–11. STANDARDS FOR FATNESS FOR MEN AND WOMEN IN PERCENT BODY FAT

Category	Men (% body fat)	Women (% body fat)
Most athletes	5–13	12–22
Optimal health	10–25	18–30
Optimal fitness	12–18	16–25
Obesity	>25	>30

Adapted with permission from Physician and Sportsmedicine. Roundtable—Body Composition. Physician Sportsmed. Copyright 1986;14(3):144–162. New York, NY: McGraw-Hill Book Co.

TABLE 6–12. CALCULATING DESIRED BODY WEIGHT[23,52]

Case Study
A 30-year-old man weighs 200 lb with a current body fat level of 20%. A desired body fat level of 15% (ie, the average range of percent body fat selected from Table 6-10 for men aged 30 to 39 years) may be used to determine desired body weight for this 30-year-old man as follows:

A. *Calculation of Current Fat Weight*
  1. Formula: Current fat weight (lb) = Current body weight (lb) × (Current % body fat/100)
  2. Example: Current fat weight (lb) = 200 lb × (20%/100)
                        = 200 lb × 0.20
                        = 40 lb

B. *Calculation of Current Lean Body Weight (LBW)*[a]
  1. Formula: Current LBW (lb) = Current body weight (lb) − Current fat weight (lb)
  2. Example: Current LBW (lb) = 200 lb − 40 lb
                     = 160 lb

C. *Calculation of Desirable Body Weight*[b,c]
  1. Formula:
$$\text{Desired body weight (lb)} = \frac{\text{Current LBW (lb)}}{1.00 - (\text{Desired \% body fat}/100)}$$
  2. Example:
$$\text{Desired body weight (lb)} = \frac{160 \text{ lb}}{1.00 - (15\%/100)}$$
$$= 188.24 \text{ lb}$$

[a]LBW (lean body weight) = density of bone and muscle tissue.
[b]Generally, desired body weight, ideal body weight, and playing weight (in athletes) may be used synonymously.
[c]Katch and McArdle[39] recommend prescribing a range for attaining desired body weight. For example, in this case study, a target desired body fat range of 15% to 17% would correspond to approximately 188.24 to 192.77 lb desired body weight, respectively.

NAME: _____ DATE: _____

AGE: _____   SEX: M   F

HEIGHT: _____ in _____ cm   WEIGHT: _____ lb _____ kg

	Skinfolds (mm)			
	Trial 1	Trial 2	Trial 3	Average
Men: Method 1				
1. Chest	_____	_____	_____	_____
2. Abdomen	_____	_____	_____	_____
3. Thigh	_____	_____	_____	_____
Men: Method 2				
1. Chest	_____	_____	_____	_____
2. Triceps	_____	_____	_____	_____
3. Subscapula	_____	_____	_____	_____
Women: Method 1				
1. Triceps	_____	_____	_____	_____
2. Suprailium	_____	_____	_____	_____
3. Thigh	_____	_____	_____	_____
Women: Method 2				
1. Triceps	_____	_____	_____	_____
2. Abdomen	_____	_____	_____	_____
3. Suprailium	_____	_____	_____	_____

Total: _____

CALCULATIONS:

RESULTS:

	Males	Females
Measured percent fat	_____	_____
Classification	_____	_____
Desired body weight range	_____	_____
Desired percent fat range	_____	_____

COMMENTS:

_____

_____

_____

Figure 6–1. Sample data sheet for skinfold measures.

REFERENCES

1. Adams GM. *Exercise Physiology Laboratory Manual*. Dubuque, Iowa: Wm C Brown Publishers; 1990.
2. American Alliance for Health, Physical Education, Recreation and Dance. *Norms for College Students*. Reston, Va: American Alliance for Health, Physical Education, Recreation and Dance; 1985.
3. American Alliance for Health, Physical Education, Recreation and Dance. *Physical Best*. Reston, Va: American Alliance for Health, Physical Education, Recreation and Dance; 1988.
4. Andres R. Mortality and obesity: The rationale for age-specific height-weight tables. In: Bierman EL, Hazzard WR, eds. *Principles of Geriatric Medicine*. New York, NY: McGraw-Hill Book Co; 1985.
5. Baun WB, Baun MR, Raven PB. A nomogram for the estimate of percent body fat from generalized equations. *Res Q Exerc Sport*. 1981;52(3):380–384.
6. Beach RB. Measurement of extremity volume by water displacement. *Phys Ther*. 1977;57:286.
7. Behnke AR, Wilmore JH. *Evaluation and Regulation of Body Build and Composition*. Englewood Cliffs, NJ: Prentice-Hall; 1974.
8. Boileau RA, Lohman TG, Slaughter MH. Exercise and body composition of children and youth. *Scand J Sports Sci*. 1985;7:17–27.
9. Brannon FJ, Geyer MJ, Foley NW. *Cardiac Rehabilitation*. Philadelphia, Pa: FA Davis Co; 1988.
10. Brooks GA, Fahey TD. *Exercise Physiology: Bioenergetics and Its Application*. New York, NY: John Wiley & Sons, Inc; 1984.
11. Brozek J, Keys A. The evaluation of leanness–fatness in man: Norms and intercorrelations. *Br J Nutr*. 1951;5:194-205.
12. Buskirk ER, Mendez J. Sports science and body composition analysis: Emphasis on cell and muscle mass. *Med Sci Sports Exerc*. 1984;16:584–593.
13. Callaway CW, Chumlea WC, Bouchard C, et al. Circumferences. In: Lohman TG, Roche AF, Martorell R, eds. *Anthropometric Standardization Reference Manual*. Champaign, Ill: Human Kinetics Publishers, Inc; 1988.
14. Cambridge Scientific Industries. *Lange Skinfold Caliper Operator's Manual*. Cambridge, Md: Cambridge Scientific Industries; 1985.
15. Cameron JR, Sorenson J. Measurement of bone mineral in-vivo: An improved method. *Science*. 1963;142:230–232.
16. Conway JM, Norris KH, Bodwell CE. A new approach for the estimation of body composition: Infrared interactance. *Am J Clin Nutr*. 1984;40:1123–1130.
17. Day J. *Perspectives in Kinanthropometry: 1984 Olympic Scientific Congress Proceedings*. Champaign, Ill: Human Kinetics Publishers, Inc; 1986;1.
18. Durnin JV, Womersly J. Body fat assessed from total body density and its estimation from skinfold thickness: Measurements on 481 men and women aged from 16 to 72 years. *Br J Nutr*. 1974;32:77–97.
19. Finberg L. Clinical assessment of total body water. In: Roche AF, ed. *Body Composition Assessments in Youth and Adults*. Columbus, Ohio: Ross Laboratories; 1985.
20. Fleck SJ. Determination of body fat via skinfold measurements. *Nat Strength Condit Assoc J*. 1981;3(5):56.
21. Forsyth HS, Sinning WE. The anthropometric estimation of body density and lean body weight of male athletes. *Med Sci Sports*. 1973;5:174–180.
22. Garrow JS. New approaches to body composition. *Am J Clin Nutr*. 1982;35:1152–1158.
23. Gettman LR. Fitness testing. In: Blair SN, Painter P, Pate RR, et al, eds. *Resource Manual for Guidelines for Exercise Testing and Prescription* (American College of Sports Medicine). Philadelphia, Pa: Lea & Febiger; 1988.
24. Golding LA, Myers CR, Sinning WE. *The Y's Way to Physical Fitness: The Complete Guide to Testing and Instruction*. 3rd ed. Champaign, Ill: Human Kinetics Publishers, Inc; 1989.
25. Gruber JJ, Pollock ML, Graves JE, et al. Comparison of Harpenden and Lange calipers in predicting body composition. *Res Q Exerc Sport*. 1990;61:184–190.
26. Heymsfield SB. Clinical assessment of lean tissues: Future directions. In: Roche AF, ed. *Body Composition Assessments in Youth and Adults*. Columbus, Ohio: Ross Laboratories; 1985.

27. Heyward VH. *Designs for Fitness: A Guide to Physical Fitness Appraisal and Exercise Prescription*. Minneapolis, Minn: Burgess Publishing Co; 1984.

28. Heyward VH. *Advanced Fitness Assessment and Exercise Prescription*. 2nd ed. Champaign, Ill: Human Kinetics Publishers, Inc; 1991.

29. Hodgdon JA, Beckett MB. Prediction of percent body fat for U.S. Navy men from body circumferences and height (Report No. 84-11). San Diego, Calif: Naval Health Research Center; 1984.

30. Hodgdon JA, Beckett MB. Prediction of percent body fat for U.S. Navy women from body circumferences and height (Report No. 84-29). San Diego, Calif: Naval Health Research Center; 1984.

31. Hodgdon JA, Beckett MB. Technique for measuring body circumferences and skinfold thicknesses (Report No. 84-39). San Diego, Calif: Naval Health Research Center; 1984.

32. Jackson AS, Pollock ML. Generalized equations for predicting body density of men. *Br J Nutr*. 1978;40:497–504.

33. Jackson AS, Pollock ML. Practical assessment of body composition. *Physician Sportsmed*. 1985;13(5):76–90.

34. Jackson AS, Pollock ML, Ward A. Generalized equations for predicting body density of women. *Med Sci Sports Exerc*. 1980;12(3):175–182.

35. Katch FI. Reliability and individual differences in ultrasound assessment of subcutaneous fat: Effects of body position. *Hum Biol*. 1983;55:789.

36. Katch FI. Assessment of lean body tissues by radiography and bioelectrical impedance. In: Roche AF, ed. *Body Composition Assessments in Youth and Adults*. Columbus, Ohio: Ross Laboratories; 1985.

37. Katch FI, Behnke AR. Arm x-ray assessment of body fat in men and women. *Med Sci Sports Exerc*. 1984;16:316.

38. Katch FI, McArdle WD. Prediction of body density from simple anthropometric measurements in college-age men and women. *Hum Biol*. 1973;45:445–454.

39. Katch FI, McArdle WD. *Nutrition, Weight Control and Exercise*. 3rd ed. Philadelphia, Pa: Lea & Febiger; 1988.

40. Khaled MA, McCutcheon MJ, Reddy S, et al. Electrical impedance in assessing human body composition: The BIA method. *Am J Clin Nutr*. 1988;47:789–792.

41. Lee J, Kolonel LN, Hinds MW. Relative merits of the weight-corrected-for-height indices. *Am J Clin Nutr*. 1981;34:2521–2529.

42. Lohman TG, Pollock ML, Slaughter MH, et al. Methodological factors and the prediction of body fat in female athletes. *Med Sci Sports Exerc*. 1984;16:92–96.

43. Lohman TG, Roche AF, Martorell R, eds. *Anthropometric Standardization Reference Manual*. Champaign, Ill: Human Kinetics Publishers, Inc; 1988.

44. Lohman TG, Roche AF, Martorell R, eds. *Anthropometric Standardization Reference Manual*, abridged ed. Champaign, Ill: Human Kinetics Publishers, Inc; 1991.

45. Lukaski HC, Bolonchuk WW, Hall CB, et al. Validation of tetrapolar bioelectrical impedance method to assess human body composition. *J Appl Physiol*. 1986;60:1327–1332.

46. Lukaski HC, Johnson PE, Bolonchuk WW, et al. Assessment of fat-free mass using bioelectrical impedance measurements of the human body. *Am J Clin Nutr*. 1985; 41:810–817.

47. Lukaski HC, Mendez J, Buskirk ER, et al. A comparison of methods of assessment of body composition including neutron activation analysis of total body nitrogen. *Metabolism*. 1981;30:777–782.

48. Marcus JB, ed. *Sports Nutrition: A Guide for the Professional Working with Active People*. Chicago, Ill: American Dietetic Association; 1986.

49. McArdle WD, Katch FI, Katch VL. *Exercise Physiology: Energy, Nutrition and Human Performance*. 3rd ed. Philadelphia, Pa: Lea & Febiger; 1991.

50. Mendez J, Lukaski HC, Buskirk ER. Fat-free mass as a function of maximal oxygen consumption and 24-hour urinary creatinine and 3-methylhistidine excretion. *Am J Clin Nutr*. 1984;39:710–715.

51. Metropolitan Life Insurance Company. New weight standards for men and women. *Statistical Bulletin Metropolitan Life Insurance Company*. 1959;40:1–4.

52. Miller DK. *Measurement by the Physical Educator: Why and How*. Carmel, Ind: Benchmark Press; 1988.

53. Minor MAD, Minor SD. *Patient Evaluation Methods for the Health Professional*. Reston, Va: Reston Publishing Company, Inc (A Prentice-Hall Company); 1985.

54. Moore M. New height-weight tables gain pounds, lose status. *Physician Sportsmed*. 1983;11:25.

55. Nieman DC. *The Sports Medicine Fitness Course*. Palo Alto, Calif: Bull Publishing Co; 1986.

56. Peterson M, Peterson K. *Eat to Compete: A Guide to Sports Nutrition*. Chicago, Ill: Year Book Medical Publishers, Inc; 1988.

57. Pollock ML, Jackson AS. Research progress in validation of clinical methods of assessing body composition. *Med Sci Sports Exerc*. 1984;16:606–613.

58. Pollock ML, Wilmore JH. *Exercise in Health and Disease: Evaluation of Prescription for Prevention and Rehabilitation*. 2nd ed. Philadelphia, Pa: WB Saunders Co; 1990.

59. Presta E, Casullo AM, Costa R, et al. Body composition in adolescents: Estimation by total body electrical conductivity. *J Appl Physiol*. 1987;63:937–941.

60. Roche AF, ed. *Body Composition Assessments in Youth and Adults*. Columbus, Ohio: Ross Laboratories; 1985.

61. Ross WD, Marfell-Jones MJ. Kinanthropometry. In: MacDougall JD, Wenger HA, Green HJ, eds. *Physiological Testing of the High-Performance Athlete*. 2nd ed. Champaign, Ill: Human Kinetics Publishers, Inc; 1991.

62. Segal KR, Gutin B, Presta E, et al. Estimation of human body composition by electrical impedance methods: A comparative study. *J Appl Physiol*. 1985;58:1565–1571.

63. Segal KR, VanLoan M, Fitzgerald PI, et al. Lean body mass estimation by bioelectrical impedance analysis: A four-site cross-validation study. *Am J Clin Nutr*. 1988;47:7–14.

64. Seidell JC, Bakker CJG, van der Kooy K. Imaging techniques for measuring adipose-tissue distribution: A comparison between computed tomography and 1.5-T magnetic resonance. *Am J Clin Nutr*. 1990;51:953–957.

65. Siri WE. Body composition from fluid spaces and density. In: Brozek J, Henschel A, eds. *Techniques for Measuring Body Composition*. Washington, DC: National Academy of Science; 1961.

66. Sloan AW. Estimation of body fat in young men. *J Appl Physiol*. 1967;23:311–315.

67. Sloan AW, Burt JJ, Blyth CS. Estimation of body fat in young women. *J Appl Physiol*. 1962;17:967–970.

68. Sloan AW, Shapiro M. A comparison of skinfold measurements with three standard calipers. *Hum Biol*. 1972;44:29–36.

69. Sloan AW, Weir JB. Nomograms for prediction of body density and total body fat from skinfold measurements. *J Appl Physiol*. 1970;28:221–222.

70. Stein J, ed. *The Random House College Dictionary*, revised ed. New York, NY: Random House; 1984.

71. Thompson JK, Grist BM, Shoemake RL. An inexpensive hand volume tank. *Phys Ther*. 1975;55:766.

72. Tokunaga K. A novel technique for the determination of body fat by computed tomography. *Int J Obesity*. 1983;7:437.

73. Tran ZV, Weltman A. Generalized equation for predicting body density of women from girth measurements. *Med Sci Sports Exerc*. 1989;21:101–104.

74. Wilmore JH. *Sensible Fitness*. 2nd ed. Champaign, Ill: Human Kinetics Publishers, Inc; 1986.

75. Wilmore JH, Buskirk ER, DiGirolamo M, et al. Roundtable—Body composition. *Physician Sportsmed*. 1986;14(3):144–162.

76. Wilmore JH, Costill DL. *Training for Sport and Activity: The Physiological Basis of the Conditioning Process*. 3rd ed. Dubuque, Iowa: Wm C Brown Publishers; 1988.

77. Wilmore JH, Frisancho RA, Gordon CC, et al. Body breadth equipment and measurement techniques. In: Lohman TG, Roche AF, Martorell R, eds. *Anthropometric Standardization Reference Manual*, abridged ed. Champaign, Ill: Human Kinetics Publishers, Inc; 1988.

Sport Performance Testing

METHODS OF TESTING

AEROBIC POWER

Table 7–1 outlines specific testing protocols for the measurement of aerobic power. For specific treadmill and bicycle ergometer testing procedures, the reader should refer to Chapter 5, Cardiovascular Endurance Testing and substitute the specific aerobic power testing protocols.

ANAEROBIC POWER AND CAPACITY

Table 7–2 outlines specific testing protocols for the measurement of anaerobic power and capacity.

Short-Term Anaerobic Test Procedure

Short-term anaerobic tests are designed to evaluate primarily the alactic anaerobic capacity of the involved muscles and usually last about 10 seconds or less.[17]

Name of Test

Margaria Staircase (Power) Test

Introduction

1. The test is designed to measure muscular power by having the client run up a flight of stairs as quickly as possible.[56]
2. The power score in the stair-sprinting test is influenced by the person's body mass. The heavier person will have a higher power score if several individuals achieve the same speed.[56]
3. This test may be better suited for testing individuals of similar body mass or for testing individuals before and after an anaerobic training program.[56]

Equipment

1. Staircase consisting of at least nine steps
2. Two switch mats connected to a time recorder with a sensitivity of 0.01 second

TABLE 7–1. AEROBIC POWER TESTING PROTOCOLS

Maximal Treadmill Protocols
1. Costill and Fox protocol[a,22,36]
2. Maksud and Coutts protocol[a,36,52]
3. Modified Åstrand protocol[a,36,66]
4. Taylor protocol[b,36,79]
5. Thoden protocol[a,81]

Maximal Leg Cycle Ergometer Protocol
1. Thoden protocol[b,81]

Additional Protocols
1. Various sports may be tested through sport-specific protocols
   (eg, rowing, paddling, cycling, swimming, cross-country skiing)[81]

[a]Continuous tests.
[b]Discontinuous tests.

3. Approximately a 6-m run-up path
4. White tape to mark the third, sixth, and ninth steps

Test Administration

1. Make sure all equipment is properly calibrated.
2. Make sure the client prepares with a proper warm-up and stretching routine.
3. Place a switch mat at the third step to start the timer and a second switch mat at the ninth step to stop the timer. Make sure the switch mats are properly secured on the steps.
4. The client stands 6 m in front of the stairs and then runs up the stairs as rapidly as possible, taking three steps at a time. Make sure that the runup pathway does not have a slippery surface and that there are no obstacles in the path of the client.
5. Repeat the test several times for the best score or average the best three trials.

TABLE 7–2. ANAEROBIC POWER AND CAPACITY TESTING PROTOCOLS

Short-term Anaerobic Tests
1. 50-Yard dash test (with a football)[2]
2. Margaria staircase test[17,54]
3. Maximal isokinetic tests[17]
4. Power ice skating test[39]
5. Quebec 10-second test[17,76]
6. Treadmill sprint tests (at 15, 30, 45, and 60 seconds)[82]

Intermediate-term Anaerobic Tests
1. De Bruyn-Prévost constant-load test[17,25,26]
2. Maximal isokinetic tests[17]
3. 30-Second Wingate test[1,8,9,17,30,31,37,65]

Long-term Anaerobic Tests
1. Cunningham and Faulkner treadmill test[17,24]
2. Maximal isokinetic tests[17]
3. 120-Second maximal test[17,45]
4. Quebec 90-second test[17]
5. 60-Second vertical jump test[16,17]

Additional Tests
1. Anaerobic power step test[1]
2. Jumping jacks test[46]
3. Line drill test[73]
4. 300-Yard shuttle run test[42]
5. Treadmill anaerobic power tests[1]

Adapted from Bouchard C, Taylor AW, Simoneau J-A, et al. Testing anaerobic power and capacity. In: MacDougall JD, Wenger HA, Green HJ, eds. Physiological Testing of the High-Performance Athlete. 2nd ed. Champaign, Ill: Human Kinetics Publishers, Inc; 1991.

Calculations

1. The power output is calculated by using the following formula:

$$P = \frac{F \times D}{T}$$

where P = power in kg $\cdot$ m $\cdot$ s^{-1}
F = weight of the person in kilograms
D = vertical distance between the third and ninth steps in meters (usually about 1.05 m)
T = time from the third to the ninth step in seconds

2. For specific norms for classifying men and women in terms of alactic anaerobic capacity, refer to Kalamen,[43] Margaria, Aghemo, and Rovelli,[54] and Mathews and Fox.[55]

Special Consideration

1. As an alternative, the switch mats may be placed on the second and sixth steps, thus requiring the client to take only two steps at a time. The same formula may be used; however, the distance between the two stairs would need to be measured. No standards or norms are available for the test when this procedure is used.

Intermediate-Term Anaerobic Test Procedure

Intermediate-term anaerobic tests are designed primarily to assess the lactic anaerobic power and capacity of the involved muscles and usually last about 20 to 50 seconds.[17]

Name of Test

30-Second Wingate Test

Introduction

1. This test is a means of evaluating anaerobic power output in the legs and has been adapted to test the anaerobic performance of the arms.

Equipment

1. Leg test may be performed on a Fleisch ergometer or a modified Monark cycle ergometer
2. Arm test may be performed on a Fleisch ergometer or a specially modified Monark cycle ergometer
3. Stopwatch

Test Administration

1. The client performs a 2- to 4-minute warm-up on the cycle ergometer at an intensity sufficient to elevate the heart rate to 150 to 160 beats per minute and then rests for a 3- to 5-minute interval.[67]
2. The client is instructed to pedal as fast as possible without resistance on the flywheel. After the client reaches full pedaling speed (usually within 3 to 4 seconds), the resistance is adjusted and the timer and revolution counter are activated for a period of exactly 30 seconds.
3. In the leg test, the resistance load is about 45 g/kg body weight for a Fleisch ergometer and about 75 g/kg body weight for a Monark ergometer. In the arm test, the resistance load is about 30 g/kg body weight for a Fleisch ergometer and about 50 g/kg body weight for a Monark ergometer.[17] Resistance values must be increased when testing power-trained athletes. Other researchers[67] have cited alternative methods for determining the flywheel resistance.
4. Record the pedal rate every 5 seconds for the total duration of the 30-second test.

Calculations

1. The following performance indicators may be used for determining lactic anaerobic power and capacity:[17]
   a. Mean power—work output over a 30-second period
   b. Peak power—highest power output in a 5-second period
   c. Fatigue index—difference between the peak power and the lowest 5-second power output divided by peak power
2. For specific norms for classifying various male and female athletes in terms of lactic anaerobic power and capacity, refer to Bouchard, Taylor, Simoneau, et al.[17]

Long-Term Anaerobic Test Procedure

Long-term anaerobic tests are designed primarily to evaluate the total anaerobic capacity and the ability to maintain a high power output when a large anaerobic energy component is present and usually last about 60 to 120 seconds.[17]

Name of Test

60-Second Vertical Jump Test.

Equipment

1. Ergojump (an electronic instrument designed to measure the time in contact with the platform and the flight time)[15-17]
2. Stopwatch

Test Administration

1. Make sure the client prepares with a proper warm-up and stretching routine.
2. The client is instructed to perform consecutive and maximal effort vertical jumps (with the knees bent to about 90 degrees and the hands kept on the hips to minimize horizontal and lateral displacement) for a 60-second period.[17]
3. The flight time during each jump is recorded and summed up over the 60-second period.

Calculations

1. The power output is calculated by using the following formula:[17]

$$W = \frac{9.8 \times Tf \times 60}{4N\,(60 - Tf)}$$

where W = mechanical power in $W \cdot kg^{-1}$
   9.8 = normal acceleration of gravity in $m \cdot s^{-2}$
   Tf = sum of total flight time of all jumps
   N = number of jumps during 60 seconds

MUSCULAR POWER

Table 7–3 outlines specific testing protocols for the measurement of muscular power.

TABLE 7–3. MUSCULAR POWER TESTING PROTOCOLS

Upper-Body Tests
1. Kneeling overhead throw test[57]
2. Medicine ball throw or put test[12,46]

Lower-Body Tests
1. Standing broad jump test[4,59]
2. Vertical jump test[1,12,46,59,70,74]

Upper-Body Test Procedure

Name of Test
Medicine Ball Put Test

Introduction
1. The objective of this test is to put a weighted object for a maximal distance with the arms in order to measure muscular power of the upper extremities.

Equipment
1. 6- or 9-lb medicine ball
2. 100-ft tape measure

Test Administration
1. Make sure the client prepares with a proper warm-up and stretching routine.
2. The client assumes a position behind a restraining line with the shoulders in line with the test course (the side opposite the throwing arm is facing in the direction of the throw).[12]
3. The medicine ball is tucked under the chin, and from a standing position, the client squats back without moving the feet in order to gather momentum and puts the medicine down the test course.[12]

Calculations
1. The score is the distance of the put measured from the furthest point of the back foot to the point of contact of the medicine ball after the put.
2. Measurements are generally taken to the last half-foot.

Special Considerations
1. Alternatives for this test are as follows:
   a. Use of a 4- to 12-lb shot put
   b. Use of a seated position on a chair or on the ground
   c. Use of one or two arms
2. Concentric circles drawn 1 ft apart may be used to simplify the scoring by eliminating the need for measuring the distance of each put.

Lower-Body Test Procedure

Name of Test
Vertical Jump Test

Equipment
1. A wall of sufficient height
2. Yardstick or tape measure
3. Chalk

Test Administration
1. Make sure the client prepares with a proper warm-up and stretching routine.
2. A yardstick or tape measure may be taped to the wall in order to measure the distance between the two chalk marks.
3. The client stands with the dominant side toward the wall and the feet flat on the floor.
4. The client applies ample chalk powder on the fingertips of the dominant hand and reaches as high as possible against the wall to make a mark with the fingertips at the highest reach position.
5. To execute the jump, the client squats and jumps as high as possible, making another mark at the highest point of the jump. The client should not walk or step into the jump.
6. The client should practice the jump before attempting the test.

TABLE 7–4. SPEED TESTING PROTOCOLS

1. Flying start 40-, 50-, 100-, 300-, and 440-yard sprint tests[27]
2. Stationary start 40-, 50-, and 60-yard sprint tests[123,27,28,67]
3. Stride length test[27,28]
4. Stride rate test[27]

Calculations

1. The vertical jump height is measured by taking the distance between the standing and jumping heights.
2. Measurements should be taken to the last inch.
3. The best jump score is the test score.
4. For specific norms for classifying males and females ages 10 through 17, refer to Baumgartner and Jackson[12] and Miller.[59]

SPEED

Table 7–4 outlines specific testing protocols for the measurement of speed.

Speed Test Procedures

Name of Test

Stationary Start 40-Yard Dash Test [27,28]

Equipment

1. Stop watches accurate to 0.1 second
2. An accurately measured 40-yard running course on a track with sufficient room for stopping after the test
3. Finish tape

Test Administration

1. Make sure the client prepares with a proper warm-up and stretching routine.
2. The client assumes a stationary start position in either a crouched track stance or in a standing "wide receiver" stance.
3. The clinician gives the commands of "runners to your mark, get set, and go."
4. On the command "go," the client sprints with maximal effort through the finish tape.
5. Timers (usually one to three) are placed at the finish line and start their watches on the command of "go" and stop their watches when the client breaks the tape.

Special Considerations

1. A starter's gun may be used for starting the test, which would give the client and timers auditory and visual feedback (ie, the smoke of the gun).
2. Electronic devices may be used for more accurate measures of 40-yard sprint times.
3. The client may be instructed to run on a line on the track in order to avoid side-to-side displacement.
4. Testing should be performed on a day with minimal or no headwind or tailwind.

Name of Test

Flying Start 40-Yard Dash Test[27,28]

Equipment

1. Stop watches accurate to 0.1 second
2. An accurately measured 40-yard running course on a track with sufficient room for stopping after the test
3. Finish tape

Test Administration

1. Make sure the client prepares with a proper warm-up and stretching routine.
2. Place two markers 40 yards apart.
3. The client starts 15 yards behind the first marker.
4. The client accelerates to maximum speed prior to reaching the first marker and then, while at full speed, the client continues to run between the two markers (placed 40 yards apart).
5. The timers start their watches upon the client arriving at the starting tape (ie, first marker) and stop their watches at the finishing tape (ie, second marker).

Name of Test

Stride Length Test

Equipment

1. Tape measure
2. A surface that will leave an imprint of the foot while running (eg, cinder, sand, dirt)

Test Administration

1. Make sure the client prepares with a proper warm-up and stretching routine.
2. Place two markers 25 yards apart on the running surface.
3. The client starts 50 yards behind the first marker.
4. The client accelerates to maximum speed prior to reaching the first marker and then, while at full speed, the client continues to run between the two markers (placed 25 yards apart).
5. The clinician notes the imprints left on the running surface and measures the two longest strides from the tip of the toe of the back leg to the tip of the toe of the front leg.
6. Repeat the test two to three times and record the average of the strides to the nearest inch.

Calculations

1. For specific norms for classifying males and females regarding ideal stride lengths by age, refer to Dintiman and Ward.[28]

Name of Test

Stride Rate Test

Test Administration

1. Make sure the client prepares with a proper warm-up and stretching routine.
2. Determine the client's flying 40-yard dash time as previously described.
3. Determine the client's stride length as previously described.

Calculations

1. For specific stride rate norms, refer to Dintiman and Ward.[28]

BALANCE

Table 7–5 outlines specific testing protocols for the measurement of balance.

TABLE 7–5. BALANCE TESTING PROTOCOLS

Static Tests
1. Bass stick test[41,59]
2. Stork stand test[59]

Dynamic Tests
1. Balance beam walk test[38,59]
2. Johnson modification of the Bass test[41,59]
3. Modified sideward leap[59,69]

Static Test Procedure

Name of Test
Bass Stick Test[12,59]

Equipment

1. Wooden stick with dimensions of 1 in × 1 in × 12 in
2. Adhesive tape
3. Stopwatch

Test Administration

1. Tape the wooden stick to the floor.
2. The client places the foot lengthwise on the stick (ie, the ball of the foot and heel are in contact with the stick).
3. On the command "go," the client lifts the opposite foot from the floor and attempts to hold this position for a maximum time of 60 seconds.
4. The clinician informs the client of the elapsed time at every 5-second interval.
5. The test is terminated when the following occurs:
   a. Either foot touches the floor.
   b. Balance is maintained for 60 seconds.
6. The client is given three practice trials on each foot. The score is the total time in seconds for all six trials.

Calculations

1. For specific static test norms, refer to Johnson and Nelson.[41]

Special Considerations

1. The test may be administered with the eyes open or closed.
2. The test may be administered with the ball of the foot being placed crosswise on the stick.

Dynamic Test Procedure

Name of Test
Balance Beam Walk Test[59]

Equipment

1. Balance beam (16-ft long, 4-in wide and with a height less than 1 ft to ensure safety)
2. Stopwatch

Test Administration

1. The client stands on one end of the balance beam and then proceeds to walk the full length of the beam.
2. The client pauses for 5 seconds, turns around, and walks back to the starting point.

Special Considerations

1. The test difficulty may be increased as follows:
   a. Using a smaller width balance beam
   b. Using a longer balance beam
   c. Setting a time limit for the test

AGILITY
Table 7–6 outlines specific testing protocols for the measurement of agility.

TABLE 7–6. AGILITY TESTING PROTOCOLS

1. AAHPERD shuttle run test[4,59]
2. Barrow zigzag run test[10,59]
3. Right-boomerang run test[33,59]
4. Semo agility test[47,59]
5. Squat thrust (Burpee) test[59]
6. T-test[72]

Agility Test Procedure

Name of Test
Squat Thrust (Burpee) Test

Equipment

1. Stopwatch

Test Administration

1. On the command "go," the client is to complete as many squat thrusts as possible in 10 seconds.
2. A squat thrust sequence is described as follows:
   a. The client squats and places the hands in front of the feet from a standing position.
   b. The client thrusts the legs backward and assumes a push-up type position.
   c. The client returns to a squat position with the hands placed in front of the feet.
   d. The client rises to a standing position.

Calculations

1. Scores for partial squat thrusts are as follows:
   a. ¼ for touching the hands to the floor
   b. ½ for thrusting the legs backward and assuming a push-up type position
   c. ¾ for returning to the squat position
2. The final score is the total number of complete and partial squat thrusts performed in 10 seconds.
3. A one-point penalty is assigned when any of the following occur:
   a. The feet are thrust backward before the hands touch the floor.
   b. The feet are not thrust back so that the body is in a front-leaning position.
   c. The hands leave the floor before the return to a squat position.
   d. The body is not erect with the head up while in a standing position.
4. For specific norms for grades elementary to senior high school, refer to Miller.[59]

SPORT SKILLS

Table 7–7 outlines specific testing protocols for the measurement of various sport skills.

Sport Skill Test Procedure

Name of Test
Clevett's Putting Test [20,59]

Equipment

1. Putter
2. Golf balls
3. Smooth carpet 20-ft long and 27-in wide

TABLE 7–7. SPORT SKILLS TESTING PROTOCOLS

1. Archery[12,59,75]
2. Badminton[12,51,59]
3. Basketball[12,59,60]
4. Bowling[63]
5. Field hockey[18,59]
6. Football[3,12,59]
7. Golf[12,34,59]
8. Gymnastics[12,40]
9. Handball[12,21,59]
10. Racquetball[12,44,59]
11. Soccer[12,35,59]
12. Softball[32,59]
13. Swimming[12,68]
14. Tennis[7,12,59]
15. Volleyball[12,50,59]
16. Wrestling[12,48,49]

Test Administration

1. The carpet is placed on a level and smooth surface.
2. The carpet is divided into three equal 9-in sections running the full length of the putting surface (refer to Figure 7–1).
3. Beginning 8 ft from the starting point, mark off 48 scoring areas with each scoring area being a 9-in square.
4. An imaginary hole, which is located 15 ft from the starting line, is designated as square 10 (a hole may be cut in this square to make the test more realistic).
5. The client attempts 10 putts.

Calculations

1. Each putt receives a numerical score based on the square on which the ball stops. Balls that stop exactly on a line between two squares are given the higher point value.
2. The final score is the total number of points for the 10 putts.

PSYCHOLOGIC DIMENSIONS IN PHYSICAL EDUCATION

Table 7–8 outlines specific testing protocols for the measurement of various psychologic dimensions in physical education and sport.

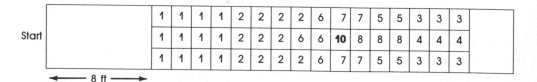

Figure 7–1. Clevett's putting test. *(Adapted from Miller, DK. Measurement by the Physical Educator: Why and How. Carmel, Ind: Benchmark Press; 1988.)*

TABLE 7–8. PSYCHOLOGICAL TESTING PROTOCOLS

1. Body cathexis scale[71]
2. Physical estimation and attraction scales (PEAS)[78]
3. Rate of perceived exertion (RPE) scale[14]
4. Self-motivation inventory (SMI)[29]
5. Semantic differential scale[77]

TABLE 7–9. HEALTH-RELATED TESTING PROTOCOLS

1. AAHPERD Health-Related Physical Fitness Test[5]
2. Manitoba Physical Fitness Performance Test[53]
3. Physical Best Program[6]
4. South Carolina Test[64]
5. Texas Test[80]

HEALTH-RELATED DIMENSIONS IN PHYSICAL EDUCATION

Table 7–9 outlines specific testing protocols for the measurement of various health-related dimensions in physical education and sport.

CLASSIFYING

Tables 7–10 to 7–12 may be used by clinicians seeking various limits to human performance. These tables, as well as other sources,[19,61] provide clinicians with a general guide for comparing the values of elite performers with those values obtained during sport performance testing of high school and college athletes.

TABLE 7–10. LIMITS OF CARDIOVASCULAR PERFORMANCE[12,42]

	$\dot{V}O_2$ max value $(mL \cdot kg^{-1} \cdot min^{-1})$
Scandinavian cross-country skier (highest value ever recorded in any athlete)	93
Male runner (highest reported value)	85
Female runner (highest reported value)	77

TABLE 7–11. LIMITS OF STRENGTH PERFORMANCE[a]

Powerlifting World Records				
		Amount Lifted		
Class—Men	**Type of Lift**	**kg**	**lb**	**Year**
82.5 kg/182 lb	Squat	379.5	836	1982
	Bench press	240	529	1981
	Deadlift	357.5	788	1980
125+ kg/275+ lb	Squat	445	981	1982
	Bench press	300	661	1981
	Deadlift	406	895	1988
		Amount Lifted		
Class—Women	**Type of Lift**	**kg**	**lb**	**Year**
60 kg/132 lb	Squat	200.5	442	1983
	Bench press	105.5	232	1989
	Deadlift	213	469	1983
90+ kg/198 lb	Squat	262.5	579	1987
	Bench press	137.5	303	1989
	Deadlift	237.5	523	1987

TABLE 7–11. (Continued)

	Olympic Lifting World Records (Men)			
		Amount Lifted		
Bodyweight Class	**Name of Lift**	**kg**	**lb**	**Year**
Light-heavyweight (82.5 kg/181¾ lb)				
	Snatch	183	403¾	1986
	Clean and jerk	225	496	1986
Super-heavyweight (110 kg/242½ lb)				
	Snatch	216	476	1987
	Clean and jerk	266	586¼	1988

*Pound values have been approximated.
Adapted from McFarlan D, ed. The Guiness Book of World Records. New York, NY: Bantam Books; 1991.

TABLE 7–12. LIMITS OF SPEED AND POWER PERFORMANCE

Track and Field World Records		
Men's Running Events	**min s**	**Year**
100 meters[a]	9.92	1988
200 meters	19.72	1979
400 meters	43.29	1988
800 meters	1:41.73	1981
1500 meters	3:29.46	1985
1 mile	3:46.32	1985
4 × 100 meter relay	37.83	1984
Marathon	2 hr. 6:50.00	1988

Men's Field Events	**m**	**ft**	**in**	**Year**
High jump	2.44	8	0	1989
Long jump	8.90	29	2½	1968

Women's Running Events	**min s**	**Year**
100 meters	10.49	1988
200 meters	21.34	1988
400 meters	47.60	1985
800 meters	1:53.28	1983
1500 meters	3:52.47	1980
1 mile	4:15.61	1989
4 × 100 meter relay	41.37	1985
Marathon	2 hr. 21:06.00	1985

Women's Field Events	**m**	**ft**	**in**	**Year**
High jump	2.09	6	10¼	1987
Long jump	7.52	24	8¼	1988

*The peak speed attained during the men's 100-meter sprint final at the 1988 Olympics has been shown to be 26.95 mph.
Adapted from McFarlan D, ed. The Guiness Book of World Records. New York, NY: Bantam Books; 1991.

REFERENCES

1. Adams GM. *Exercise Physiology Laboratory Manual.* Dubuque, Iowa: Wm C Brown Publishers; 1990.
2. American Association for Health, Physical Education and Recreation. *Skills Test Manual: Football.* Washington, DC: American Association for Health, Physical Education and Recreation; 1965.

3. American Association for Health, Physical Education and Recreation. *Football Skills Test Manual*. Washington, DC: American Association for Health, Physical Education and Recreation; 1966.

4. American Association for Health, Physical Education, Recreation and Dance. *Youth Fitness Test Manual*. Reston, Va: American Alliance for Health, Physical Education, Recreation and Dance; 1976.

5. American Association for Health, Physical Education, Recreation and Dance. *Health-Related Physical Fitness Manual*. Washington, DC: American Association for Health, Physical Education, Recreation and Dance; 1980.

6. American Association for Health, Physical Education, Recreation and Dance. *Physical Best*. Washington, DC: American Association for Health, Physical Education, Recreation and Dance; 1988.

7. Avery C, Richardson P, Jackson A. A practical tennis serve test: Measurement of skill under simulated game conditions. *Res Q*. 1979;50:554–564.

8. Ayalon A, Inbar O, Bar-Or O. Relationships among measurements of explosive strength and anaerobic power. In: Nelson RC, Morehouse CA, eds. *International Series on Sports Sciences* (Vol 1, Biomechanics IV): *Proceedings of the Fourth International Seminar on Biomechanics*. Baltimore, Md: University Park Press; 1974.

9. Bar-Or O, Dotan R, Inbar O. A 30 second all-out ergometric test: Its reliability and validity for anaerobic capacity. *Israel J Med Sci*. 1977;13:126.

10. Barrow HM, McGee R, Tritschler KA. *Practical Measurement in Physical Education and Sport*. 4th ed. Philadelphia, Pa: Lea & Febiger; 1989.

11. Bass RI. An analysis of the components of tests of semi-circular canal function and of static and dynamic balance. *Res Q*. 1939;10:33–52.

12. Baumgartner TA, Jackson AS. *Measurement for Evaluation in Physical Education and Exercise Science*. 4th ed. Dubuque, Iowa: Wm C Brown Publishers; 1991.

13. Bergh U. *Physiology of Cross-Country Skiing*. Champaign, Ill: Human Kinetics Publishers, Inc; 1982.

14. Borg G. Psychophysical bases of perceived exertion. *Med Sci Sports Exerc*. 1982;14:371–381.

15. Bosco C, Komi PV, Tihanyi J, et al. Mechanical power test and fiber composition of human leg extensor muscles. *Eur J Appl Physiol*. 1983;51:129–135.

16. Bosco C, Luhtanen P, Komi PV. A simple method for measurement of mechanical power in jumping. *Eur J Appl Physiol*. 1983;50:273–282.

17. Bouchard C, Taylor AW, Simoneau J-A, et al. Testing anaerobic power and capacity. In: MacDougall JD, Wenger HA, Green HJ, eds. *Physiological Testing of the High-Performance Athlete*. 2nd ed. Champaign, Ill: Human Kinetics Publishers, Inc; 1991.

18. Chapman N. Chapman ball control test-field hockey. *Res Q*. 1982;53:239–242.

19. Clarke DH, Eckert HM, eds. *Limits of Human Performance* (Number 18, The American Academy of Physical Education). Champaign, Ill: Human Kinetics Publishers, Inc; 1985.

20. Clevett MA. An experiment in teaching methods of golf. *Res Q*. 1931;2:104–112.

21. Cornish C. A study of measurement ability in handball. *Res Q*. 1949;20:215–222.

22. Costill DL, Fox EL. Energetics of marathon running. *Med Sci Sports*. 1969;1:81–86.

23. Crews TR, Meadors WJ. Analysis of reaction time, speed and body composition of college football players. *J Sports Med Phys Fitness*. 1978;18:169–172.

24. Cunningham DA, Faulkner JA. The effect of training on aerobic and anaerobic metabolism during a short exhaustive run. *Med Sci Sports*. 1969;1(2):65–69.

25. De Bruyn-Prévost P. Determination of anaerobic physical fitness (anaerobic endurance). In: Ostyn M, Beunen G, Simons J, eds. *International Series on Sport Sciences: Kinanthropometry II*. Baltimore, Md: University Park Press; 1980.

26. De Bruyn-Prévost P, Sturbois X. Physiological response of girls to aerobic and anaerobic endurance tests. *J Sports Med Phys Fitness*. 1984;24:149–154.

27. Dintiman GB. *How to Run Faster*. West Point, NY: Leisure Press; 1984.

28. Dintiman GB, Ward RD. *Sport Speed*. Champaign, Ill: Leisure Press; 1988.

29. Dishman RK, Ickes W. Self-motivation and adherence to therapeutic exercise. *J Behavioral Med*. 1981;4:21–36.

30. Dotan R, Bar-Or O. Load optimization for the Wingate anaerobic test. *Eur J Appl Physiol*. 1983;51:409–417.

31. Evans JA, Quinney HA. Determination of resistance settings for anaerobic power testing. *Can J Appl Sport Sci*. 1981;6:53–56.

32. Fox MG, Young OG. A test of softball batting ability. *Res Q*. 1954;25:26–27.

33. Gates DP, Sheffield RP. Tests of change of direction as measurement of different kinds of motor ability in boys of 7th, 8th and 9th grades. *Res Q.* 1940;11:136–147.

34. Green KN, East WB, Hensley LD. A golf skill test battery for college males and females. *Res Q Exerc Sport.* 1987;58:72–76.

35. Heath ML, Rogers EG. A study in the use of knowledge and skill tests in soccer. *Res Q.* 1932;3:33–53.

36. Heyward VH. *Advanced Fitness Assessment and Exercise Prescription.* 2nd ed. Champaign, Ill: Human Kinetics Publishers, Inc; 1991.

37. Inbar O, Bar-Or O. Changes in arm and leg anaerobic performance in laboratory and field tests following vigorous physical training. In: Simri U, ed. *Art and Science of Coaching: Proceedings of the International Seminar on Art and Science in Coaching.* Israel: Wingate Institute; 1980.

38. Jensen CR, Hirst CC. *Measurement in Physical Education and Athletics.* New York, NY: Macmillan Publishing Co; 1980.

39. Jette M, Thoden JS, Reed A. Les bases scientifiques de l'évaluation périodique [The scientific basis of periodic evaluation]. [Special hockey issue]. *Mouvement.* 1975;2:99–104.

40. Johnson BL. A screening test for pole vaulting and selected gymnastic events. *J Health Phys Education Recreation.* 1973;44:71–72.

41. Johnson BL, Nelson JK. *Practical Measurements for Evaluation in Physical Education.* 4th ed. Minneapolis, Minn: Burgess Publishing Co; 1986.

42. Jones A. 300-yard shuttle run. *Nat Strength Condit Assoc J.* 1991;13(2):56–57.

43. Kalamen J. Measurement of maximum muscular power in man. Unpublished doctoral dissertation, Ohio State University, 1968.

44. Karpman M, Isaacs L. An improved racquetball skills test. *Res Q.* 1979;50:526–527.

45. Katch V, Weltman A. Interrelationship between anaerobic power output, anaerobic capacity and aerobic power. *Ergonomics.* 1979;22:325–332.

46. Kibler WB. *The Sport Preparticipation Fitness Examination.* Champaign, Ill: Human Kinetics Publishers, Inc; 1990.

47. Kirby RF. A simple test of agility. *Coach and Athlete.* 1971;(June):30–31.

48. Klinzing JE, Karpowicz W. A test to measure the performance capabilities of wrestlers. *Nat Strength Condit Assoc J.* 1983;5(4):40.

49. Kraft GC. The construction and standardization of a wrestling knowledge test for college men. P.E.D. Dissertation. Bloomington, Ind: Indiana University; 1971.

50. Liba MR, Stauff MR. A test for the volleyball pass. *Res Q.* 1963;34:56–63.

51. Lockhart A, McPherson FA. The development of a test of badminton playing ability. *Res Q.* 1949;20:402–405.

52. Maksud MG, Coutts KD. Comparison of a continuous and discontinuous graded treadmill test for maximal oxygen uptake. *Med Sci Sports.* 1971;3:63–65.

53. Manitoba Department of Education. *Manitoba Physical Fitness Performance Test Manual and Fitness Objectives.* Manitoba, Canada; 1977.

54. Margaria R, Aghemo P, Rovelli E. Measurement of muscular power (anaerobic) in man. *J Appl Physiol.* 1966;21:1662–1664.

55. Mathews DK, Fox EL. *The Physiological Basis of Physical Education and Athletics.* 2nd ed. Philadelphia, Pa: WB Saunders Co; 1976.

56. McArdle WD, Katch FI, Katch VL. *Exercise Physiology: Energy, Nutrition and Human Performance.* 3rd ed. Philadelphia, Pa: Lea & Febiger; 1991.

57. McBride J. The kneeling overhead throw. *Nat Strength Condit Assoc J.* 1991;13(1):49–50.

58. McFarlan D, ed. *The Guinness Book of World Records.* New York, NY: Bantam Books; 1991.

59. Miller DK. *Measurement by the Physical Educator: Why and How.* Carmel, Ind: Benchmark Press; 1988.

60. Miller WK. Achievement levels in basketball skills for women physical education majors. *Res Q.* 1954;25:450–455.

61. Murphy P. Longer, higher, faster: Athletes continue to reach new heights. *Physician Sportsmed.* 1986;14(8):140.

62. Noakes T. *Lore of Running: Discover the Science and Spirit of Running.* 3rd ed. Champaign, Ill: Human Kinetics Publishers, Inc; 1991.

63. Olson JK, Liba MR. A device for evaluating spot bowling ability. *Res Q.* 1967;38:193–210.

64. Pate RR, ed. *South Carolina Physical Fitness Test Manual.* Columbia, SC: Governor's Council on Physical Fitness; 1978.

65. Patton JF, Murphy MM, Frederick FA. Maximal power outputs during the Wingate anaerobic test. *Int J Sports Med.* 1985;6:82–85.

66. Pollock ML, Wilmore JH, Fox SM. *Health and Fitness through Physical Activity*. New York, NY: John Wiley & Sons, Inc; 1978.

67. Powers SK, Howley ET. *Exercise Physiology: Theory and Application to Fitness and Performance*. Dubuque, Iowa: Wm C Brown Publishers; 1990.

68. Rosentswieg J. A revision of the power swimming test. *Res Q*. 1968;39:818–819.

69. Safrit MJ. *Introduction to Measurement in Physical Education and Exercise Science*. St. Louis, Mo: Times Mirror/Mosby College Publishing; 1986.

70. Sargent DA. The physical test of a man. *Am Phys Ed Rev*. 1921;26(4):188–194.

71. Secord PF, Jourard SM. The appraisal of body cathexis: Body cathexis and the self. *J Consulting Psychology*. 1953;17:343–347.

72. Semenick D. The T-test. *Nat Strength Condit Assoc J*. 1990;12(1):36–37.

73. Semenick D. The line drill test. *Nat Strength Condit Assoc J*. 1990;12(2):47–49.

74. Semenick D. The vertical jump. *Nat Strength Condit Assoc J*. 1990;12(3):68–69.

75. Shifflett B, Schuman B. A criterion-reference test for archery. *Res Q*. 1982;53:330–335.

76. Simoneau J-A, Lortie G, Boulay MR, et al. Tests of anaerobic alactacid and lactacid capacities: Description and reliability. *Can J Appl Sport Sci*. 1983;8:266–270.

77. Snider JG, Osgood CE. *Semantic Differential Technique: A Source Book*. Chicago, Ill: Aldine; 1969.

78. Sonstroem RJ. Physical estimation and attraction scales: Rationale and research. *Med Sci Sports*. 1978;10:97–102.

79. Taylor HL, Buskirk E, Henschel A. Maximal oxygen intake as an objective measure of cardiorespiratory performance. *J Appl Physiol*. 1955;8:73–80.

80. Texas Governor's Commission on Physical Fitness. *Physical Fitness–Motor Ability Test*. Austin, Tex; 1973

81. Thoden JS. Testing aerobic power. In: MacDougall JD, Wenger HA, Green HJ, eds. *Physiological Testing of the High-Performance Athlete*. 2nd ed. Champaign, Ill: Human Kinetics Publishers, Inc; 1991.

82. Thomson JM, Garvie KJ. A laboratory method for determination of anaerobic energy expenditure during sprinting. *Can J Appl Sport Sci*. 1981;6:21–26.

Chapter Eight 8
Work Performance Testing*

GUIDELINES FOR TESTING

Table 8–1 outlines guidelines for functional testing that will assist the clinician in administering various functional tests. Table 8–2 outlines various indications that may be used for stopping functional tests, and Table 8–3 outlines sample precautions that may be used as a screening guide prior to initiating functional testing.

METHODS OF TESTING

Standing Test Procedure[2-4,9,10,14,15,21,31,32,35]

Introduction

1. This is an indirect form of measurement.

Equipment

1. Valpar 8, Valpar 4, Crawford Small Parts, Full Body ROM, or other support surface set at or above waist height or other light-repeated activity tests
2. Heart rate monitor, blood pressure cuff, and stethoscope
3. Stopwatch

Test Administration

1. The clinician instructs the client in the proper procedure and allows for practice (if necessary) as follows:
   a. The client is to stand in one place performing the test procedure but is allowed to weight shift or change position as he or she would normally do at work.
2. The clinician records the client's total time and single longest duration in standing.
3. The suggested time for the test is 30 minutes.

---

*This chapter has been adapted from Slane SM. *Functional Capacities Assessment in Work Hardening*. Thorofare, NJ: SLACK, Inc; in prep.

TABLE 8–1. GUIDELINES FOR FUNCTIONAL TESTING

1. The clinician should determine the specific duration, intensity, and frequency of each test based on specific job requirements and demands.
2. The clinician should record the client's rating of perceived exertion (RPE) during and after the test procedure (see Chapter 5 for RPE measurement procedures).
3. The clinician should record the client's heart rate and blood pressure pre- and post-test and at other appropriate time intervals (eg, 1-minute intervals during a walking test, 5-minute intervals during a standing test).
4. The clinician should record the client's heart rate and blood pressure recovery rates (eg, at 1-, 3-, 5-, or 10-minute intervals) for tests that specifically stress the cardiovascular system.
5. The clinician should note the following while testing the client:
   a. Frequent, extreme, or awkward body postures and positioning
   b. Facial grimacing
   c. Leaning or the use of supportive postures and body positioning
   d. Pace, rhythm, and quality of work
   e. Errors or missteps
   f. Deviation in movement patterns (eg, gait problems, favoring of one arm or leg)
   g. Deviation from instructed test procedure (eg, the client lifting with a straight leg posture)
   h. Hazardous situations (eg, loss of balance, inappropriate use of momentum, inability to control a load)
   i. Inability to maintain proper footing or traction
   j. Excessive use of muscle substitution
   k. Gradual decrease in range of motion and strength
6. The clinician should note any cardiovascular changes (eg, increased heart rate or blood pressure, shortness of breath) while testing the client.
7. The clinician should note the client's subjective reports of pain (ie, type, intensity, frequency, and duration). The clinician may obtain a pain rating by asking the client to identify his or her pain level on a scale of 0 to 10 with 0 being classified as no pain and 10 being classified as maximum pain.

TABLE 8–2. INDICATIONS FOR STOPPING A FUNCTIONAL TEST

1. The client requests to stop.
2. Failure of the monitoring system.
3. The testing clinician stops the test at his or her own discretion.
4. The client cannot maintain specific test-related postures or positions.
5. The client displays objective signs of distress (eg, diaphoresis, increased respiration, excessive weight shifting).
6. The client demonstrates abnormal cardiovascular changes (eg, shortness of breath, severe elevation of heart rate or blood pressure or both from resting levels).
7. The client is unable to complete the task within a designated time frame or other specified criteria (eg, number of repetitions, number of cycles).
8. The client completes the designated time frame or other specified criteria (eg, number of repetitions, number of cycles).
9. The client complains of pain or other subjective symptoms that prevent continuation of the test in a safe manner.
10. The client demonstrates unsafe body mechanics during the test (eg, favoring of one extremity, inability to maintain proper footing or traction, inability to maintain balance and control of a load, muscle substitution).
11. The client demonstrates a gradual decrease in range of motion and strength.

TABLE 8–3. PRECAUTIONS TO FUNCTIONAL TESTING

1. The clinician determines if the client is physically able to perform the test based on a musculoskeletal evaluation.
2. The client demonstrates severe position shifting, awkward positioning, gait abnormalities, or balance problems or attempts to sit or lean on objects consistently prior to or during the musculoskeletal evaluation.
3. The client has a significant current medical history (eg, limited weight-bearing tolerance, repeated buckling or giving away of the knees).
4. The client has a significant past medical history (eg, high blood pressure, cardiac abnormalities, diabetes, seizure disorders).

Walking Test Procedure[2-4,9,10,14,15,21,35]

Introduction

1. This is a direct form of measurement.

Equipment

1. Treadmill or 1-mile course (the client should be observable at all points on the course)
2. Heart rate monitor, blood pressure cuff, and stethoscope
3. Stopwatch

Test Administration

1. The clinician instructs the client in the proper procedure and allows for practice (if necessary) as follows:
   a. On a treadmill, the client attempts to walk for a prescribed distance at a comfortable pace, preferably 2 to 3 mph or faster (the client is given the option of controlling the walking pace so that it is natural and comfortable). The client is not allowed to lean or support his or her body on the equipment or support bars while performing the test.
   b. On a track, the client walks a prescribed distance as far as he or she is able at a pace of 2 to 3 mph or faster.
2. Timing is started when the client begins walking and ends when the client completes the prescribed course, distance, or time or can no longer continue walking.
3. The clinician notes the elapsed time, distance walked, and the speed of gait (if the test is performed on a treadmill).
4. The clinician records heart rate and blood pressure recovery rates at 1-, 3-, 5-, and 10-minute intervals.
5. The suggested time for the test is 30 minutes.

Special Consideration

1. If the walking test is conducted on a treadmill, results should be compared and correlated with treadmill submaximal cardiovascular testing.

Sitting Test Procedure[2,3,9,10,14,15,21,31,32,35]

Introduction

1. This is an indirect form of measurement.

Equipment

1. Straight-back or backless chair (based on job requirements)
2. Heart rate monitor, blood pressure cuff, and stethoscope
3. Suggested test equipment: Valpar 8, Valpar 4, Pennsylvania Bi-Manual Work Sample, Crawford Small Parts, WEST Activity Sort, Minnesota Rate of Manipulation, EAS-9 Test. Table or support surface set at approximately 30-in height
4. Stopwatch

Test Administration

1. Initial portion of the sitting tolerance examination starts during the intake interview. The time is recorded as soon as the client is seated. If the client stands for any reason, timing is stopped and recorded. Timing resumes when the client is reseated. If the client does not complete the test for the prescribed time, he or she should be allowed to repeat the test while aware of observation.
2. If the client is performing a standardized test (eg, Valpar 8), instructions should be given to remain seated for the entire duration of the test. If the

client should stand for any reason, timing is stopped and recorded. Timing resumes when the client is reseated.

3. The clinician records the client's total time and the single longest duration in sitting.
4. The suggested time for the test is 30 minutes.

Balance Test Procedure[15,33,35]

Introduction

1. This is a direct form of measurement.

Equipment

1. Balance beam (16-ft long, 6-in wide, and with a height less than 1 ft to ensure safety)
2. Heart rate monitor, blood pressure cuff, and stethoscope
3. Stopwatch

Test Administration

1. The clinician instructs the client in the proper procedure and allows for practice (if necessary) as follows:
   a. The client starts the test on a 6-in-wide balance beam. The client is to walk the length of the beam, turn around, and walk back to the starting position with a heel-toe gait. This sequence should be completed for four repetitions.
   b. If successful in attempt (a), the client is to walk the length of the beam and back to the starting position backwards. This sequence should be completed for four repetitions.
   c. If successful in attempt (b), the client is to walk the length of the beam and back to the starting position in a sideways pattern. This sequence should be completed for four repetitions.
   d. If successful in attempt (c), the client can perform the above sequence on a 4-in-wide balance beam.
2. The clinician should record the time of each subtest and the number of steps taken.
3. The client is to attempt to perform these tests without errors, missteps, or falling.

Stair Climbing Test Procedure[3,7,14,15,21,23,27]

Introduction

1. This is a direct form of measurement.

Equipment

1. Flight of stairs (minimum recommended number of steps is eight)
2. Heart rate monitor, blood pressure cuff, and stethoscope
3. Stopwatch

Test Administration

1. The clinician instructs the client in the proper procedure and allows for practice (if necessary) as follows:
   a. The client is to ascend and descend stairs at a comfortable pace continuously for a maximum time of 5 minutes.
   b. The client is allowed to use the handrail only for light balance and safety.

2. The clinician should begin timing as the client starts to ascend the first step.
3. The clinician should note any excessive use of the handrail.
4. The clinician should note if the client ascends the steps in a reciprocal or nonreciprocal pattern. If the client uses a nonreciprocal or some other type of abnormal climbing pattern, verbal cues should be used and the client should be allowed to attempt a more "normal" climbing pattern.
5. The clinician records the total number of steps climbed and the number of steps climbed in each 1-minute period.
6. The clinician records heart rate and blood pressure recovery rates at 1-, 3-, 5-, and 10-minute intervals.

Crawling Test Procedure[3,7,15,35]

Introduction

1. This is a direct form of measurement.

Equipment

1. An area of floor mapped off for 14 ft
2. Knee pads or padding for the floor, as needed
3. Heart rate monitor, blood pressure cuff, and stethoscope
4. Stopwatch

Test Administration

1. The clinician instructs the client in the proper procedure and allows for practice (if necessary) as follows:
   a. The client is to assume the all fours position.
   b. The client is to crawl in the designated 14-ft area forwards and backwards for a total of four repetitions.

Repetitive Forward Bending Test Procedure[23]

Introduction

1. This is a direct form of measurement.

Equipment

1. Adjustable-height shelving (chest height and below knee)
2. Heart rate monitor, blood pressure cuff, and stethoscope
3. Stopwatch
4. Optional equipment: video recorder assessment device

Test Administration

1. The clinician measures the height of the client's chest level and knee level. Two shelves or platforms are set at chest height and just below the knee level.
2. The clinician instructs the client in the proper procedure and allows for practice (if necessary) as follows:
   a. The client is to move objects from the chest-height level to the knee level. After all the objects are transported, the reverse procedure is utilized, transporting from the low to the high surface.
   b. The client should maintain a smooth, steady rhythm throughout the test. It is not recommended that the client perform the repetitions quickly. The rate should be in the range of 10 to 20 repetitions per minute.
   c. If the client's number of repetitions per minute is below 10, he or she should be given the opportunity to try again. If the frequency decreases again, verbal cues can be given to facilitate an increase in speed, if possible.
3. The suggested time for the test is 5 minutes.

4. The total number of repetitions completed during the test are recorded along with the number of repetitions per 1-minute segment.

Sustained Stoop Test Procedure[3,15,35]

Introduction

1. This is a direct form of measurement.

Equipment

1. Full Body Range of Motion (platform set at knee height), WEST Busbench, or Valpar Work Sample #4
2. Heart rate monitor, blood pressure cuff, and stethoscope
3. Stopwatch

Test Administration

1. The clinician instructs the client in the proper procedure and allows for practice (if necessary) as follows:
   a. The clinician positions the test activity at the client's knee level.
   b. The client must maintain the stooped position (ie, to bend the head and shoulders or the body generally, forward and downward from an erect position at the trunk) without bending his or her knees in order to properly complete the test.
2. The suggested time for the test is 5 minutes.

Static Grasp Test Procedure[2,3,14,15,22,35]

Introduction

1. This is a direct form of measurement.

Equipment

1. Jamar dynamometer

Test Administration

1. The client is instructed to sit for all the static grasp strength tests.
2. Total grip strength is measured as follows:
   a. Strength measurements are recorded at each of the five grip positions, starting with position 1 (closest to the dynamometer) and advancing to position 5 (furthest from the dynamometer).
   b. The client holds the dynamometer with the arm against the side, the elbow flexed to 90 degrees, and the forearm in a neutral position.
   c. The client is instructed to exert the maximum grip force for a duration of 5 seconds.
   d. The client alternates between the dominant and nondominant hands until all five positions have been assessed.
3. Peak force grip strength is measured as follows:
   a. The clinician adjusts the handle width to position 2 (theoretically, the position of maximum strength) for maximum force production.
   b. The client holds the dynamometer with the arm against the side, the elbow flexed to 90 degrees, and the forearm in a neutral position.
   c. The client is instructed to exert the maximum grip force for a duration of 5 seconds.
4. The clinician records all grip strength readings, plotting all five position forces on a linear graph and averaging the three trials for a peak grip force. It is assumed that the client has exerted maximal effort in testing if the five-position test, on graphing of data, demonstrates a bell-shaped curve with a peak force at position 2 or 3.

5. Normative data from Mathiowetz[22] may be utilized to determine strength percentiles.
6. The clinician should note if the client avoids contact with any part of his or her hand.
7. The clinician should note any use of muscle substitution.

Unburdened Total Body Range of Motion/Manipulation Test Procedure[21,34,35]

Introduction

1. This is a direct form of measurement.

Equipment

1. WEST II Brief Tool Use
2. Heart rate monitor, blood pressure cuff, and stethoscope
3. Stopwatch

Test Administration

1. Follow the standardized Brief Tool Use Evaluation Procedure for the WEST II apparatus.
2. The clinician records the time for assembly and disassembly at each level.
3. The clinician notes the following regarding the client throughout the test:
   a. Standing posture and lower extremity weight-bearing status.
   b. Upper extremity range of motion and patterns of use.
   c. Postures utilized when performing assemblies and disassemblies at all levels.
   d. Techniques utilized for assuming and maintaining a squatting or kneeling position.
   e. Unusual movement patterns or techniques.
4. The clinician should note the levels completed (indicated in inches from the floor) as well as the time intervals between the levels for assembly and disassembly.

Dynamic Repetitive Push/Pull Test Procedure[5,11,16-19,28,35]

Introduction

1. This is a direct form of measurement.

Equipment

1. Push Trainer-One (PT-One) from Ergonomic Assessment Strength Training (EAST)
2. Heart rate monitor, blood pressure cuff, and stethoscope
3. Stopwatch

Test Administration

1. The clinician instructs the client in the proper procedure and allows for practice (if necessary) as follows:
   a. During the trial repetitions, the client is to practice the release of the locking mechanism in order to understand the safety principles.
   b. The client is to stand on the track surface facing the push/pull handle.
   c. The client is to grasp the handle with a shoulder-width grip, squeezing the release mechanism.
   d. The client leans forward into the bar with the chest against the bar and the back extended.
   e. The client is to the push the bar the entire length of the track to the end, stop, and slowly return to the starting position. One to three repetitions

are completed at each level to ensure safety in the performance of the task at that level.

f. The client starts with a 10-lb load, with the resistance being increased in 10-lb increments until the client is unable to safely perform the activity or refuses to attempt the test procedure.

g. When the client reaches a level he or she cannot safely attempt, the weight is lowered by 10 lb and the procedure is retested. From this point, the weight is increased in 2½-lb increments until a maximum level is reached.

h. After completion of the push assessment, a brief rest period is provided to allow for heart rate and blood pressure to return to near resting levels.

i. Upon heart rate and blood pressure returning to near resting levels, a pulling assessment is initiated (if applicable in the job requirements). Follow the same procedure as in the push test; however, in this case the client leans backward and pulls in a slow, progressive manner without "jerking" or using rapid acceleration maneuvers.

2. The clinician records the maximum safely completed level for pushing and pulling.
3. The clinician notes any deviations from the instructed "normal" push/pull postures.
4. Heart rate is taken after each level and blood pressure after every third level.

Dynamic Vertical Pull Test Procedure[5,11,16-19,28]

Introduction

1. This is a direct form of measurement.

Equipment

1. High pulley apparatus (attached 15 to 20 ft above the ground), rope, and weights
2. Heart rate monitor, blood pressure cuff, and stethoscope
3. Stopwatch

Test Administration

1. The clinician instructs the client in the proper procedure and allows for practice (if necessary) as follows:
   a. The client is to stand below and just off to one side of the pulley assembly.
   b. The client is to grasp the rope, with the right hand held above head height and the left hand positioned at shoulder height.
   c. The client is to pull the rope down with the right arm, using the left arm for support. As the right hand reaches shoulder height, the left arm is positioned overhead to initiate another downward pulling force. The client is to pull the weight all the way up to the top portion of the pulley assembly.
   d. At the completion of the motion, the client is to return the weight to the starting position, using the reverse procedure.
   e. The client is allowed to practice the test procedure without resistance.
   f. The client starts with a 10-lb load, with the resistance being increased in 10-lb increments until the client is unable to safely perform the activity or refuses to attempt the test procedure.
   g. When a weight is reached that the client cannot complete, the resistance is lowered by 10 lb and the procedure is repeated. The resistance is then increased in 2½-lb increments until a maximum level is reached.
2. The clinician records the maximum safely completed level for pulling.
3. The clinician notes the amount of time required to complete each level.

4. As a safety precaution, the maximum weight tested should not exceed the client's lowest recorded grip strength.
5. Heart rate is taken after each level and blood pressure after every third level.

Dynamic Lifting Test Procedure—West II[13,20,21,34,35]

Introduction

1. This is a direct form of measurement.

Equipment

1. WEST II
2. Heart rate monitor, blood pressure cuff, and stethoscope
3. Stopwatch

Test Administration

1. The following test procedure is based on the use of the WEST II. Baseline measurements are recorded for the following positions:
   a. Anatomic heights
      (1) Head
      (2) Eye
      (3) Shoulder
      (4) Knuckle
      (5) Knee
   b. Functional heights
      (1) Full reach
      (2) Lowest reach
      (3) Carrying (hand position at 90 degrees elbow flexion)
   c. Minimal horizontal distance from the load
      (1) Load positioned at carrying height. The client stands facing the load with the load against the abdomen. The distance from the medial malleoli to the load is recorded.
2. The clinician instructs the client in the proper procedure and allows for practice (if necessary) as follows:
   a. A starting weight of 5 lb is placed on a table with a surface height of 30 in and positioned 8 to 10 ft in front of the WEST apparatus.
   b. The client lifts the weight, turns 180 degrees, and walks toward the WEST apparatus, hanging the weight on the frame at waist height.
   c. The client lifts the load through 6-in increments from waist height to an overhead reach height.
   d. After completing the reach height portion, the client lowers the weight directly to waist-height level, and then starts lowering the weight through 6-in increments down to the lowest position of 6 in from the floor.
   e. After reaching the lowest position, the client lifts the weight from the lowest position of 6 in up to the reach height. The client then lowers the weight through the entire range of motion back down to the lowest position of 6 in from the floor.
   f. The client completes the lift by returning the weight from the 6-in position to the waist-height position.
   g. To complete the sequence, the client returns the weight apparatus back to the starting position on the table.
3. The weights are increased in 5-lb increments until the client is unable to complete the lift safely or refuses to continue.
4. When the client reaches a level he or she cannot safely attempt, the weight is lowered to the level of the last successful attempt and the lift is retested. From

this point, the weight is increased in 2½-lb increments until a maximum level is reached.

5. The clinician records the time required for each level.
6. The clinician rates the client's safe lifting biomechanics based on the following areas:
   a. Horizontal distance
   b. Spinal torque
   c. Stance position
   d. Pace and control of the lift
   e. Body mechanics
7. The clinician records the maximum safely completed level at the following heights:
   a. Knuckle
   b. Shoulder
   c. Reach
8. Heart rate is taken after each level and blood pressure after every third level.

Dynamic Lifting Test Procedure—Box Lift[2,3,20,35]

Introduction

1. This is a direct form of measurement.

Equipment

1. Containers to lift
2. Adjustable-height shelving unit
3. Heart rate monitor, blood pressure cuff, and stethoscope
4. Stopwatch

Test Administration

1. Baseline measurements are recorded for the following positions:
   a. Anatomic height
      (1) Knuckle
   b. Functional heights
      (1) Full reach
      (2) Lowest reach
      (3) Carrying (hand position at 90 degrees elbow flexion)
2. The clinician instructs the client in the proper procedure utilizing the Blankenship-style boxes[2,3] and allows for practice (if necessary) as follows:
   a. The client is instructed in the proper lifting technique (ie, with a straight back and bent leg position). The client is to pick up the box and lower it to floor level and, after a brief pause, the box is lifted back to the table surface.
   b. The client starts lifting with the empty box. The weight is gradually increased in 5-lb increments until the client cannot maintain proper form (ie, with a straight back and bent leg position) or the client refuses to continue.
   c. The client is tested in the following lifts:
      (1) Floor to knuckle
      (2) Knuckle to shoulder
      (3) Shoulder to reach

3. The clinician rates the client's safe lifting biomechanics based on the following areas:
   a. Horizontal distance
   b. Spinal torque
   c. Stance position
   d. Pace and control of the lift
   e. Body mechanics
4. The clinician records the maximum safely completed level at the following heights:
   a. Knuckle
   b. Shoulder
   c. Reach
5. The clinician records the time required for each level.
6. Heart rate is taken after each level and blood pressure after every third level.

Carrying Test Procedure[2,3,15,21,25,35]

Introduction

1. This is a direct form of measurement.

Equipment

1. Carrying container with dimensions consistent with the job demands
2. Table with a surface height of 30 to 36 in (depending upon job requirements)
3. Unmarked test weights (eg, bar stock, lead shot)
4. Heart rate monitor, blood pressure cuff, and stethoscope
5. Stopwatch

Test Administration

1. The clinician determines the carrying distance for the test based upon job demands.
2. The clinician measures and marks the distance for the test.
3. The clinician instructs the client in the proper procedure and allows for practice (if necessary) as follows:
   a. Carry the container with elbows flexed to 90 degrees and the container against the abdomen. The back is to be maintained in a straight position, with no excessive flexion or extension.
   b. The client is to pick up the container, turn 180 degrees, and walk the prescribed test distance. The client then turns 180 degrees, returns to the table, and sets the weight down.
   c. The client is to take normal strides (running or fast walking is not allowed).
4. The client starts with an empty container (weight of 5 to 10 lb).
5. The weight is increased in 5-lb increments for females and 10-lb increments for males until the maximum safe level is reached (determined by the client losing proper body mechanics).
6. The clinician records the maximum safely completed weight.
7. The clinician also records the following:
   a. The type and size of the container
   b. The distance traveled
   c. The total number of steps taken with each trial
   d. The time for each trial and the total time of the test
8. Heart rate is taken after each carry and blood pressure after every third carry.

CLASSIFYING

Tables 8–4 and 8–5 may be used for classifying a client based on physical demand levels of work.[12,21,25,26,29] Other clinicians have also attempted to classify work in terms of energy expenditure and heart rate.[1,6,8,24]

Figure 8–1 may be used as a sample return-to-work recommendation form, and Figure 8–2 may be used as a sample data sheet for functional testing.

TABLE 8–4. PHYSICAL DEMAND LEVELS OF WORK[a]

Classifications	Occasional[b]	Frequent[b]	Constant[b]
Very heavy[c]	Over 100 lb	Over 50 lb	Over 20 lb
Heavy[c]	Up to 100 lb	Up to 50 lb	Up to 20 lb
Medium[c]	Up to 50 lb	Up to 20 lb	Up to 10 lb
Light[d]	Up to 20 lb	Up to 10 lb	Negligible
Sedentary[e]	Up to 10 lb	Negligible	Negligible

[a]For specific definitions and guidelines, refer to US Department of Labor.[29,30]
[b]"Occasionally" defines an activity or condition that exists up to one-third of the time. "Frequently" defines an activity or condition that exists one-third to two-thirds of the time. "Constantly" defines an activity or condition that exists two-thirds or more of the time.
[c]Force required to move objects.
[d]Force required to move objects. Usually requires walking or standing to a significant degree. However, if the use of arm or leg controls requires exertion of forces greater than that for Sedentary Work and the worker sits most of the time, the job is rated for light work.
[e]Force required to lift, carry, push, pull, or otherwise move objects, including the human body. Sedentary work involves sitting most of the time but may involve walking or standing for brief periods of time. Jobs are sedentary if walking and standing are required only occasionally and all other sedentary criteria are met.
Adapted from US Department of Labor. Dictionary of Occupational Titles. 4th ed (Suppl). Washington, DC: US Government Printing Office; 1986.

TABLE 8–5. ADDITIONAL PHYSICAL DEMAND LEVELS OF WORK

Classifications	Walking/Carrying
Very heavy	3.5 mph with 50-lb or more load
Heavy	3.5 mph with 50-lb or less load
Medium-heavy	3.5 mph, 0% grade, with 35-lb load or 115-lb wheelbarrow, 2.5 mph, 0% grade
Medium	3.5 mph, 0% grade or slower speed with 25-lb or less load
Light-medium	3.0 mph, 0% grade or slower speed with 20-lb or less load
Light	2.5 mph, 0% grade or slower speed with 10-lb or less load
Sedentary-light	Intermittent self-paced, no load
Sedentary	None

Adapted with permission from Matheson LN, Niemeyer LO. Work Capacity Evaluation: Systematic Approach to Industrial Rehabilitation. Anaheim, Calif: Employment and Rehabilitation Institute of California; 1987: Appendix 10.

COMPANY NAME: _____
PATIENT'S NAME: (Last) _____ (First) _____
AGE: _____   GENDER: M   F   DATE OF INJURY/ILLNESS: _____
DIAGNOSIS/CONDITION (Brief Explanation): _____
_____

This patient was seen and treated on (Date) _____ and based on the above description of the patient's current medical problem, I have made the following recommendations:

1. ☐ His/her return to work with no limitations on (Date) _____.

2. ☐ He/she may return to work on (Date) _____ with the restrictions identified in the following chart. These restrictions are in effect until (Date) _____ or until the patient is re-evaluated on (Date) _____.

		Never (0% of workday)	Occasional (1–33% of workday)	Frequent (34–66% of workday)	Constant (67–100% of workday)
☐ Very heavy work					
☐ Heavy work	Lift	☐	☐	☐	☐
☐ Medium-heavy work	Carry	☐	☐	☐	☐
	Walk	☐	☐	☐	☐
☐ Medium work	Stand	☐	☐	☐	☐
	Sit	☐	☐	☐	☐
☐ Light-medium work	Push	☐	☐	☐	☐
	Pull	☐	☐	☐	☐
☐ Light work	Bend	☐	☐	☐	☐
	Twist	☐	☐	☐	☐
☐ Sedentary-light work	Squat	☐	☐	☐	☐
	Climb	☐	☐	☐	☐
☐ Sedentary work	Reach	☐	☐	☐	☐

OTHER INSTRUCTIONS AND/OR RESTRICTIONS (INCLUDING PRESCRIBED MEDICATIONS) ARE AS FOLLOWS:
_____
_____

3. ☐ Patient be re-evaluated on (Date) _____ since he/she is totally incapacitated at this time.

4. ☐ Patient referral to:

   ☐ None

   ☐ Family physician: Dr. _____

   ☐ Consulting physician: Dr. _____

   ☐ Further diagnostic testing: _____

   ☐ Work hardening and/or functional capacity evaluation at: _____

   ☐ _____

Attending Physician's Signature: _____ Date: _____

I hereby authorize my attending physician and/or medical facility to release any information or copies thereof required in the course of my examination or treatment for the injury identified above to my employer or his representative.

Patient's Signature: _____ Date: _____

Figure 8–1. Sample return-to-work recommendation record form. *(Adapted from Zenz C. Occupational Medicine: Principles and Practical Applications. 2nd ed. St. Louis, Mo: Mosby–Year Book; 1988.)*

NAME: _____   DATE: _____

AGE: _____ SEX: M   F

HEIGHT: _____ in _____ cm   WEIGHT: _____ lb _____ kg

MATERIAL HANDLING ACTIVITIES

	Max (lb)	5–RM (lb)	10–RM (lb)
Floor-to-knuckle lifting	_____	_____	_____
Floor-to-shoulder lifting	_____	_____	_____
Floor-to-reach lifting	_____	_____	_____
Waist-to-shoulder lifting	_____	_____	_____
Waist-to-reach lifting	_____	_____	_____
Bilateral carrying	_____	_____	_____
Unilateral carrying right	_____	_____	_____
Unilateral carrying left	_____	_____	_____
Horizontal pushing	_____	_____	_____
Horizontal pulling	_____	_____	_____
Vertical pulling	_____	_____	_____
_____	_____	_____	_____

FUNCTIONAL TOLERANCES

	Total Time (hours:minutes)
Sitting	_____
Standing	_____
Walking	_____
Driving	_____
Crawling	_____
Bending	_____
Kneeling	_____
Squatting	_____
Climbing	_____
Reaching horizontal	_____
Reaching overhead	_____
_____	_____

SPECIAL TESTS

_____

_____

_____

COMMENTS:

_____

_____

_____

Figure 8–2. Sample data sheet for functional testing.

REFERENCES

1. Åstrand P-O, Rodahl K. *Textbook of Work Physiology: Physiological Bases of Exercise*. 3rd ed. New York, NY: McGraw-Hill Book Co; 1986.
2. Blankenship KL. *Functional Capacity Evaluation: The Procedure Manual*. Macon, Ga: American Therapeutics, Inc; 1986.
3. Blankenship KL. *Industrial Rehabilitation II: A Seminar Syllabus*. Macon, Ga: American Therapeutics; 1990.
4. Chaffin DB, Andersson G. *Occupational Biomechanics*. 2nd ed. New York, NY: John Wiley & Sons, Inc; 1991.
5. Chaffin DB, Andres RO, Garg A. Volitional postures during maximal push/pull exertions in the sagittal plane. *Human Factors*. 1983;25(5):541–550.
6. Christensen EH. Physiological evaluation of work in the Nykroppa iron works. In: Floyd WF, Welford AT, eds. *Ergonomics Society Symposium on Fatigue*. London, England: Lewis; 1953.
7. Davis PO, Dotson CO, Maria DLS. Relationship between simulated fire fighting tasks and physical performance measures. *Med Sci Sports Exerc*. 1982;14(1):65–71.
8. Durnin JVGA, Passmore R. *Energy, Work and Leisure*. London, England: Heinemann Educational Books Ltd; 1967.
9. Field TF. Criteria for physical assessments. *The Field Report*. 1989;4(2):1–5.
10. Field TF, Pettit L. *Measuring Physical Capacities*. Athens, Ga: VSB, Inc; 1985.
11. Grieve DW. The influence of posture on power output generated in single pulling movements. *Appl Ergonomics*. 1984;15.2:115–117.
12. Harrand G. *The Harrand Guide of Developing Physical Capacity Evaluations*. Menomonie, Wis: Materials Development Center, Stout Vocational Rehabilitation Institute; 1982.
13. Havranek JE. *Physical Capacity Assessment and Work Hardening Therapy: Procedures and Applications*. Athens, Ga: Elliott and Fitzpatrick, Inc; 1988.
14. Isernhagen S. *Work Injury: Management and Prevention*. Gaithersburg, Md: Aspen Publishers, Inc; 1988.
15. Isernhagen S. *Functional Capacities Evaluation: The Kinesiophysical Approach*. Duluth, Minn: Isernhagen and Associates; 1990.
16. Kroemer KHE. Horizontal push and pull forces exertable when standing in working positions on various surfaces. *Appl Ergonomics*. 1974;5.2:94–102.
17. Kroemer KHE. Development of "liftest," a dynamic technique to assess the individual capability to lift material. NIOSH report 210-79-0041, February 1982.
18. Kroemer KHE. An isoinertial technique to assess individual lifting capability. *Human Factors*. 1983;25:493–506.
19. Kroemer KHE, Howard JM. Toward standardization of muscle strength testing. *J Med Sci Sports*. 1970;2(4):224–230.
20. Matheson LN. Guidelines for the evaluation of manual materials handling capacity of disabled workers. *Industrial Rehabil Q*. 1988;1(2).7–8.
21. Matheson LN, Niemeyer LO. *Industrial Rehabilitation Resource Book, Performance Assessment and Capacity Testing*. Mission Viejo, Calif: Matheson and Niemeyer; 1989.
22. Mathiowetz V. Grip and pinch strength measurements. In: Amundsen LR, ed. *Muscle Strength Testing: Instrumented and Non-Instrumented Systems*. New York, NY: Churchill Livingstone; 1990.
23. Mayer TG, Gatchel RJ. *Functional Restoration for Spinal Disorders: The Sports Medicine Approach*. Philadelphia, Pa: Lea & Febiger; 1988.
24. McArdle WD, Katch FI, Katch VL. *Exercise Physiology: Energy, Nutrition and Human Performance*. 3rd ed. Philadelphia, Pa: Lea & Febiger; 1991.
25. National Institute for Occupational Safety and Health (NIOSH). *Safety in Manual Materials Handling*. Cincinnati, Ohio: Department of Health and Human Services; 1978.
26. National Institute for Occupational Safety and Health (NIOSH). *Work Practices Guide for Manual Lifting*. Cincinnati, Ohio: Department of Health and Human Services; 1981.
27. O'Connell ER, Thomas PC, Cady LE, et al. Energy costs of simulated stair climbing as a job related task in fire fighting. *J Occup Med*. 1986;28(4):282–284.
28. Pheasant ST, Grieve DW, Rubin T, et al. Vector representations of human strength in whole body exertions. *Appl Ergonomics*. 1982;13(2):139–144.

29. US Department of Labor. *Dictionary of Occupational Titles*. 4th ed. Washington, DC: US Government Printing Office; 1977.
30. US Department of Labor. *Selected Characteristics of Occupation Defined in the Dictionary of Occupational Titles*. Washington, DC: US Government Printing Office; 1981.
31. *Valpar Upper Extremity Range of Motion Work Sample*. Valpar International Corporation, Tucson, Ariz.
32. *Valpar Upper Extremity Repetitive Task Work Sample*. Valpar International Corporation, Tucson, Ariz.
33. Venditti PP. Functional and work capacity evaluation. In: White AH, Anderson R. *Conservative Care of Low Back Pain*. Baltimore, Md: Williams & Wilkins; 1991.
34. *WEST 2 Work Capacity Evaluation Device Users Manual*. Huntington Beach, Calif: Work Evaluation Systems Technology; 1985.
35. *Wx: Work Capacities, Inc Training Manual. Functionally Fit for Work Analysis, Basic Skills in Work Capacity Services and On-Site Ergonomic Job Analysis*. Westwood, Kan: Wx: Work Capacities, Inc; 1988.
36. Zenz C. *Occupational Medicine: Principles and Practical Applications*. 2nd ed. St. Louis, Mo: Mosby-Year Book; 1988.

Section Three 3

Clinical Guidelines for Exercise Prescription and Rehabilitation

Exercise Prescription for Flexibility and Range of Motion

PRECAUTIONS, CONTRAINDICATIONS, AND GUIDELINES

Tables 9–1 to 9–3 provide the clinician with precautions, contraindications, and guidelines for stretching.

GUIDELINES FOR EXERCISE PRESCRIPTION

Modes of Flexibility Training

Table 9–4 has been presented so that the reader may compare the various modes of flexibility, range of motion, joint mobilization, and muscle energy techniques. At times, these concepts are erroneously used by interchanging the terms and techniques. These techniques and methods may have a common denominator; the clinician should not use them interchangeably, however.

This section specifically focuses on flexibility training, with specific prescription parameters for static stretching.

Static Stretching

1. Advantages of static flexibility over dynamic flexibility include the following:[8]
   a. Less danger of exceeding normal ranges of motion
   b. Lower energy requirements
   c. Less muscle soreness

Ballistic (Dynamic) Stretching

1. Research remains unclear; however, potential advantages may include the following:
   a. Simulates sport-specific skills during training (eg, a pitcher on a baseball team progressively increases his range and speed of pitching motion after

TABLE 9–1. PRECAUTIONS FOR STRETCHING

1. Do not passively force a joint beyond its normal range of motion. Remember, normal range of motion varies among normal individuals.
2. Newly united fractures should be protected by stabilization between the fracture site and the joint where the motion takes place.
3. Use extra caution in patients with known or suspected osteoporosis due to disease, prolonged bed rest, age, or prolonged use of steroids.
4. Avoid vigorous stretching of muscles and connective tissues that have been immobilized over a long period of time. Connective tissues (tendons and ligaments) lose their tensile strength after prolonged immobilization.
   a. High-intensity, short-duration procedures tend to cause more trauma and resulting weakness of soft tissues than low-intensity, long-duration stretch.
   b. Strengthening exercises should be added to a stretching program at some point so that a patient will be able to develop an appropriate balance between flexibility and strength.
5. If a patient experiences joint pain or muscle soreness lasting more than 24 hours, too much force has been used during stretching. Patients should experience no more residual discomfort than a transitory feeling of tenderness.
6. Avoid stretching edematous tissue, as it is more susceptible to injury than normal tissue. Continued irritation of edematous tissues usually causes increased pain and edema.
7. Avoid overstretching weak muscles, particularly those that support body structures in relation to gravity.

Reprinted with permission from Kisner C, Colby LA. Therapeutic Exercise: Foundations and Techniques. 2nd ed. Philadelphia, Pa: FA Davis Co; 1990:129. Data from Agre,[1] Basmajian and Wolf,[5] Beaulieu,[7] Evjenth and Hamberg,[9] Fox and Matthews,[10] Hlasney,[11] and Kottke.[16]

TABLE 9–2. CONTRAINDICATIONS TO STRETCHING

1. When a bony block limits joint motion
2. After a recent fracture
3. Whenever there is evidence of an acute inflammatory or infectious process (heat and swelling) in or around joints
4. Whenever there is sharp, acute pain with joint movement or muscle elongation
5. When a hematoma or other indication of tissue trauma is observed
6. When contractures or shortened soft tissues are providing increased joint stability in lieu of normal structural stability or muscle strength
7. When contractures or shortened soft tissues are the basis for increased functional abilities, particularly in patients with paralysis or severe muscle weakness

Reprinted with permission from Kisner C, Colby LA. Therapeutic Exercise: Foundations and Techniques. 2nd ed. Philadelphia, Pa: FA Davis Co; 1990;129.

TABLE 9–3. GENERAL GUIDELINES FOR STRETCHING

1. A warm-up should precede a stretching program.[20]
2. The client should start out with simple stretches and gradually progress to more advanced levels.
3. The client should start out with a few stretches for each muscle group and gradually progress, paying particular attention to "problem" regions.
4. The client should be instructed not to compare his or her own level of flexibility with others.
5. During stretching exercises, the client should breathe in a slow and rhythmical manner.
6. The client should dress in comfortable and loose clothing in order to avoid restrictions in movement.

    formal static flexibility exercises have been completed for the shoulder and arm)

    b. Simulates sport-specific skill during competition (eg, a kicker on a football team simulates ballistic kicking motions after he has performed static flexibility exercises for his hamstrings)

2. Disadvantages include the following:
   a. Predisposes an individual to muscle strain-type injuries
   b. A rapidly stretched muscle may increase intrafusal muscle spindle activity, reflexively causing a protective muscle contraction of the activated muscles[18]
   c. Potential for higher levels of muscle soreness, which may be a result of small tears in connective tissue and muscle
   d. Fails to provide tissues an adequate time to adapt to a stretch.[2]

TABLE 9–4. MODES OF FLEXIBILITY, RANGE OF MOTION, JOINT MOBILIZATION, AND MUSCLE ENERGY

Flexibility Training[14]
1. Static stretching
2. Ballistic (dynamic) stretching
3. Passive stretching
   a. Manual stretching
   b. Prolonged mechanical stretching
   c. Cyclic mechanical stretching
   d. Self-stretching
4. Active stretching
5. Proprioceptive neuromuscular facilitation (active inhibition)
   a. Contract–relax (hold–relax) technique
   b. Contract relax–contract (hold–relax–contract) technique
   c. Agonist contraction

Range of Motion Exercise[14]
1. Passive range of motion
2. Active range of motion
3. Active-assistive range of motion

Joint Mobilization[14]
1. Mobilization
   a. Physiologic movements
   b. Accessory movements (component motions and joint play)
2. Manipulation
   a. Thrust
   b. Manipulation under anesthesia

Muscle Energy Techniques[17,21]

Passive Stretching

1. Optimal passive stretching is obtained only when all voluntary and reflex muscular resistance is eliminated.[20]
2. A disadvantage of this method may be that the clinician or stretching partner will apply the external force incorrectly (ie, too rapidly or with too much force).[2]
3. Types of passive stretching include:
   a. Manual stretching[11]
   b. Prolonged mechanical stretching[14]
   c. Cyclic mechanical stretching[11]
   d. Self-stretching

Active Stretching

1. Disadvantages of this method include:
   a. Higher energy requirements compared to passive and static stretching
   b. May initiate the stretch reflex[2]
   c. The client may perform the stretch improperly

Proprioceptive Neuromuscular Facilitation (Active Inhibition

1. Types of proprioceptive neuromuscular facilitation (PNF) include the following:
   a. Contract–relax (hold–relax) technique[14,15,22]:
      (1 The client starts with a specified muscle or muscle group in a comfortably lengthened position.
      (2 The client performs an isometric contraction of the same muscle or muscle group against substantial resistance for 5 to 10 seconds.
      (3 The client voluntarily relaxes the muscle or muscle group.
      (4 The clinician lengthens the muscle or muscle group by passively moving the extremity through the gained range.
   b. Contract–relax–contract (hold–relax–contract) technique[14,15,22]:
      (1 The client starts with a specified muscle or muscle group in a comfortably lengthened position.
      (2 The client performs an isometric contraction of the same muscle or muscle group against substantial resistance for 5 to 10 seconds.
      (3 The client voluntarily relaxes the muscle or muscle group.
      (4 The client actively contracts the antagonist of the muscle or muscle group and actively moves the joint through the gained range.
2. Disadvantages include the following:
   a. May be time-consuming
   b. May require the assistance of a partner

Intensity of Training

The following may be used as guidelines for prescribing the intensity of static stretching:

1. The American College of Sports Medicine[3] states that the degree of a stretch should not be so extreme as to cause significant pain.
2. The intensity of training may be gauged by stretching just below the pain threshold.
3. The client should gradually ease into and out of a stretch.
4. The stretch should be performed slowly with no "jerking" or bouncing movements.
5. The stretch should be performed in a "comfort zone" where there is tension in a muscle without pain.[19]

Frequency of Training

The following may be used as guidelines for prescribing the frequency of static stretching for each individual exercise:

1. Moffatt[18] states that one should perform two to six repetitions of each stretch.
2. The American College of Sports Medicine[3] states that one should perform three to five repetitions of each stretch.

The following may be used as guidelines for prescribing the frequency of static stretching on a weekly basis:

1. Moffatt[18] states that a maintenance program may be conducted three to four times per week.
2. The American College of Sports Medicine[3] states that a stretching program should be performed at least three times per week and may be included in the warm-up or cool-down or both.

Duration of Training

The following may be used as guidelines for prescribing the duration of static stretching for each individual exercise:

1. Beaulieu[6] states that a stretch may be held for 10 to 15 seconds at first and gradually, over a period of several weeks, increased to 45 to 60 seconds.
2. Anderson[4] states one should begin with an "easy" stretch for 10 to 30 seconds, followed by a "developmental" stretch for an additional 10 to 30 seconds.
3. Moffatt[18] states that one should maintain a stretching position for about 8 to 12 seconds.
4. The American College of Sports Medicine[3] states that a stretch should be sustained for 10 to 30 seconds.

The following may be used as guidelines for prescribing the duration of static stretching for the total exercise session:

1. Beaulieu[6] states that stretching exercises as part of a conditioning program may range from a period of 10 to 20 minutes for each session.
2. Thirty minutes of static stretching performed two times per week will improve flexibility within five weeks.[8]

DESIGNING TRAINING AND REHABILITATION PROGRAMS

Figure 9–1 may be used for designing a flexibility program, and Figures 9–2 to 9–39 illustrate sample stretching exercises for the upper and lower extremity.[12,13]

NAME: _____ DATE: _____
AGE: _____ SEX: M   F
WEIGHT: _____ lb _____ kg   HEIGHT: _____ in _____ cm
RESTING HR: _____ RESTING BP: _____/_____

PRE-EXERCISE WARM-UP EXERCISES

UPPER BODY
1. _____
2. _____
3. _____

LOWER BODY
1. _____
2. _____
3. _____

PRE-EXERCISE STRETCHING EXERCISES

UPPER BODY
1. _____
2. _____
3. _____

LOWER BODY
1. _____
2. _____
3. _____

POST-EXERCISE COOL-DOWN EXERCISES

UPPER BODY
1. _____
2. _____
3. _____

LOWER BODY
1. _____
2. _____
3. _____

POST-EXERCISE STRETCHING EXERCISES

UPPER BODY
1. _____
2. _____
3. _____

LOWER BODY
1. _____
2. _____
3. _____

SPECIAL INSTRUCTIONS

_____
_____

Figure 9–1. Sample form for designing flexibility programs.

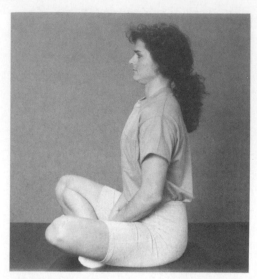

Figure 9–2. Chin tuck exercise. While in a seated position, make a "double chin" without cervical flexion, extension, lateral flexion, or rotation.

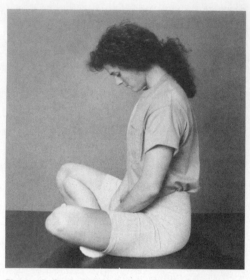

Figure 9–3. Cervical flexion static stretch. While in a seated position, fully flex the neck forward.

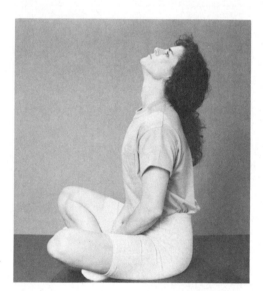

Figure 9–4. Cervical extension static stretch. While in a seated position, fully extend the neck backward.

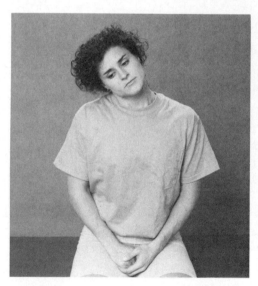

Figure 9–5. Cervical lateral flexion static stretch. While in a seated position, bring the ear to the shoulder while avoiding cervical rotation, flexion, and extension.

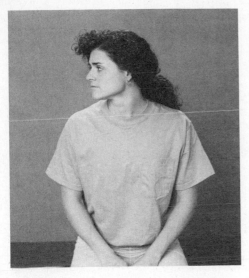

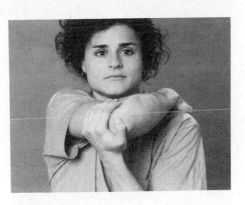

Figure 9–7. Posterior shoulder/upper back static stretch. While in a seated position, horizontally adduct one arm fully across the chest while applying a force to the elbow with the other arm into horizontal adduction.

Figure 9–6. Cervical rotation static stretch. While in a seated position, fully rotate (attempting to look over the shoulder) the neck without cervical flexion or extension.

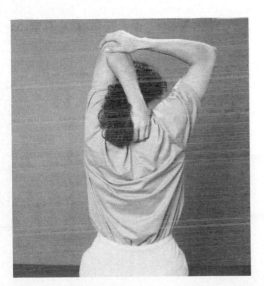

Figure 9–8. Inferior shoulder static stretch. While in a seated position, lift one arm behind the neck to full abduction while applying a force to the elbow into shoulder abduction.

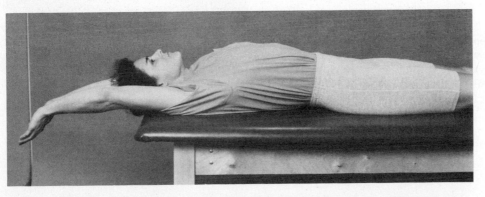

Figure 9–9. Inferior shoulder/upper back static stretch. While in a supine position, fully flex both shoulders (thus, both arms are overhead) and let gravity provide a stretching force.

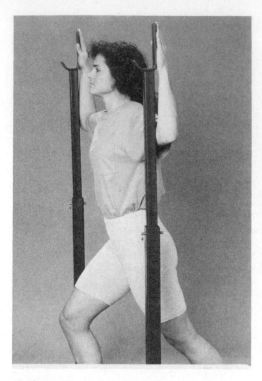

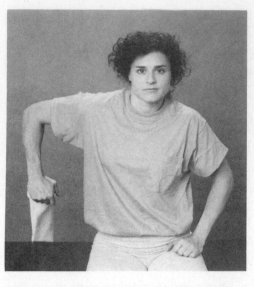

Figure 9–11. Shoulder internal rotation static stretch. While in a seated position, bend the elbow to 90 degrees of flexion, abduct one arm to approximately 90 degrees, and fully rotate the arm internally by holding onto a towel of appropriate length that is fixed at one end to the table. Sitting or leaning forward will increase the stretch.

Figure 9–10. Anterior shoulder/chest static stretch. While in a standing position, abduct both arms using ranges from 90 to 120 degrees while braced against a fixture (eg, doorway) and apply a stretching force by leaning forward with the upper body.

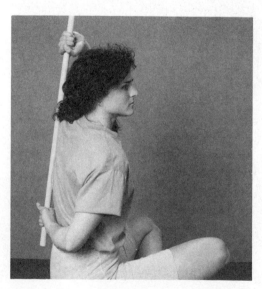

Figure 9–12. Shoulder internal rotation static stretch. While in a seated position, bend the elbow to 90 degrees of flexion, place the forearm behind the back, and fully rotate the arm internally with the use of an assistive device.

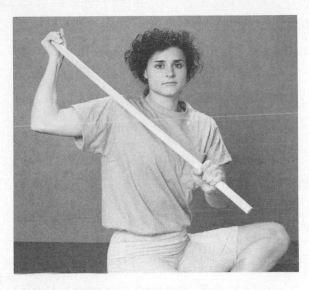

Figure 9–13. Shoulder external rotation static stretch. While in a seated position, bend the elbow to 90 degrees of flexion, abduct the arm to approximately 90 degrees, and fully rotate the arm externally with the use of an assistive device.

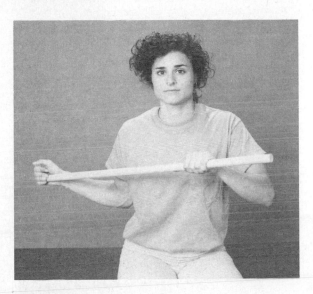

Figure 9–14. Shoulder external rotation static stretch. While in a seated position, bend the elbow to 90 degrees of flexion, keep the arm adducted by the side, and fully rotate the arm externally with the use of an assistive device.

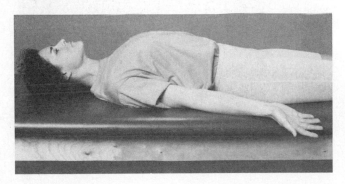

Figure 9–15. Chest (pectoralis minor) static stretch. While in a supine position, with the arms beside the body, rotate the arms externally while retracting both scapulae.

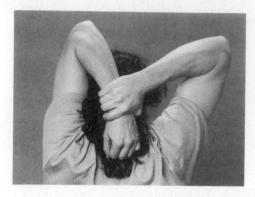

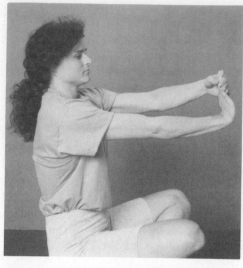

Figure 9–16. Tricep static stretch. While in a seated position, lift one arm behind the neck, fully abduct the shoulder, and flex the elbow. Apply a force with the opposite arm at the wrist in the direction of elbow flexion and shoulder abduction of the arm being stretched.

Figure 9–17. Wrist flexor static stretch. While in a seated position, fully extend one wrist and elbow and apply a force into extension at the fingertips with the other hand.

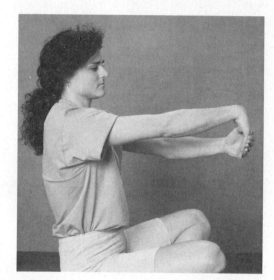

Figure 9–18. Wrist extensor static stretch. While in a seated position, fully flex one wrist and extend the elbow and apply a force into flexion at the fingertips with the other hand.

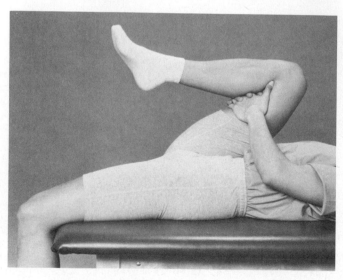

Figure 9–19. Hip flexor and extensor static stretch. While in a supine position, hang one leg over the edge of a table and pull the opposite knee to the chest with both arms (keep hand placement behind the knee in order to prevent excessive compressive forces).

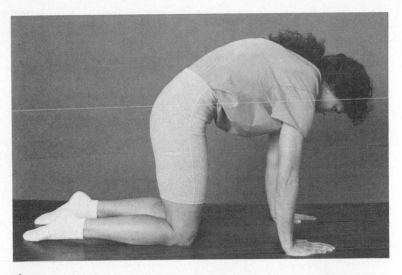

A

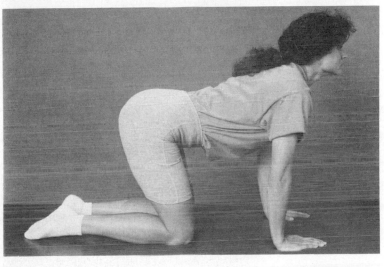

B

Figure 9–20. Back static stretch. While in a hands-and-knees position,
(A) arch the back, decreasing lumbar lordosis (lumbar flexion);
(B) arch the back, increasing lumbar lordosis (lumbar extension).

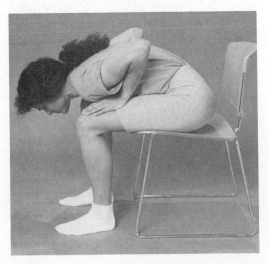

Figure 9–21. Low back flexion static stretch.
While in a seated position, flex the trunk
forward, with the hands supporting the upper
body on the knees.

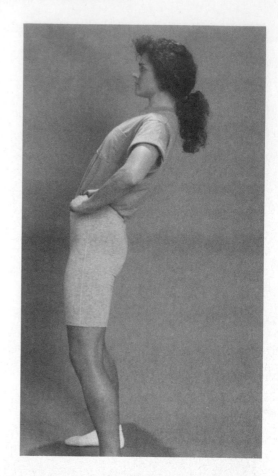

Figure 9–22. Low back extension static stretch. While in a standing position, extend the trunk backward, with hands placed on the hips and feet spaced slightly wider than shoulder width apart.

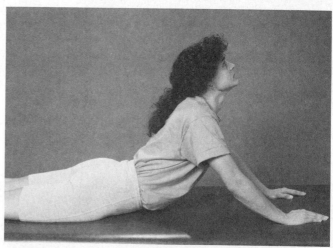

Figure 9–23. Low back extension static stretch. While in a prone position, extend the arms out in front, exerting a pushing force into trunk extension.

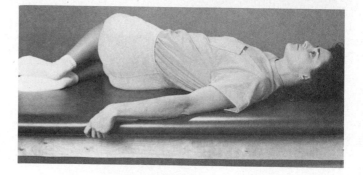

Figure 9–24. Low back rotation static stretch. While in a supine position, flex both knees and hips, and rotate both knees to one side while keeping the upper back flat.

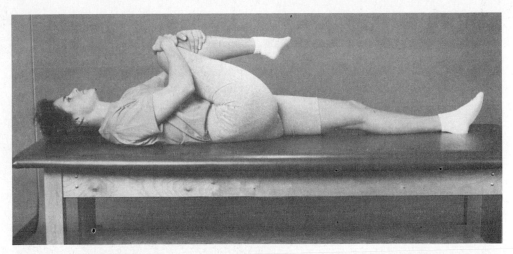

Figure 9–25. Piriformis static stretch. While in a supine position, keep one leg straight and fully flex the other leg toward the opposite shoulder while applying a diagonal pulling force on the outer portion of the knee.

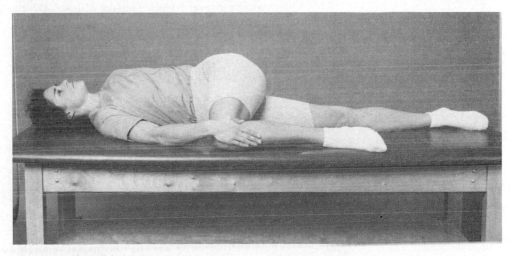

Figure 9–26. Piriformis static stretch. While in a side-lying position, keep the leg next to the table straight and the top leg flexed to approximately 90 degrees. A slight stabilizing force is applied with one arm to the outer portion of the knee while the top shoulder is rotated slightly backward.

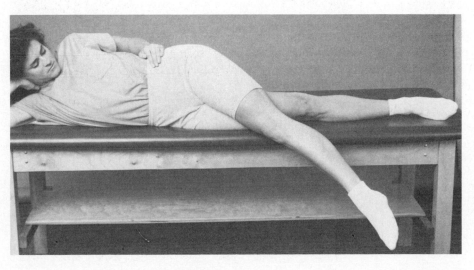

Figure 9–27. Iliotibial band static stretch. While in a side-lying position, drop the top leg in front of the table, thus allowing gravity to provide a stretching force. (*Note*: The Ober test position is probably a more effective stretch; however, it is harder to perform for some individuals.)

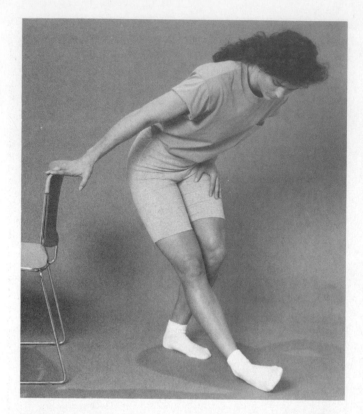

Figure 9–28. Iliotibial band static stretch. While in a standing position, with one knee flexed and the upper body supported with the arms, the leg being stretched is kept straight and rotated outward. Apply a squatting-type force with the body to increase the stretch.

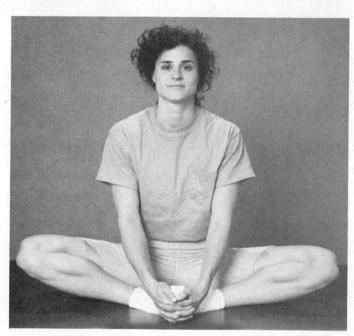

Figure 9–29. Adductor static stretch. While in a seated position, bring both feet together by flexing the hips and knees. To increase the stretch, apply a downward force with the arms to the inner portion of the legs.

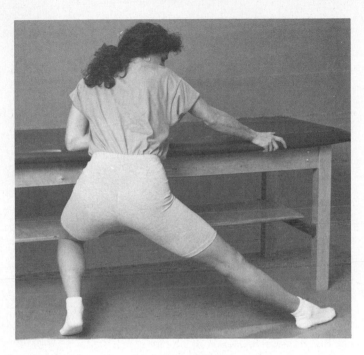

Figure 9–30. Adductor static stretch. While in a standing position, brace the upper body against a table, bend one knee, and extend the other leg. Lean toward the bent leg to provide a stretch to the adductor muscles of the straight leg.

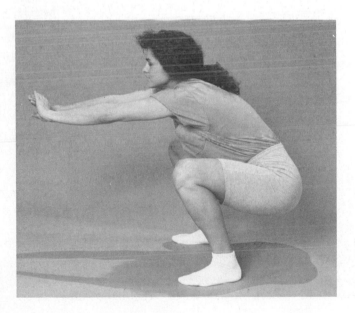

Figure 9–31. Squat static stretch. While in a standing position, space feet slightly wider than shoulder width apart and attempt to assume a squat position (where the thighs are slightly below the parallel position) while keeping the heels on the floor and the arms outstretched in front.

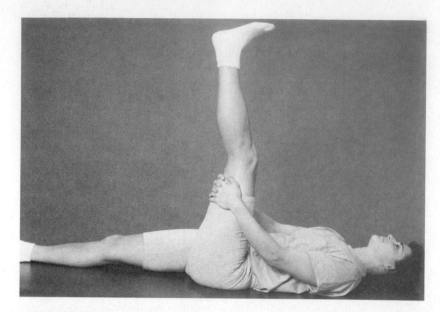

Figure 9–32. Hamstring static stretch. While in a supine position, keep one leg straight, flex the other hip to 90 degrees, and slowly extend the knee, with hand placement behind the knee. (*Note*: Simultaneous dorsiflexion of the foot of the leg being stretched applies a stretching force to the gastrocnemius muscle.)

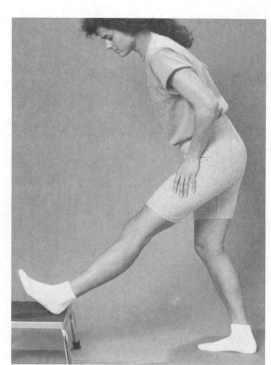

Figure 9–33. Hamstring static stretch. While in a standing position, keep one leg slightly flexed and place the other leg on a surface height appropriate for flexibility level. (*Note*: Stability may be increased by bracing against an object with one or both hands.)

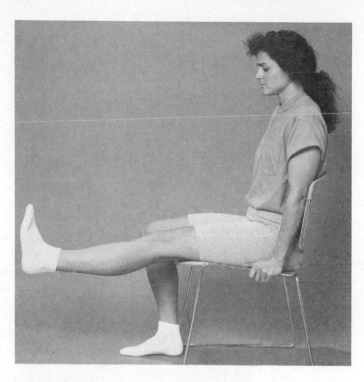

Figure 9–34. Hamstring static stretch. While in a seated position, flex the hip and knee of one leg while keeping the other leg extended out in front. While keeping the back straight, a stretching force is applied by flexing the trunk forward.

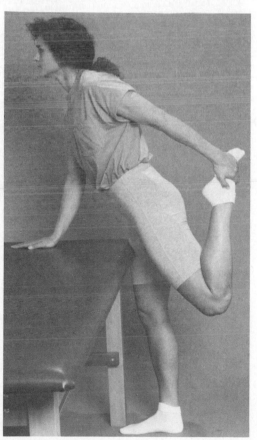

Figure 9–35. Quadricep static stretch. While in a standing position, fully flex one knee while applying a mild force into knee flexion and hip extension with hand placement at the ankle. (*Note:* Avoid an excessive knee flexion force.)

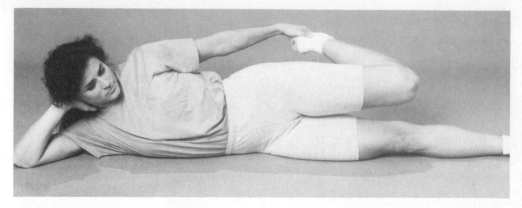

Figure 9–36. Quadricep static stretch. While in a side-lying position, fully flex the top leg while applying a mild force into knee flexion and hip extension. (*Note:* Avoid an excessive knee flexion force.)

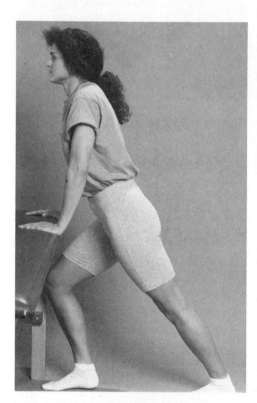

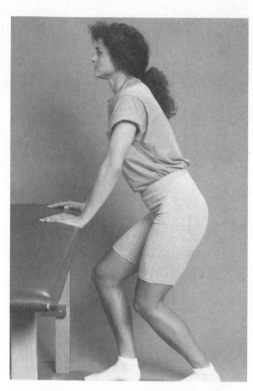

Figure 9–37. Gastrocnemius static stretch. While in a standing position, brace the upper body against a wall or an object and extend the leg that is to be stretched. Place the leg slightly behind the body. With the heel on the floor and the foot pointing forward, lean forward with the upper body to increase the stretch.

Figure 9–38. Soleus static stretch. While in a standing position, brace the upper body against a wall or an object and flex the leg that is to be stretched. Keep the leg directly underneath the body. With the heel on the floor and the foot pointing forward, apply a squatting-type force with the body to increase the stretch.

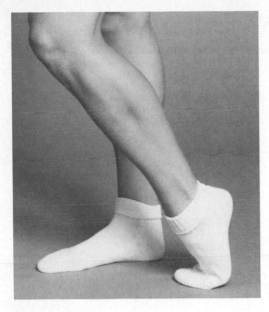

Figure 9–39. Great toe flexor static stretch.
While in a standing position, place the great toe on the floor in a fully extended position and apply an extension force to increase the stretch.

REFERENCES

1. Agre JC. Static stretching for athletes. *Arch Phys Med Rehabil*. 1978;59:561.
2. Alter MJ. *Sport Stretch*. Champaign, Ill: Human Kinetics Publishers, Inc; 1990.
3. American College of Sports Medicine. *Guidelines for Exercise Testing and Prescription*. 4th ed. Philadelphia, Pa: Lea & Febiger; 1991.
4. Anderson B. *Stretching*. Bolinas, Calif: Shelter Publications; 1980.
5. Basmajian JV, Wolf SL, eds. *Therapeutic Exercise*. 5th ed. Baltimore, Md: Williams & Wilkins; 1990.
6. Beaulieu JE. *Stretching for All Sports*. Pasadena, Calif: The Athletic Press; 1980.
7. Beaulieu JE. Developing a stretching program. *Physician Sportsmed*. 1981;9:59.
8. deVries H. Evaluation of static stretching procedures for improvement of flexibility. *Res Q*. 1962;33:222–229.
9. Evjenth O, Hamberg J. *Muscle Stretching in Manual Therapy—A Clinical Manual*. Alfta, Sweden: Alfta Rehab; 1984;1.
10. Fox E, Matthews D. *The Physiological Basis of Physical Education and Athletics*. Philadelphia, Pa: Saunders College Publishing; 1981.
11. Hlasney J. Effect of flexibility exercises on muscle strength. *Phys Ther Forum*. 1988;7:3.
12. Kaplan PE, Tanner ED. *Musculoskeletal Pain and Disability*. Norwalk, Conn: Appleton & Lange; 1989.
13. Kendall FP, McCreary EK. *Muscles: Testing and Function*. 3rd ed. Baltimore, Md: Williams & Wilkins; 1983.
14. Kisner C, Colby LA. *Therapeutic Exercise: Foundations and Techniques*. 2nd ed. Philadelphia, Pa: FA Davis Co; 1990.
15. Knott M, Voss D. *Proprioceptive Neuromuscular Facilitation*. 2nd ed. New York, NY: Harper & Row; 1968.
16. Kottke F. Therapeutic exercise. In: Krusen F, Kottke F, Ellwood M. *Handbook of Physical Medicine and Rehabilitation*. 2nd ed. Philadelphia, Pa: WB Saunders Co; 1971.
17. Mitchell F, Moran P, Pruzzo N. *An Evaluation and Treatment Manual of Osteopathic Muscle Energy Procedures*. Valley Park, Mich: Mitchell, Moran and Pruzzo Assoc; 1979.
18. Moffatt RJ. Strength and flexibility considerations for exercise prescription. In: Blair SN, Painter P, Pate RR, et al, eds. *Resource Manual for Guidelines for Exercise Testing and Prescription* (American College of Sports Medicine). Philadelphia, Pa: Lea & Febiger; 1988.
19. Ross RM, Jackson AS. *Exercise Concepts, Calculations and Computer Applications*. Carmel, Ind: Benchmark Press; 1990.
20. Sapega AA, Quedenfeld TC, Moyer RA, et al. Biophysical factors in range-of-motion exercise. *Physician Sportsmed*. 1981;9(12):57–65.

21. Saunders HD. *Evaluation, Treatment and Prevention of Musculoskeletal Disorders*. Eden Prairie, Minn: Educational Opportunities; 1985.
22. Wallin D, Ekblom B, Grahn R, et al. Improvement of muscle flexibility. *Am J Sports Med*. 1985;13:263.

Exercise Prescription for Muscular Strength and Endurance

PRECAUTIONS, CONTRAINDICATIONS, AND GUIDELINES

Tables 10–1 and 10–2 outline various precautions and contraindications to resistance training, and Table 10–3 outlines general guidelines for lifting.

GUIDELINES FOR EXERCISE PRESCRIPTION

ISOMETRIC

Modes of Training

1. Manual resistance (eg, self or clinician applied)
2. Body resistance (eg, flexed arm hang from a pull-up bar)
3. Free weight resistance (used with range stops)
4. Pulley/cable resistance (used with range stops)
5. Machine resistance (eg, Cybex)

Table 10–4 outlines various advantages and disadvantages of isometric training.

Intensity, Frequency, and Duration of Training
Table 10–5 outlines isometric training protocols.

ISOTONIC

Modes of Training

1. Manual resistance (eg, self or clinician applied)
2. Body resistance (eg, push-ups, pull-ups)

TABLE 10–1. PRECAUTIONS FOR RESISTANCE TRAINING

1. Avoid sustained handgripping in order to not evoke an excessive increase in blood pressure.
2. Avoid breath holding during lifting activities (ie, Valsalva's maneuver). As a general rule, the client should exhale on the most strenuous portions of the exercise.
3. Use spotters for heavy weights and potentially dangerous exercises (eg, bench press, squats).
4. Use collars at the end of barbells to prevent the weights from slipping.
5. Start slowly with a predetermined weight suitable to the client's strength based on strength testing (eg, 1-RM, 10-RM).

TABLE 10–2. CONTRAINDICATIONS TO RESISTANCE TRAINING

1. When a muscle or joint is inflamed or swollen[14]
2. If a client experiences severe joint or muscle pain during resistance exercise or for more than 24 hours after exercise[14]
3. If a client has joint instability[10]
4. The client has uncontrolled hypertension or other cardiovascular complications

TABLE 10–3. GENERAL GUIDELINES FOR LIFTING

1. Maintain a wide base of support (feet wider than hips).
2. Bend at the knees, not at the waist.
3. Tighten the abdominal and gluteal muscles during lifting.
4. Keep items as close to the body as possible.
5. Avoid twisting at the waist when carrying or lifting any item. Instead, use the feet to position the body correctly. (Basic rule: "The nose should follow the toes.")
6. Keep the back straight and the head in a neutral position (looking forward with the chin parallel to the floor) during lifting.
7. See if an item can be pushed, slid, or maneuvered with a dolly. If possible, get the assistance of another person before attempting to lift and carry a very heavy item.
8. Determine how an item should be positioned in order to get the best grip and handling possible.
9. Consider potential obstacles during the carrying route and clear them, if possible.
10. Test the weight of an item before lifting and moving it long distances.
11. Take rest "breaks" while carrying a heavy item long distances.
12. Do not lift with quick and sudden movements.
13. Use both arms to lift, when possible.
14. Attempt to distribute the weight equally between the arms.
15. Warm up and stretch for 10 minutes before starting the workday.
16. Stretch the legs and back for 30 to 60 seconds after sitting or standing for prolonged periods of time.
17. Wear nonskidsoled shoes that support the feet properly.
18. Wear "tackified" gloves for additional grip support during the handling of potentially slippery items.
19. Concentrate on the task at all times.

3. Free weight resistance (eg, barbells, dumbbells)
4. Machine resistance (eg, Eagle, Nautilus, Universal, Keiser, N-K Unit)
5. Elastic resistance (eg, Thera-Band, surgical tubing)
6. Pulley/cable resistance (eg, wall-mounted system, Elgin Exercise Unit)
7. Water resistance (eg, swimming pool)
8. Arm cycle ergometer resistance (eg, UBE)
9. Leg cycle ergometer resistance (eg, Monark)
10. Accessory resistance (eg, weighted vests, ankle weights, hand-held weights, weight boots)
11. Air resistance (eg, wind tunnel)
12. Sport-specific resistance (eg, throwing a shot put)
13. Work-specific resistance (eg, using a sledge hammer)

Table 10–6 outlines various advantages and disadvantages of isotonic training.

TABLE 10–4. ADVANTAGES AND DISADVANTAGES OF ISOMETRIC TRAINING

Advantages
1. It is an inexpensive method of training.[11]
2. Preparatory time is minimal.
3. Potential for injury is minimized since there are no moving devices or weights that may be dropped.[11]
4. It can aid in the strength development of individuals immobilized in a cast or when it is necessary to restrict movement secondary to a painful arc of motion.[9]
5. It may be easily adapted for a home exercise program.
6. It is easy to teach.
7. It is usually safe postoperatively and thus may be utilized during the early stages of rehabilitation.

Disadvantages
1. Strength gains are specific to the angle of training.[11]
2. Training through a full range of motion will require the use of multiple angles, which may be time-consuming.[11]
3. There is a lack of feedback regarding the amount of force being applied, although some machines may provide a display of static force.[11]
4. It is not directly applicable to sport or work performance activities.
5. It is not functional or skill related.
6. Cardiovascular stresses may result from Valsalva's maneuver.

TABLE 10–5. ISOMETRIC TRAINING PROTOCOLS[a]

Static Strength

Intensity	Duration	Repetitions	Frequency
100% MVC[b]	5 s/contraction	5–10	5 days/week

Static Endurance

Intensity	Duration	Repetitions	Frequency
60% MVC or less	Until fatigued	1/session	5 days/week

[a]Physiologic overflow occurs a total of 20 degrees from the training angle (ie, 10 degrees in either direction).[15]
[b]Maximum voluntary contraction.
From "Designing muscular fitness programs" in Advanced Fitness Assessment and Exercise Prescription. *2nd ed. (Table 5.1, p 122) by Vivian H. Heyward, 1991. Champaign, Il: Human Kinetics. Copyright 1991 by Vivian H. Heyward. Adapted by permission. Data from Hettinger and Müller[12] and Liberson.[18]*

TABLE 10–6. ADVANTAGES AND DISADVANTAGES OF ISOTONIC TRAINING

Advantages
1. The client can visualize the work being performed and the progress in strength.[11]
2. The client works accessory and stabilization muscles when using free weights.[11]
3. Costs are usually more reasonable when purchasing free weights.
4. Isotonic training offers more exercise variability within training sessions.
5. A variety of training equipment is available.
6. This may be adapted for a home exercise program.

Disadvantages
1. When using free weights, safety is a factor since all lifting requires proper technique.
2. This may require the use of a training partner or spotter.
3. This may be time-consuming since there is a setup time for each exercise.
4. This usually requires time for the client to learn the test procedure.
5. Cardiovascular stresses may result from Valsalva's maneuver.

Intensity, Frequency, and Duration of Training

Tables 10–7 to 10–12 outline isotonic training protocols, and Table 10–13 provides sample guidelines for prescribing isotonic training programs.

TABLE 10–7. DELORME AND WATKINS PROTOCOL[a,6-8]

Sets	Repetitions	Percentage of RM
1st	10	50% of 10 RM
2nd	10	75% of 10 RM
3rd	10	100% of 10 RM

[a]Progressive resistance exercise (PRE).

TABLE 10–8. OXFORD PROTOCOL[23]

Sets	Repetitions	Percentage of RM
1st	10	100% of 10 RM
2nd	10	75% of 10 RM
3rd	10	50% of 10 RM

TABLE 10–9. BERGER PROTOCOL[2-4]

Sets	Repetitions	Percentage of RM
1st	6	100% of 6 RM
2nd	6	100% of 6 RM
3rd	6	100% of 6 RM

TABLE 10–10. MACQUEEN PROTOCOLS[19,21]

Protocol A

Sets	Repetitions	Percentage of RM
1st	10	100% of 10 RM
2nd	10	100% of 10 RM
3rd	10	100% of 10 RM

Protocol B[a]

Sets	Repetitions	Percentage of RM
1st	2–3	100% of 2–3 RM
2nd	2–3	100% of 2–3 RM
3rd	2–3	100% of 2–3 RM
4th	2–3	100% of 2–3 RM
(5th)	(2–3)	(100% of 2–3 RM)[b]

[a]Advanced program.
[b]Optional set.

TABLE 10–11. STONE AND KROLL PROTOCOL[20,22]

Sets	Repetitions	Percentage of RM
1st	8	50% of 4 RM
2nd	8	80% of 4 RM
3rd	6	90% of 4 RM
4th	4	95% of 4 RM
5th	4	100% of 4 RM

TABLE 10–12. DAPRE[a] PROTOCOL

Part I

Sets	Repetition	Portion of Working Weight Used
1st	10	50%
2nd	6	75%
3rd[b]	Maximum	100%
4th[c]	Maximum	Adjusted working weight

Part II

Number of Repetitions Performed During Set	Adjusted to Working Weight for 4th Set	Adjusted to Working Weight for Next Exercise Session
0–2	Decrease 5–10 lb and repeat set	Decrease 5–10 lb and repeat set
3–4	Decrease 0–5 lb	Keep weight the same
5–7	Keep weight the same	Increase 5–10 lb
8–11	Increase 5–10 lb	Increase 5–15 lb
13 to . . .	Increase 10–15 lb	Increase 10–20 lb

[a]Daily adjusted progressive resistance exercise.
[b]Adjusted working weight for the fourth set is based on the total number of repetitions of the full working weight performed during the third set (see Part II).
[c]Adjusted working weight for the next exercise session is based on the total number of repetitions performed during the fourth set (see Part II).
Adapted with permission from Knight KL. Guidelines for rehabilitation of sports injuries. In: Harvey JS, ed. Rehabilitation of the Injured Athlete [Clinics in Sports Medicine 4(3)]. Philadelphia, Pa: WB Saunders Co; 1985:413–414. Data from Knight[16] and Knight.[17]

ISOKINETIC

Mode of Training

1. Machine resistance (eg, Cybex, Biodex)

Table 10–14 outlines various advantages and disadvantages of isokinetic training.

Intensity, Frequency, and Duration of Training
Table 10–15 outlines isokinetic training protocols.

TABLE 10–13. GENERALIZED PROGRAM DESIGNS FOR ISOTONIC TRAINING[a,b]

Intensity Classification	Training Variables	Percentage of 1-RM	Repetition Range	Set Range	Rest Interval Range
Very heavy	Power	80	1–3	3–6	2–4 minutes
Heavy	Strength	80–90	3–8	3–5	2–4 minutes
Moderate	Hypertrophy	70–80	8–12	3–6	30–90 seconds
Light	Muscular endurance	60–70[c]	12–45 +	2–3	30 seconds or less

[a]Training frequency may be outlined as follows:

1. 3 days a week (eg, Monday, Wednesday, Friday or Tuesday, Thursday, Saturday) where all exercises are performed on each day. Training load may be varied by having Monday a heavy load, Wednesday a light load, and Friday a moderate load.

2. 4 days a week (eg, Monday, Tuesday, Thursday, Friday) where exercises are grouped (eg, upper body versus lower body or pushing versus pulling) and training sessions are arranged for a Monday, Thursday and Tuesday, Friday "split" program. Training load may be varied by having Monday a heavy load, Thursday a light load, and Tuesday a light load, Friday a heavy load.

[b]The American College of Sports Medicine[1] recommends the following for the average healthy adult:

1. A minimum of 8 to 10 exercises involving the major muscle groups.

2. A minimum training frequency of 2 times per week.

3. A minimum of 1 set of 8 to 12 repetitions.

4. Near fatigue intensity levels.

[c]Although it is common to see percentages of less than 60% recommended for developing muscular endurance (especially in circuit training programs), Baechle states that endurance activities associated with the sport, not strength training, should be relied on to produce the needed changes in sport-specific muscular endurance.

Adapted with permission from Baechle TR. Preseason strength training. In: Mellion MB, Walsh WM, Shelton GL, eds. The Team Physician's Handbook. Philadelphia, Pa: Hanley & Belfus, Inc; 1990:38.

TABLE 10–14. ADVANTAGES AND DISADVANTAGES OF ISOKINETIC TRAINING

Advantages

1. Maximal contraction through a full range of motion may be applied at specified speeds.[11]
2. High speeds of training may be used safely and effectively since there is only a small ballistic component.[11]
3. The equipment accommodates for a painful arc of motion.[14]
4. The exercise may be continued safely, even when fatigue sets in.[14]
5. The equipment is usually linked to computers for test and retest compatibility.

Disadvantages

1. Since the resistance may be moved easily, the client may not work at maximal intensities.[11]
2. Unless a specific gauge or recorder is available, specific gains in strength are difficult to visualize.[11]
3. The equipment is expensive and takes up a large amount of space.[14]
4. The equipment cannot be used for a home exercise program.[14]
5. With this training it takes longer to set up an exercise program for various muscle groups.[14]
6. This training usually requires time for the client to learn the test procedure (ie, generating maximal force in the specified direction).
7. Cardiovascular stresses may result from Valsalva's maneuver.
8. This training requires time to train the staff in order to administer the test accurately.

TABLE 10–15. ISOKINETIC TRAINING PROTOCOLS[a]

Isokinetic Strength

Sets	Intensity	Repetitions	Speed[b]	Frequency
3	Maximum contraction	2–15	24–180 degrees/s	3–5 days/week

Isokinetic Endurance

Sets	Intensity	Repetitions	Speed	Frequency
1	Maximum contraction	Until fatigued	At least 180 degrees/s	3–5 days/week

[a]Some clinicians have suggested that training effects only carry over 15 degrees per second from the training velocity utilized.[6,13]

[b]A common exercise session may include training at 60, 120, and 180 degrees per second or 60, 150, and 240 degrees per second.[14]

From "Designing muscular fitness programs" in Advanced Fitness Assessment and Exercise Prescription. *2nd ed. (Table 5.3, p 125), by Vivian H. Heyward, 1991. Champaign, Ill: Human Kinetics. Copyright 1991 by Vivian H. Heyward. Adapted by permission.*

DESIGNING TRAINING AND REHABILITATION PROGRAMS

Figure 10–1 may be used for designing a generalized strength conditioning program, and Figures 10–2 to 10–40 illustrate sample muscular strength and endurance exercises for the upper and lower extremities utilizing manual, free-body, elastic, dumbbell, barbell, and machine resistance.

NAME: _____

WEIGHT: _____ lb _____ kg   HEIGHT: _____ in _____ cm   RESTING HR: _____   RESTING BP: _____/_____

AGE: _____   SEX: M   F   DATE: _____

DATE: _____

EXERCISES	Sets/Reps Weight	Sets/Reps Weight	Sets/Reps Weight	Sets/Reps Weight	Sets/Reps Weight	Sets/Reps Weight	Sets/Reps Weight	Sets/Reps Weight
1.	___/___ ___	___/___ ___	___/___ ___	___/___ ___	___/___ ___	___/___ ___	___/___ ___	___/___ ___
2.	___/___ ___	___/___ ___	___/___ ___	___/___ ___	___/___ ___	___/___ ___	___/___ ___	___/___ ___
3.	___/___ ___	___/___ ___	___/___ ___	___/___ ___	___/___ ___	___/___ ___	___/___ ___	___/___ ___
4.	___/___ ___	___/___ ___	___/___ ___	___/___ ___	___/___ ___	___/___ ___	___/___ ___	___/___ ___
5.	___/___ ___	___/___ ___	___/___ ___	___/___ ___	___/___ ___	___/___ ___	___/___ ___	___/___ ___
6.	___/___ ___	___/___ ___	___/___ ___	___/___ ___	___/___ ___	___/___ ___	___/___ ___	___/___ ___
7.	___/___ ___	___/___ ___	___/___ ___	___/___ ___	___/___ ___	___/___ ___	___/___ ___	___/___ ___
8.	___/___ ___	___/___ ___	___/___ ___	___/___ ___	___/___ ___	___/___ ___	___/___ ___	___/___ ___
9.	___/___ ___	___/___ ___	___/___ ___	___/___ ___	___/___ ___	___/___ ___	___/___ ___	___/___ ___
10.	___/___ ___	___/___ ___	___/___ ___	___/___ ___	___/___ ___	___/___ ___	___/___ ___	___/___ ___
11.	___/___ ___	___/___ ___	___/___ ___	___/___ ___	___/___ ___	___/___ ___	___/___ ___	___/___ ___
12.	___/___ ___	___/___ ___	___/___ ___	___/___ ___	___/___ ___	___/___ ___	___/___ ___	___/___ ___

Figure 10–1. Sample form for designing generalized resistance training programs.

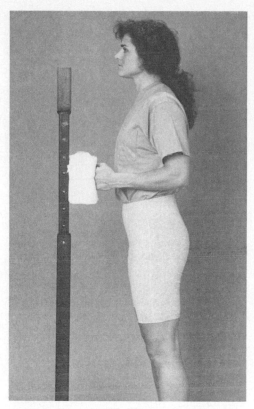

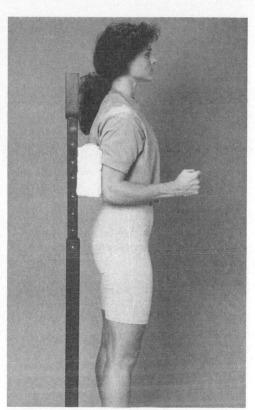

Figure 10–2. Anterior shoulder isometric exercise. While in a standing position, apply a forward force with the hand into an immovable object.

Figure 10–3. Posterior shoulder isometric exercise. While in a standing position, apply a backward force with the elbow into an immovable object.

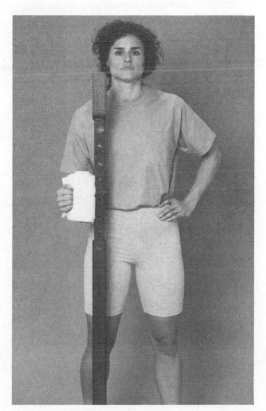

Figure 10–4. Shoulder internal rotation isometric exercise. While in a standing position, apply an internal rotation force with the hand into an immovable object.

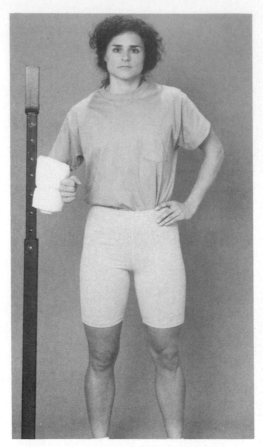

Figure 10–5. Shoulder external rotation isometric exercise. While in a standing position, apply an external rotation force with the hand into an immovable object.

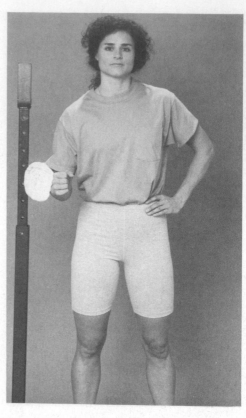

Figure 10–6. Shoulder abduction isometric exercise. While in a standing position, apply an outward force with the elbow into an immovable object.

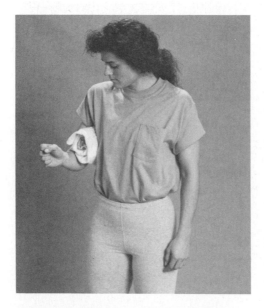

Figure 10–7. Shoulder adduction isometric exercise. While in a standing position, apply an inward force with the elbow into a towel.

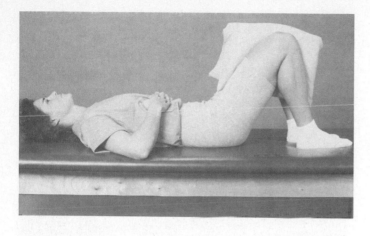

Figure 10–8. Hip adductor isometric exercise. While in a supine position, flex both the knees and hips and place a pillow between the knees for applying a force into adduction (ie, squeeze the pillow).

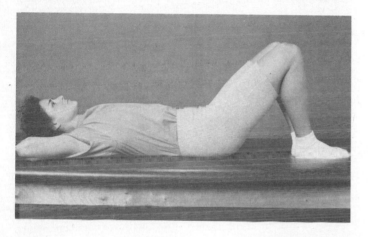

Figure 10–9. Pelvic tilt isometric exercise. While in a supine position, flex both the knees and hips and attempt to reduce lumbar lordosis by flattening the back into the table using the abdominal and not the gluteal muscles. The arms may be placed behind the neck or by the side.

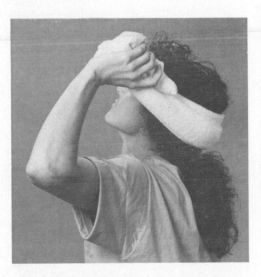

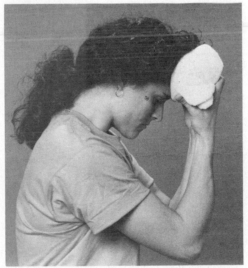

Figure 10–10. Cervical extension isotonic exercise. While in a seated position, place both hands or a towel behind the head and apply an extension force throughout the range of motion.

Figure 10–11. Cervical flexion isotonic exercise. While in a seated position, place both hands or a towel on the forehead and apply a flexion force throughout the range of motion.

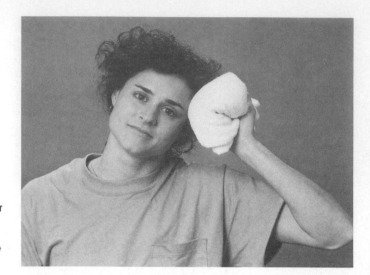

Figure 10–12. Cervical lateral flexion isotonic exercise. While in a seated position, place one hand or a towel on the side of the head and apply a lateral flexion force throughout the range of motion.

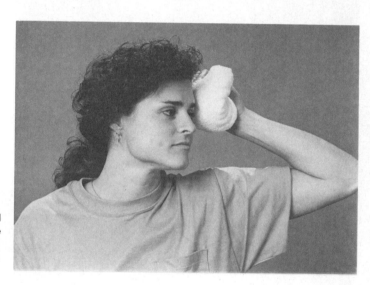

Figure 10–13. Cervical rotation isotonic exercise. While in a seated position, place one hand or a towel at the temple region of the head and apply a rotation force throughout the range of motion.

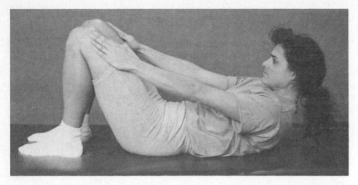

A

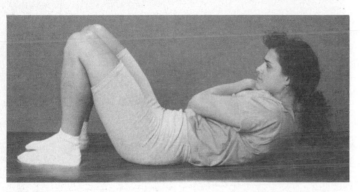

B

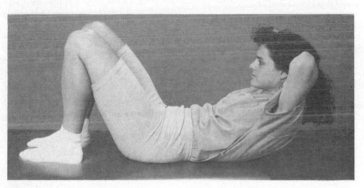

C

Figure 10–14. Abdominal curl-up isotonic exercise. While in a supine position, flex both knees and hips. The exercise may be performed at the following three levels of increasing difficulty. (**A**) Raise the shoulders, with the hands placed on the thighs. (**B**) Raise the shoulders, with the hands crossed on the chest. (**O**) Raise the shoulders, with the hands placed behind the neck.

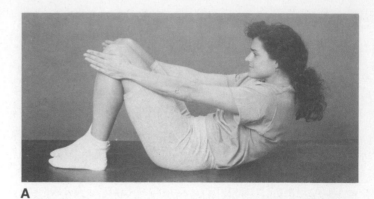

A

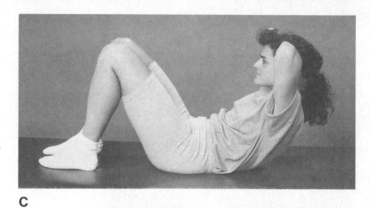

B

Figure 10–15. Partial abdominal sit-up isotonic exercise. While in a supine position, flex both knees and hips. The exercise may be performed at the following three levels of increasing difficulty. **(A)** Raise the trunk, with the hands placed on the thighs. **(B)** Raise the trunk, with the hands crossed on the chest. **(C)** Raise the trunk, with the hands placed behind the neck.

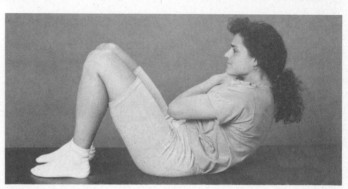

C

Figure 10–16. Pull-up isotonic exercise. While in a standing position, place the hands slightly wider than shoulder width apart and pull the body up until the chin crosses the bar using a supinated grip. (*Note:* A pronated grip may also be used depending on the conditioning goal.)

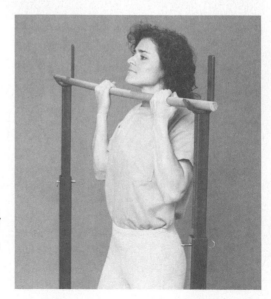

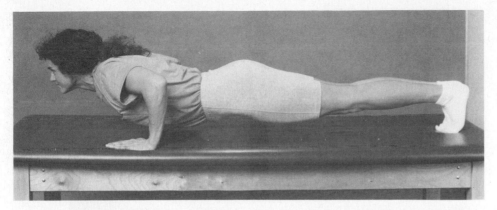

Figure 10–17. Push-up isotonic exercise. While in a prone position, place the hands slightly wider than shoulder width apart and push the body up until the elbows are in full extension. (*Note:* A modified push-up position may be used with the knees on the floor.)

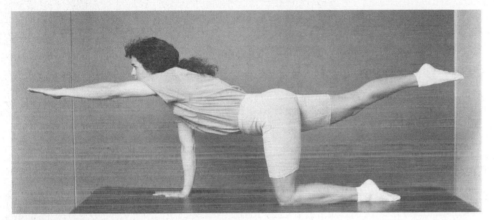

Figure 10–18. Upper and lower back isotonic exercise. While in a hands-and-knees position, extend the opposite arm and leg and return to the starting position. Repeat on the other side.

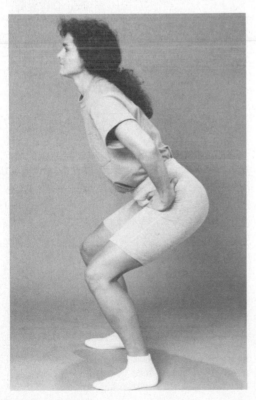

Figure 10–19. Squat isotonic exercise. While in a standing position, place both feet flat on the floor and the hands on the hips. Perform a squatting motion until the thighs are parallel to the floor.

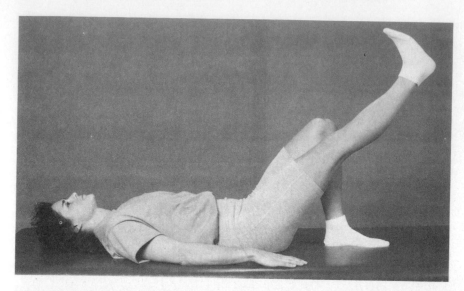

Figure 10–20. Straight leg isometric/isotonic exercise. While in a supine position, keep one knee flexed and the other leg extended. Contract the quadriceps and then raise the extended leg to the level of the flexed knee. (*Note:* Weights may be placed at the ankle according to varying strength levels.)

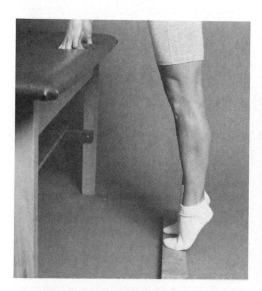

Figure 10–21. Heel raise isotonic exercise. While in a standing position, brace both hands against an object and plantarflex both feet, thus raising the heels off the floor.

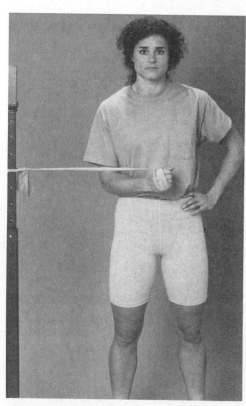

Figure 10–22. Shoulder internal rotation isotonic exercise. While in a standing position, internally rotate the arm using an elastic band.

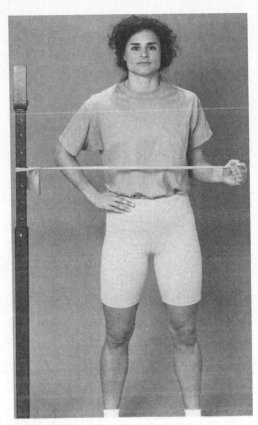

Figure 10–23. Shoulder external rotation isotonic exercise. While in a standing position, externally rotate the arm using an elastic band.

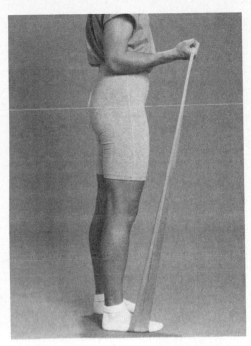

Figure 10–24. Bicep curl isotonic exercise. While in a standing position, flex the arm using an elastic band.

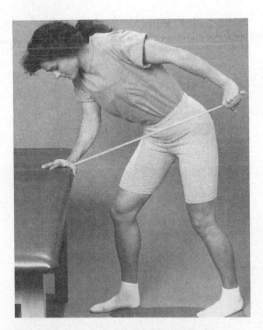

Figure 10–25. Tricep extension isotonic exercise. While in a standing position, brace one arm against a table and extend the other arm using an elastic band.

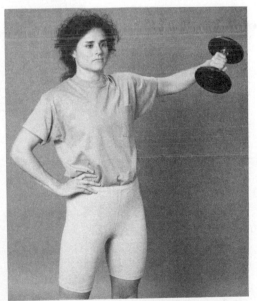

Figure 10–26. Shoulder lateral raise isotonic exercise. While in a standing position, raise one arm to approximately 90 degrees shoulder abduction with slight shoulder internal rotation using a dumbbell.

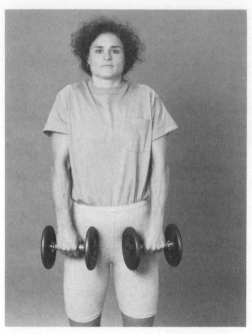

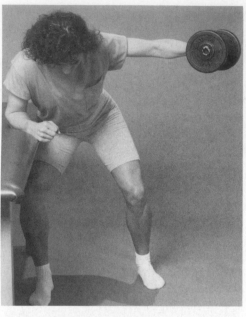

Figure 10–27. Shoulder shrug isotonic exercise. While in a standing position, shrug both shoulders upward using two dumbbells.

Figure 10–28. Posterior shoulder lateral raise isotonic exercise. While in a trunk-flexed position, brace one arm against a table and raise the other arm laterally using one dumbbell.

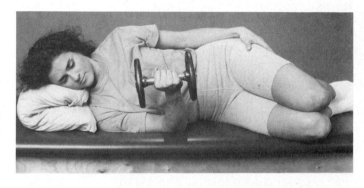

Figure 10–29. Shoulder internal rotation isotonic exercise. While in a side-lying position, internally rotate the arm using one dumbbell.

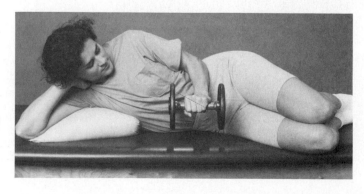

Figure 10–30. Shoulder external rotation isotonic exercise. While in a side-lying position, externally rotate the arm using one dumbbell.

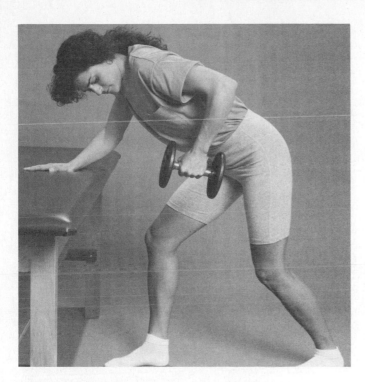

Figure 10–31. Upper back rowing isotonic exercise. While in a trunk-flexed position, brace one arm against a table and flex the other arm with a rowing-type motion using one dumbbell.

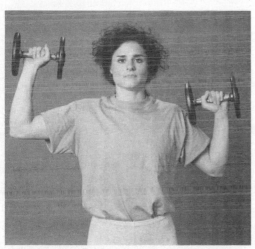

Figure 10–32. Shoulder press isotonic exercise. While in a standing position, alternately extend each arm using two dumbbells.

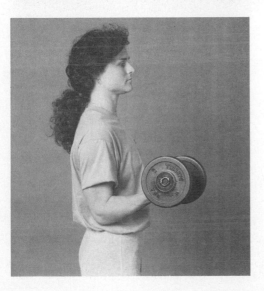

Figure 10–33. Bicep curl isotonic exercise. While in a standing position, alternately flex each arm using two dumbbells.

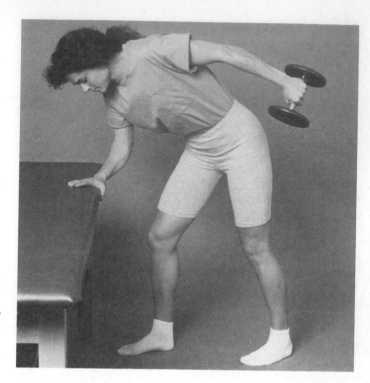

Figure 10–34. Tricep extension isotonic exercise. While in a standing position, brace one arm against a table and extend the other arm using one dumbbell.

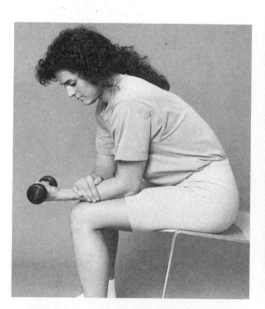

Figure 10–35. Wrist flexion isotonic exercise. While in a seated position with the forearm supinated, flex the wrist using one dumbbell.

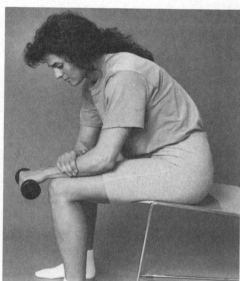

Figure 10–36. Wrist extension isotonic exercise. While in a seated position with the forearm pronated, extend the wrist using one dumbbell.

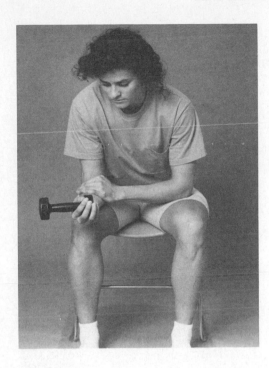

Figure 10–37. Forearm pronation and supination isotonic exercise. While in a seated position, pronate and supinate the forearm by gripping a small dumbbell by one end.

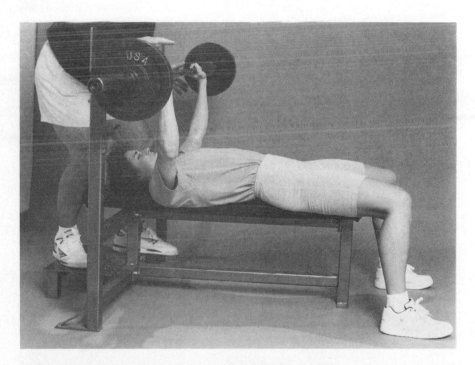

Figure 10–38. Bench press isotonic exercise. While in a supine position on the bench, lift the bar using the assistance of a spotter, if necessary. Lower the bar to the chest and then raise the barbell until the arms are in an extended position.

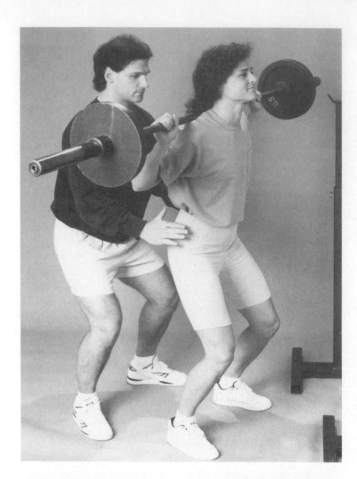

Figure 10–39. Squat isotonic exercise. While in a standing position, lift the bar using the assistance of a spotter, if necessary. Squat with the barbell until the thighs are parallel to the floor and return to a standing position.

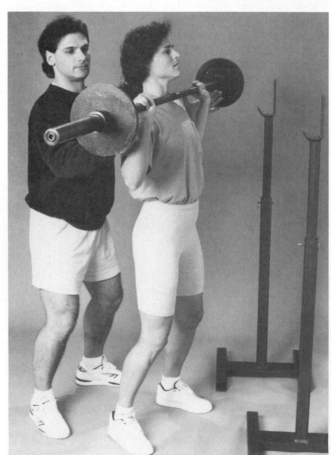

Figure 10–40. Press isotonic exercise. While in a standing position, lift the bar using the assistance of a spotter, if necessary. Lift the barbell overhead until the arms are in an extended position and return to shoulder level.

REFERENCES

1. American College of Sports Medicine. Position stand: The recommended quantity and quality of exercise for developing and maintaining cardiorespiratory and muscular fitness in healthy adults. *Med Sci Sports Exerc.* 1990;22(2):265–274.
2. Berger RA. Effects of varied weight training programs on strength. *Res Q.* 1962;33:168–181.
3. Berger RA. Optimum repetitions for the development of strength. *Res Q.* 1962;33:334–338.
4. Berger RA. Comparative effects of three weight training programs. *Res Q.* 1963;34:396–397.
5. Davies GJ. *A Compendium of Isokinetics in Clinical Usage and Rehabilitation Techniques.* 3rd ed. LaCrosse, Wis: S & S Publishers; 1987.
6. DeLorme TL. Restoration of muscle power by heavy resistance exercises. *J Bone Joint Surg (Am).* 1945;27:645.
7. DeLorme TL, Watkins AL. Techniques of progressive resistance exercise. *Arch Phys Med Rehabil.* 1948;29:263.
8. DeLorme TL, Watkins AL. *A Progressive Resistance Exercise.* New York, NY: Appleton-Century; 1951.
9. DiNubile NA. Strength training. In: DiNubile NA, ed. *The Exercise Prescription* [Clinics in Sports Medicine 10(1)]. Philadelphia, Pa: WB Saunders Co; 1991.
10. Drez D, ed. *Therapeutic Modalities for Sports Injuries.* Chicago, Ill: Year Book Medical Publishers, Inc; 1989.
11. Fisher AG, Jensen CR. *Scientific Basis of Athletic Conditioning.* 3rd ed. Philadelphia, Pa: Lea & Febiger; 1990.
12. Hettinger T, Müller EA. Muskelleistung und muskeltraining. *Eur J Appl Physiol.* 1953;15:111–126.
13. Jenkins WL, Thackaberry M, Killian C. Speed-specific isokinetic training. *J Orthop Sports Phys Ther.* 1984;6:181–183.
14. Kisner C, Colby LA. *Therapeutic Exercise: Foundations and Techniques.* 2nd ed. Philadelphia, Pa: FA Davis Co; 1990.
15. Knapik JJ, Mawadsley RH, Ramos MU. Angular specificity and test mode specificity of isometric and isokinetic strength training. *J Orthop Sports Phys Ther.* 1983;5:58–65.
16. Knight KL. Knee rehabilitation by the daily adjustable progressive resistive exercise technique. *Am J Sports Med.* 1979;7:336–337.
17. Knight KL. Quadriceps strengthening with DAPRE technique: Case studies with neurological implications. *Med Sci Sports Exerc.* 1985;17:636.
18. Liberson WT. Brief isometric exercise. In: Basmajian JV, ed. *Therapeutic Exercise.* 3rd ed. Baltimore, Md: Williams & Wilkins; 1978.
19. MacQueen IJ. Recent advances in the technique of progressive resistance. *Br Med J.* 1954;11:1193.
20. Sanders MT. Weight training and conditioning. In: Sanders B, ed. *Sports Physical Therapy.* Norwalk, Conn: Appleton & Lange; 1990.
21. Sanders MT, Sanders B. Mobility: Active-resistive training. In: Gould JA, ed. *Orthopaedic and Sports Physical Therapy.* 2nd ed. St Louis, Mo: CV Mosby Co; 1990.
22. Stone WJ, Kroll WA. *Sports Conditioning and Weight Training: Programs for Athletic Competition.* 3rd ed. Dubuque, Iowa: Wm C Brown Publishers; 1991.
23. Zinovieff AN. Heavy resistance exercise: The Oxford technique. *Br J Phys Med.* 1951;14:129.

Chapter Eleven

Exercise Prescription for Cardiovascular Endurance

GUIDELINES FOR EXERCISE PRESCRIPTION

Modes of Training

When selecting a mode of training, the clinician should vary the program activities as follows in order to minimize injuries and eliminate boredom:

1. High-impact (eg, running/jogging) versus low-impact (eg, walking) activities
2. Individual (eg, swimming) versus group (eg, volleyball) activities
3. Indoor (eg, stationary cycling) versus outdoor (eg, outdoor leisure cycling) activities
4. Skilled (eg, tennis) versus nonskilled (eg, walking) activities

Generally, cardiovascular endurance training may be categorized as follows:

1. Continuous training
2. Interval training
3. Circuit training
4. Fartlek training

This chapter will focus on continuous training parameters in prescribing cardiovascular endurance programs. Interval, circuit, and fartlek training are more often associated with sport performance and, therefore, will be presented in *Chapter 12*.

Continuous Training

1. Continuous training imposes a submaximal energy requirement that is consistent throughout the training session.[4]
2. The following is a list of continuous training activities that utilize large muscle groups, can be maintained for prolonged periods of time, and are rhythmic and aerobic in nature[4]:
   a. Walking
   b. Running/jogging
   c. Cycling
      (1) Outdoor leisure cycling

       (2) Standard cycling apparatus
       (3) Standard cycling apparatus with upper body variation
       (4) Recumbent cycling apparatus
    d. Swimming
       (1) Swimming laps in pool
       (2) Stationary swimming apparatus
    e. Treadmill
       (1) Standard treadmill apparatus
       (2) Low-impact treadmill apparatus (ie, treadmill has "trampoline-type" surface)
       (3) Aquatic treadmill apparatus
    f. Upper body exercise (UBE) cycle
    g. Stair climbing
       (1) Piston option
       (2) Revolving option
    h. Rowing
       (1) Rowing in water
       (2) Stationary rowing apparatus
    i. Skiing
       (1) Outdoor cross-country skiing
       (2) Stationary cross-country skiing apparatus
       (3) Stationary skiing apparatus
    j. Mountain climbing
       (1) Outdoor mountain climbing
       (2) Stationary mountain climbing apparatus
    k. Ladder-climbing apparatus
       (1) Stationary ladder-climbing apparatus
    l. Hiking
    m. Trampoline
       (1) Mini-rebounder apparatus
    n. Step training apparatus
    o. Aerobic dance/calisthenics
       (1) Regular aerobic dance
       (2) Low-impact aerobic dance
       (3) High-impact aerobic dance
       (4) Aerobic water calisthenics
       (5) Aerobic dance routines with heavy hands
    p. Dancing
       (1) Folk/ballroom dancing
       (2) Modern dancing
    q. Ice or roller skating
    r. Rope skipping
    s. Aerobic games (eg, modified basketball and volleyball designed for sustained and low-intensity activity)

Intensity of Training

The intensity of cardiovascular endurance training may vary from 55% to 90% of maximal heart rate (HRmax) or 40% to 85% of maximal oxygen uptake ($\dot{V}O_2$ max) or HRmax reserve.[3,4] Training (or exercise) intensity may be prescribed by heart rate (see Figure 11–1 and Tables 11–1, 11–2, and 11–3), METs (see Table 11–4), or ratings of perceived exertion (RPE) (*see Table 5–14*).

Prescription by Heart Rate

This method is based on the assumption that there exists a relatively linear relationship between heart rate and exercise intensity.[4] The following are methods for calculating appropriate heart rate ranges:

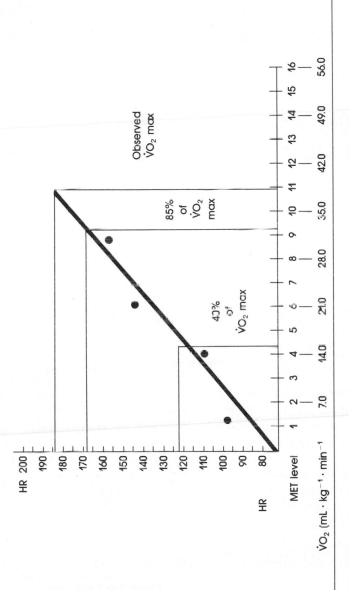

Figure 11–1. Plotting target heart rate range. After performing a maximal exercise test, plot the heart rates corresponding to various exercise intensities in $\dot{V}O_2$ or METs on the graph. Draw a line that best fits through these data points. For example, in a hypothetical testing situation, a client's $\dot{V}O_2$ max was observed to be 38 mL · kg⁻¹ · min⁻¹ (10.9 METs) with a maximal heart rate of 184 beats per minute. The target heart rate range would then be determined by finding the heart rates that correspond to 40% and 85% of $\dot{V}O_2$ max. Thus, 40% of $\dot{V}O_2$ max would be approximately 15 mL · kg⁻¹ · min⁻¹ (4.3 METs) and 85% of $\dot{V}O_2$ max would be approximately 32 mL · kg⁻¹ · min⁻¹ (9.1 METs). The approximate target heart rate range for this client would then be 120 to 168 beats per minute. Adapted from the American College of Sports Medicine. Guidelines for Exercise Testing and Prescription. 4th ed. Philadelphia, Pa: Lea & Febiger; 1991.

TABLE 11–1. KARVONEN OR HEART RATE RESERVE METHOD[a,b]

	Target Heart Rate Range[c]	
	Lower Limit	Upper Limit
Maximal heart rate[d]	200	200
Resting heart rate	− 70	− 70
Heart rate reserve[e]	130	130
Conditioning intensity (%)	× .60	× .80
	78	104
Resting heart rate	+ 70	+ 70
Target heart rate	148	174

[a]60% to 80% of heart rate reserve is approximately equal to 60% to 80% $\dot{V}O_2$ max.

[b]A criticism of this method is the variability of resting heart rate (see *Chapter 5* for measuring heart rate). However, a 10 beat per minute error in resting heart rate affects the heart rate max reserve value by only 2% to 3%.[23]

[c]A target heart rate range or training zone is defined when an upper and a lower limit range is specified, and a target rate is defined when a specified percentage of maximal limit is recommended.[23]

[d]Maximal heart rate may be obtained during testing or by using the age-adjusted estimate (220 − age). Without the actual measurement of heart rate max, one should be aware of the general variations secondary to the population, apparatus utilized, protocol utilized, health status, fitness level, and the effects of medications.[23]

[e]Heart rate reserve = maximal heart rate minus resting heart rate.

Adapted from the American College of Sports Medicine. Guidelines for Exercise Testing and Prescription. 4th ed. Philadelphia, Pa: Lea & Febiger; 1991.

1. Maximal exercise test method uses the results obtained on graded exercise test (See Figure 11–1).
2. Karvonen or heart rate reserve method uses a formula for calculating heart rate ranges (See Table 11–1).
3. Percentage of maximal heart rate method uses a formula for calculating heart rate ranges (See Table 11–2 and 11–3).
4. McArdle, Katch, and Katch[16] note that an exercise heart rate of 70% maximum is frequently referred to as "conversational exercise" because it is sufficient to stimulate a training effect yet it is not so strenuous as to limit an individual from talking during a workout session.

Prescription by METs

1. Once a client's functional aerobic capacity has been determined from a graded exercise test, appropriate conditioning intensities may be prescribed. For example, if a client's functional aerobic capacity is 10 METs (35 mL · kg^{-1} · min^{-1}), then a training frequency of 60% to 70% would correspond to 6 to 7 METs. Therefore, the client would perform activities (see Table 11–4) that produce an average intensity of 6 to 7 METs.[13] Average intensity may be obtained by alternating equal time intervals at 6 and 7 METs, thus yielding an average rate of energy expenditure within this desired range.[4]

TABLE 11–2. PERCENTAGE OF MAXIMAL HEART RATE METHOD[a,b,12,23]

	Target Heart Rate Range	
	Lower Limit	Upper Limit
Maximal heart rate[c]	200	200
Conditioning intensity (%)[d]	× .70	× .85
Target heart rate	140	170

[a]There exists a variability of heart rate max at any given age (standard deviation of 12 beats per minute).

[b]Since this method underestimates the target heart rate, it has been recommended to add 10% to 15% to the training heart rate obtained from this method.[2,17,20,22,23]

[c]Maximal heart rate may be obtained during testing or by using the age-adjusted estimate (220 − age). Without the actual measurement of heart rate max, one should be aware of the general variations secondary to the population, apparatus utilized, protocol utilized, health status, fitness level, and the effects of medications.[23]

[d]70%, 80%, and 85% of maximal heart rate is approximately equal to 56%, 70%, and 78% of $\dot{V}O_2$ max, respectively.[16,24]

TABLE 11–3. AGE-PREDICTED HEART RATES[a,b,c]

Age	100%	85%	75%	70%	Age	100%	85%	75%	70%
20	200	170	150	140	43	177	150	133	124
21	199	169	149	139	44	176	150	132	123
22	198	168	148	139	45	175	149	131	122
23	197	167	148	138	46	174	148	130	122
24	196	167	147	137	47	173	147	130	121
25	195	166	146	136	48	172	146	129	120
26	194	165	146	136	49	171	145	128	120
27	193	164	145	135	50	170	144	128	119
28	192	163	144	134	51	169	144	127	118
29	191	162	143	134	52	168	143	126	118
30	190	162	142	133	53	167	142	125	117
31	189	161	142	132	54	166	141	124	116
32	188	160	141	132	55	165	140	124	116
33	187	159	140	131	56	164	139	123	115
34	186	158	140	130	57	163	139	122	114
35	185	157	139	130	58	162	138	122	113
36	184	156	138	129	59	161	137	121	113
37	183	156	137	128	60	160	136	120	112
38	182	155	136	127	61	159	135	119	111
39	181	154	136	127	62	158	134	118	111
40	180	153	135	126	63	157	133	118	110
41	179	152	134	125	64	156	133	117	109
42	178	151	134	125	65	155	132	116	108

[a]Numbers in the 100% column are derived by taking 220 minus age in years.
[b]Numbers in the 70%, 75%, and 85% columns are derived by multiplying the numbers in the 100% column.
[c]Numbers in this table have been rounded off according to Brown and LeMay.[7]

2. Limitations of this method include:
   a. Its failure to consider variations in energy expenditure among individuals according to size, environmental factors (eg, wind, hills, sand, snow, heat, cold, humidity, altitude, pollution), physical condition, and level of skill.[4,9]
   b. Determining the oxygen uptake equivalency of a MET. The standard MET equivalent is given as 3.5 mL $O_2 \cdot kg^{-1} \cdot min^{-1}$. In upright exercise, standing rest oxygen uptake is closer to 4.0 mL $O_2 \cdot kg^{-1} \cdot min^{-1}$. The 3.5 mL $O_2 \cdot kg^{-1} \cdot min^{-1}$ value does not take into consideration the change from sitting to standing that is not part of the activity. Also, it should be noted that the 3.5 mL $O_2 \cdot kg^{-1} \cdot min^{-1}$ value is only an average and, therefore, resting $\dot{V}O_2$ should be measured (when possible) for increasing the accuracy of this method.[9]

Prescription by Ratings of Perceived Exertion (RPE)

1. During steady-state exercise, RPE may be used as a valid and reliable indicator of exercise intensity for testing and training.[5,6] RPE response to graded exercise correlates highly with $\dot{V}O_2$, heart rate, and ventilation.[4]
2. Using the 15-point (6 to 20) RPE scale (see Table 5–14), a rating of 12 to 13 ("somewhat hard") and 16 ("hard") corresponds to approximately 60% and 85% of the heart rate range, respectively.[4]
3. Using the 10-point (1 to 10) RPE scale (see Table 5–14), a rating of 4 and 6 corresponds to approximately 60% and 85% of the heart rate range, respectively.[4]
4. Since RPE is a good general indicator of fatigue, it may be used to estimate the intensity of nonsteady-state training sessions.[23]

Frequency of Training

The frequency of cardiovascular endurance training may vary from several daily sessions (for those individuals with functional capacities less than 5 METs) to 3 to 5 days per week.[4]

TABLE 11–4. ENERGY COST OF VARIOUS ACTIVITIES[a,b]

			METs[c]	Kilocalories[d,e,f] (kcal · min⁻¹)
Basketball (game)			7–12	8.5–15.0
Bicycling (recreational)			3–8	3.7–10.0
Golf (walking—carrying bag or pulling cart)			4–7	5.0–8.5
Paddleball/racquetball			8–12	10.0–15.0
Running				
mph	grade (%)	min · mi⁻¹ (min:s)		
5.5	0	10:55	8.3	10.1
6.0	0	10:00	10.0	12.0
7.0	0	8:35	11.5	14.0
8.0	0	7:30	12.8	15.6
9.0	0	6:40	14.2	17.5
10.0	0	6:00	16.0	19.6
12.0	0	5:00	20.0	24.5
Snow skiing (downhill)			5–8	6.0–10.0
Softball			3–6	3.7–7.5
Swimming			4–8	5.0–10.0
Tennis			4–9	5.0–11.0
Volleyball			3–6	3.7–7.5
Walking				
mph	grade (%)	min · mi⁻¹ (min:s)		
2.0	0	30:00	2.0	2.5
2.5	0	24:00	2.5	3.0
3.0	0	20:00	3.0	3.7
3.5	0	17:08	3.5	4.2
4.0	0	15:00	4.6	5.5
4.5	0	13:20	5.7	7.0
5.0	0	12:00	6.9	8.3

[a]For further activities (sports, exercise classes, games, and dancing) in METS and in kcal · min⁻¹, refer to the American College of Sports Medicine,[4] Fardy, Yanowitz, and Wilson,[9] Fox, Naughton, and Gorman,[10] McArdle, Katch, and Katch,[16] and Pollock and Wilmore.[23]

[b]Energy cost values are based on an individual of 154 lbs of body weight (70 kg).

[c]A kcal is a unit of measure based on heat production (1 kcal equals approximately 200 mL of oxygen consumed).

[d]A MET is the basal oxygen requirement of the body while sitting quietly (1 MET equals 3.5 mL · kg⁻¹ · min⁻¹ of oxygen consumed).

[e]In racquetball, for example, RPEs of 12 to 13 (moderate workout), 14 to 15 (moderate to hard workout), and 16 to 17 (very hard workout) correspond to 10 kcal · min⁻¹, 12.5 kcal · min⁻¹, and 15 kcal · min⁻¹, respectively.[23]

[f]To determine the total kilocalorie cost of the various activities, multiply the kilocalories per minute by the total number of minutes of participation. In sports such as racquetball, one should cut the total time by half (due to "rest" breaks) in estimating proper kilocalorie expenditure.[23]

Adapted by permission of Macmillan Publishing Company from Health and Fitness through Physical Activity by Michael L. Pollock, Jack H. Wilmore, and Samuel M. Fox III (Tables 4.3, 4.4; pp. 128–129, 134–135). Copyright 1978 (New York, NY: Macmillan Publishing Company). Data from Pollock and Wilmore.[23]

The following may be used as general guidelines for prescribing training (or exercise) frequency:

1. Individuals with functional capacities less than 3 METs may train 5 to 15 minutes, several times per day.[3,4,22,23]
2. Individuals with functional capacities between 3 and 5 METs may train one to two times per day.[4]
3. Individuals with functional capacities greater than 5 METs may train at least three times per week on alternate days.[4] V̇O₂ max improvements were noted to be similar for those individuals who trained every other day and on three consecutive days.[18]
4. Individuals on weight reduction programs may benefit from training four to five times per week.[1,23]

5. Improvement in $\dot{V}O_2$ max tends to plateau when the training frequency is increased above three days per week.[3,11,19,23]

6. Improvement in $\dot{V}O_2$ max tends to be small to not apparent when the training frequency is more than five days per week.[3,14,15,19]

7. Improvement in $\dot{V}O_2$ max generally is not significant when the training frequency is less than two days per week.[3,11,19,26,27]

8. Cardiorespiratory fitness may be maintained (once a desired level is reached) by training two to four days per week, provided that the intensity and duration are similar to those used to attain the current level of cardiorespiratory fitness.[8,13,14]

9. Those individuals training frequently (ie, four to five times or greater per week) should consider alternating between high- and low-intensity sessions as well as alternating between high-impact (eg, running/jogging), medium-impact (eg, walking), and low-impact (eg, swimming, stationary cycling, stationary stair climbing apparatus) activities in order to prevent musculoskeletal injuries.[4,21,23]

Duration of Training

The duration of cardiovascular endurance training may vary from 20 to 60 minutes (exclusive of a warm-up and cool-down period) of continuous aerobic activity. The duration of training is inversely related to the intensity of training; thus, lower intensity activity should be conducted over a longer period of time.[3,4] Since duration and intensity are closely interrelated, it should be emphasized that the total amount of work (energy cost) accomplished in a training program is an important criterion for cardiovascular improvement.[23]

The following may be used as general guidelines for prescribing training (or exercise) duration:

1. Cardiovascular improvements have been obtained with training sessions of 5 to 10 minutes' duration with an intensity of more than 90% of functional capacity. However, this type of program increases the risk of orthopedic injuries.[4]

2. During the first weeks of conditioning, training sessions of 20 to 30 minutes' duration at an intensity of 40% to 60% of functional capacity are advisable for sedentary, asymptomatic, and symptomatic individuals.[4]

3. Generally, 15 to 20 minutes of very heavy, high-intensity activity (85% of heart rate max reserve or higher), 20 to 30 minutes of heavy, high-intensity activity (75% to 84% of heart rate max reserve), or 40 to 50 minutes of moderate-intensity activity (50% to 74% of heart rate max reserve) meet the guideline standards established by the American College of Sports Medicine (see Table 11–5). Because of the problems (eg, noncompliance, injuries) asso-

TABLE 11–5. CLASSIFICATION OF INTENSITY OF EXERCISE BASED ON 30 TO 60 MINUTES OF ENDURANCE TRAINING

HRmax[a,b]	$\dot{V}O_2$ max[c] or HRmax Reserve[a]	Rating of Perceived Exertion	Classification of Intensity
< 35%	< 30%	< 10	Very light
35–59%	30–49%	10–11	Light
60–79%	50–74%	12–13	Moderate
80–89%	75–84%	14–16	Heavy
≥ 90%	≥ 85%	> 16	Very heavy

[a]Relative intensity.
[b]HRmax = maximal heart rate.
[c]$\dot{V}O_2$ max = maximal oxygen uptake.
Reprinted with permission from Pollock ML, Wilmore JH. Exercise in Health and Disease: Evaluation and Prescription for Prevention and Rehabilitation. 2nd ed. Philadelphia, Pa: WB Saunders Co; 1990:105.

NAME: _____ AGE: _____ SEX: M F DATE: _____

RESTING HR: _____ RESTING BP: _____ / _____ WEIGHT: _____ lb _____ kg HEIGHT: _____ in _____ cm

AGE-PREDICTED MAX HEART RATE: _____ 70% _____ 75% _____ 85% _____

PRE-EXERCISE WARM-UP SESSION: _____

PRE-EXERCISE STRETCHING SESSION: _____

MODE: (Sample: Walking/Running)

	INTENSITY								FREQUENCY	DURATION
min · mi⁻¹ (min:s)	Speed (mph)	Grade (%)	Rest Relief (min)	Sets and Repetitions	Heart Rate Range (bpm)	$\dot{V}O_2$ Max Range (%)	METs Range	RPE Range	Days per Week	Total Time (min)
Week 1										
Week 2										
Week 3										
Week 4										
Week 5										
Week 6										
Week 7										
Week 8										

Note: A rest relief period, along with appropriate sets and repetitions, may be prescribed for those performing interval-type training.

POST-EXERCISE COOL-DOWN SESSION: _____

POST-EXERCISE STRETCHING SESSION: _____

SPECIAL INSTRUCTIONS: _____

Figure 11–2. Sample form for designing cardiovascular endurance exercise programs.

NAME: _____ AGE: _____ SEX: M F DATE: _____

RESTING HR: _____ RESTING BP: _____ / _____ WEIGHT: _____ lb _____ kg HEIGHT: _____ in _____ cm

AGE-PREDICTED MAX HEART RATE: _____ 70% _____ 75% _____ 85% _____

PRE-EXERCISE WARM-UP SESSION: _____

PRE-EXERCISE STRETCHING SESSION: _____

MODE: (Sample: Stationary Cycling)

| | | | INTENSITY | | | | | FREQUENCY | DURATION |
	Workload kg · m · min⁻¹ (kp) (watts)	Speed (mph) (kph) (rpm)	Rest Relief (min)	Sets and Repetitions	Heart Rate Range (bpm)	V̇O₂ Mcx Range (%)	METs Range	RPE Range	Days per Week	Total Time (min)
Week 1										
Week 2										
Week 3										
Week 4										
Week 5										
Week 6										
Week 7										
Week 8										

Note: 1. A rest relief period, along with appropriate sets and repetitions, may be prescribed for those performing interval-type training.
2. When prescribing workload and speed, either kg · m · min⁻¹, kp, or watts and mph, kph, or rpm may be selected, respectively.

POST-EXERCISE COOL-DOWN SESSION: _____

POST-EXERCISE STRETCHING SESSION: _____

SPECIAL INSTRUCTIONS: _____

Figure 11–3. Sample form for designing cardiovascular endurance exercise programs.

175

ciated with attaining and maintaining very-high-intensity activity (ie, 85% of heart rate max reserve or higher), a program of 20 to 30 minutes becomes a more realistic minimal standard. For this reason, the American College of Sports Medicine is changing its minimal duration standard from 15 to 20 minutes to 20 to 30 minutes.[3,4,23,27]

4. Sharkey[25] prescribes duration in terms of calories expended during exercise. Participants in the low (less than 35 mL $\cdot$ kg^{-1} $\cdot$ min^{-1}), medium (35 to 45 mL $\cdot$ kg^{-1} $\cdot$ min^{-1}), and high (greater than 45 mL $\cdot$ kg^{-1} $\cdot$ min^{-1}) fitness categories would exercise long enough to burn 100 to 200, 200 to 400, and over 400 calories per exercise session, respectively.

DESIGNING TRAINING AND REHABILITATION PROGRAMS

Figures 11–2 and 11–3 may be used to design a cardiovascular endurance program.

REFERENCES

1. American College of Sports Medicine. Position stand: Proper and improper weight-loss programs. *Med Sci Sports Exerc.* 1983;15(1):ix–xiii.
2. American College of Sports Medicine. *Guidelines for Exercise Testing and Prescription.* 3rd ed. Philadelphia, Pa: Lea & Febiger; 1986.
3. American College of Sports Medicine. Position stand: The recommended quantity and quality of exercise for developing and maintaining cardiorespiratory and muscular fitness in healthy adults. *Med Sci Sports Exerc.* 1990;22(2):265–274.
4. American College of Sports Medicine. *Guidelines for Exercise Testing and Prescription.* 4th ed. Philadelphia, Pa: Lea & Febiger; 1991.
5. Birk TJ, Birk CA. Use of ratings of perceived exertion for exercise prescription. *Sports Med.* 1987;4:1–8.
6. Borg GV, Linderholm H. Perceived exertion and pulse rate during graded exercise in various age groups. *Acta Medica Scandinavica.* 1967;472(Suppl):194–206.
7. Brown TL, LeMay HE. *Chemistry: The Central Science.* Englewood Cliffs, NJ: Prentice-Hall; 1981.
8. Brynteson P, Sinning WE. The effects of training frequencies on the retention of cardiovascular fitness. *Med Sci Sports.* 1973;5:29–33.
9. Fardy PS, Yanowitz FG, Wilson PK. *Cardiac Rehabilitation, Adult Fitness and Exercise Testing.* 2nd ed. Philadelphia, Pa: Lea & Febiger; 1988.
10. Fox SM, Naughton JP, Gorman PA. Physical activity and cardiovascular health. The exercise prescription: Frequency and type of activity. *Mod Concepts Cardiovasc Dis.* 1972;41:25.
11. Gettman LR, Pollock ML, Durstine JL, et al. Physiological responses of men to 1, 3 and 5 day per week training programs. *Res Q.* 1976;47:638–646.
12. Hellerstein HK, Ader R. Relationship between percent maximal oxygen uptake (% max $\dot{V}O_2$) and percent maximal heart rate (% MHR) in normals and cardiacs. *Circulation.* 1971;43–44(Suppl II):76.
13. Heyward VH. *Advanced Fitness Assessment and Exercise Prescription.* 2nd ed. Champaign, Ill: Human Kinetics Publishers, Inc; 1991.
14. Hickson RC, Rosenkoetter MA. Reduced training frequencies and maintenance of increased aerobic power. *Med Sci Sports Exerc.* 1981;13:13–16.
15. Martin WH, Montgomery J, Snell PG, et al. Cardiovascular adaptations to intense swim training in sedentary middle-aged men and women. *Circulation.* 1987;75:323–330.
16. McArdle WD, Katch FI, Katch VL. *Exercise Physiology: Energy, Nutrition and Human Performance.* 3rd ed. Philadelphia, Pa: Lea & Febiger; 1991.
17. Metier CP, Pollock ML, Graves JE. Exercise prescription for the coronary artery bypass graft surgery patient. *J Cardiopul Rehabil.* 1986;6:236–242.
18. Moffatt RJ, Stamford BA, Neill RD. Placement of tri-weekly training sessions: Importance regarding enhancement of aerobic capacity. *Res Q.* 1977;48:583–591.
19. Pollock ML. The quantification of endurance training programs. In: Wilmore JH, ed. *Exercise and Sport Sciences Reviews.* New York, NY: Academic Press; 1973.

20. Pollock ML, Foster C, Rod JL, et al. Comparison of methods for determining exercise training intensity for cardiac patients and healthy adults. In: Kellerman JJ, ed. *Comprehensive Cardiac Rehabilitation*. Basel, Switzerland: Karger; 1982.
21. Pollock ML, Gettman LR, Milesis C, et al. Effects of frequency and duration of training on attrition and incidence of injury. *Med Sci Sports*. 1977;9:33–36.
22. Pollock ML, Pels AE, Foster C, et al. Exercise prescription for rehabilitation of the cardiac patient. In: Pollock ML, Schmidt DH, eds. *Heart Disease and Rehabilitation*. 2nd ed. New York, NY: John Wiley & Sons, Inc; 1979.
23. Pollock ML, Wilmore JH. *Exercise in Health and Disease: Evaluation and Prescription for Prevention and Rehabilitation*. 2nd ed. Philadelphia, Pa: WB Saunders Co; 1990.
24. Powers SK, Howley ET. *Exercise Physiology: Theory and Application to Fitness and Performance*. Dubuque, Iowa: Wm C Brown Publishers; 1990.
25. Sharkey BJ. *Physiology of Fitness*. 3rd ed. Champaign, Ill: Human Kinetics Publishers, Inc; 1990.
26. Shephard RJ. Intensity, duration and frequency of exercise as determinants of the response to a training regime. *Int Z Angew Physiol*. 1969;26:272–278.
27. Wenger HA, Bell GJ. The interactions of intensity, frequency and duration of exercise training in altering cardiorespiratory fitness. *Sports Med*. 1986;3:346–356.

Exercise Prescription for Sport Performance

PRINCIPLES AND SYSTEMS

The components of sport performance training may be outlined as follows:

1. General parameters
   a. Flexibility
   b. General muscular strength
   c. General muscular endurance
   d. General cardiovascular endurance
      (1) Continuous training
2. Sport-specific parameters
   a. Advanced muscular strength
      (1) Eccentric training
      (2) Plyometrics
   b. Advanced muscular endurance
      (1) Plyometrics
   c. Advanced cardiovascular endurance
      (1) Circuit training
      (2) Interval training
      (3) Fartlek training
   d. Speed
      (1) Resisted training
      (2) Assisted training
   e. Power
      (1) Plyometrics
      (2) Functional activities
   f. Balance
      (1) Static
      (2) Dynamic
   g. Agility

There are two systems of sport performance training, as follows:

1. Periodization
2. Cross training

The methods of sport performance preparation may be outlined as follows:

1. Physical preparation
   a. Muscular strength
   b. Muscular endurance
   c. Flexibility
   d. Cardiovascular endurance
   e. Speed
   f. Power
   g. Balance
   h. Agility
2. Psychologic preparation
   a. Visualization
   b. Hypnosis
   c. Stress management
   d. Meditation
3. Nutritional preparation
   a. Adjusting daily diet for specific nutritional requirements
   b. Adjusting diet for precompetition peaking
4. Technical preparation
   a. Skill-specific simulation activities (eg, a quarterback and wide receiver practicing pass patterns)
   b. Sport-specific simulation activities (eg, a quarterback and wide receiver practicing pass patterns in a full scrimmage)
5. Tactical preparation
   a. Pacing strategies (eg, practicing pace for a particular running event)
   b. Timing strategies (eg, practicing quarterback to wide receiver pass patterns)

GUIDELINES FOR EXERCISE PRESCRIPTION

CARDIOVASCULAR ENDURANCE

Circuit Training

Modes of Training

Circuit training programs may be designed to train for general fitness (eg, strength, flexibility, endurance), one or several components of sport-specific conditioning (eg, power, speed, coordination, balance, and agility), or one or several components of work-specific conditioning (eg, climbing, pushing, pulling, carrying, lifting).

Typically, interval training incorporates work intervals followed by relief intervals, whereas circuit training may or may not have specifically designated relief intervals. Thus, circuit-interval training is a combination of both circuit and interval training methods, incorporating specific relief intervals between the exercise modalities (ie, work intervals).[95]

The following are sample methods of circuit training:

1. Fitness Court Circuit: indoor/outdoor exercise stations arranged in a designated circuit pattern. The fitness court is ideal for sites with limited space and generally can fit into a 20 to 40-foot square with approximately 15 to 20 flexibility, endurance, and strength stations. Commercial versions (eg, Parcourse, Wells Fargo Gamefield) of these circuits may be found at parks;

however, they may also be designed according to individual specifications. Figure 12–1 illustrates a sample fitness court circuit pattern.

2. Fitness Trail Circuit: outdoor exercise stations arranged in a designated circuit pattern along a walking/running trail.[63] The fitness trail is ideal for the perimeter of a hospital, school, or park setting and is generally spread out over a ½- to 2-mile course with approximately 10 to 20 flexibility, endurance, and strength stations. Commercial versions (eg, Parcourse, Wells Fargo Gamefield, SouthWood Fit-Trail) of these circuits may be found at parks, schools, and hospitals; however, they may also be designed according to individual specifications. Figure 12–2 illustrates a sample fitness trail circuit pattern.

3. Aquatic Circuit: exercise stations arranged in a designated circuit pattern along the perimeter of an indoor or outdoor pool that incorporate stationary activities for training various muscle groups. The exercise stations may also be used in conjunction with swimming laps emphasizing various swimming techniques (eg, freestyle, backstroke, breaststroke, butterfly). Commercial versions (eg, Parcourse) of these circuits are available; however, they may also be designed according to individual specifications. Figure 12–3 illustrates a sample aquatic circuit pattern.

4. Free weight or Machine Circuit: exercise stations arranged in a designated circuit pattern utilizing any one of the numerous types of resistance machines or free weight systems that are available commercially. The circuit program may be designed by using 15 to 25 flexibility, endurance, and strength stations. Figure 12–4 illustrates a sample free weight or machine circuit pattern.

5. Sport-specific Circuit: a sample circuit for training sprinters arranged in a designated circuit pattern for emphasizing flexibility, speed skill, speed strength, and coordination. The circuit program may be performed on a track or field or in a large gymnasium by using 15 to 25 exercises. Figure 12–5 illustrates a sample sport-specific circuit pattern.

6. Work-specific Circuit: Although a work-specific circuit is not related to sports conditioning, some similarities exist when conditioning and rehabilitating a worker versus an athlete. Therefore, a sample circuit for training firefighters has been presented and may be arranged in a designated circuit pattern for emphasizing general fitness components (eg, flexibility, muscular strength, muscular endurance, cardiovascular endurance) and functional tasks (eg, carrying, pushing, pulling, jumping, lifting, crawling, climbing). The circuit program may be performed in a clinical setting or a firefighter's training center by utilizing 15 to 25 exercises. The circuit can be performed with or without the firefighter's full gear and equipment, which may vary from 50 to 120 lb.[42,97,133] Clinicians may refer to other sources for specific firefighting performance standards.[24,29,43,83,113] Figure 12–6 illustrates a sample work-specific circuit pattern for firefighters.[6]

Intensity, Frequency, and Duration of Training

For specific exercise prescription variables (ie, mode, intensity, frequency, duration) of circuit training, the clinician should refer to established guidelines and

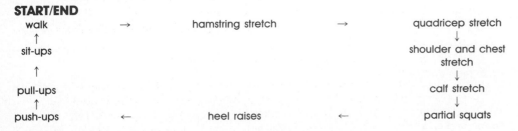

Figure 12–1. Sample fitness court circuit.

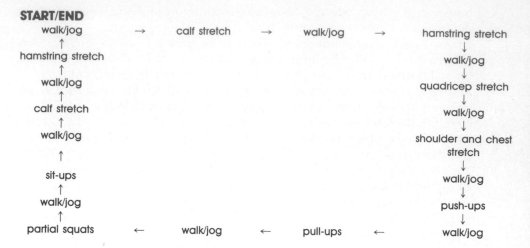

Figure 12–2. Sample fitness trail circuit.

sources.[3,61,96,108,109,115,145,157,168] In general, circuit training programs may be designed by adjusting the following variables:

1. Varying the intensity of the following:
   a. Total circuit (recommended at 40% to 60% of one-repetition maximum)[62]
   b. Individual exercises
   c. Relief interval—rest or work relief[91]
2. Varying the frequency of the following:
   a. Number of days per week the circuit is performed
   b. Number of sets of the circuit performed per exercise session (recommended at 2 to 3 circuits)[62]
   c. Number of sets of each exercise performed per station
   d. Number of repetitions of each exercise performed per station (recommended at 10 to 15 repetitions)[8]
3. Varying the duration of the following:
   a. Total circuit (recommended at 25 to 30 minutes)[62]
   b. Individual exercises (if exercise is being timed, instead of total repetitions being counted)
   c. Relief interval—rest or work relief (recommended at 15 to 30 seconds of rest relief)[8,91]
4. Varying the total number of exercises in the circuit (recommended at 8 to 12 exercises)[62,156]
5. Varying the activities between the upper and lower body

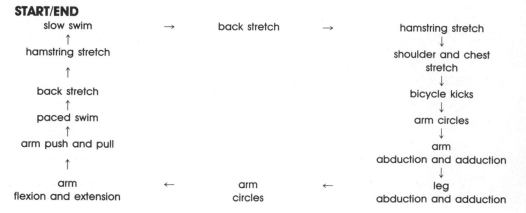

Figure 12–3. Sample aquatic court circuit.

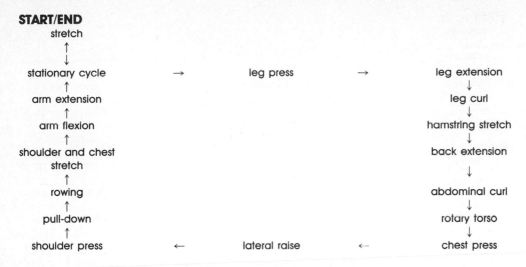

Figure 12–4. Sample free weight or machine circuit.

6. Varying the use of cardiovascular and resistance machines and calisthenic-type activities (eg, push-ups, abdominal curls)

Interval Training

Modes, Intensity, Frequency, and Duration of Training

For specific exercise prescription variables (ie, mode, intensity, frequency, duration) of interval training, the clinician should refer to established guidelines and sources.[11,22,57,73,95,118,147,157] Table 12–1 outlines guidelines for determining interval training work rates for running. In general, interval training programs may be designed by adjusting the following variables:

1. Varying the intensity of the following:
   a. Exercise or work interval (recommended at 70% to 85% of $\dot{V}O_2$ max)
   b. Relief interval—rest or work relief[91]

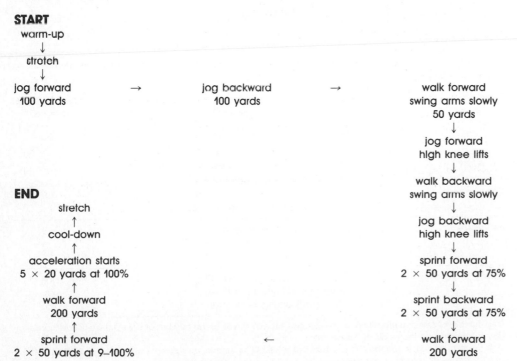

Figure 12–5. Sample sport-specific circuit.

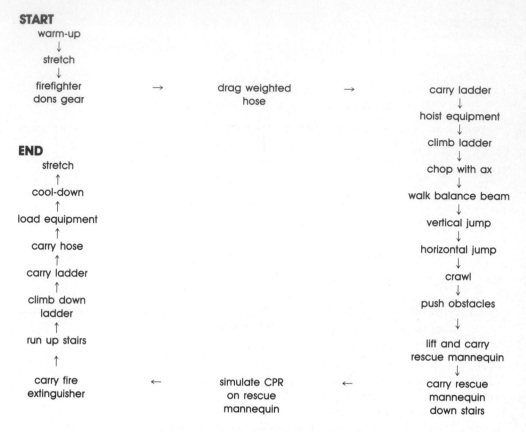

Figure 12–6. Sample work-specific circuit for firefighters.

2. Varying the frequency of the following:
   a. Number of days per week the interval training is performed
   b. Number of sets of each exercise or work interval performed per training session
3. Varying the duration of the following:
   a. Total interval training program

TABLE 12–1. GUIDELINES FOR DETERMINING INTERVAL TRAINING WORK RATES FOR RUNNING VARIOUS DISTANCES

Training Distances	Exercise Interval[a]	Work to Relief Interval[b]
55 yards	1.5 seconds slower than best time recorded from a running start	1:3
110 yards	3 seconds slower than best time recorded from a running start	1:3
220 yards	5 seconds slower than best time recorded from a running start	1:3
440 yards	1 to 4 seconds faster than the average 440-yard run times recorded during a mile run	1:2
660–1320 yards	3 to 4 seconds slower than the average 440-yard run times recorded during a mile run	1:1 or 1:1.5

[a]The number of sets and repetitions of the exercise interval as well as the number of days per week one trains may vary depending on the goals of the program.
[b]The duration of work to rest may be expressed as a ratio. For example, for a sprinter who runs a 10-second exercise interval, the relief interval would approximately be 30 seconds (thus, a 1:3 ratio).
Adapted from Fox EL, Mathews DK. Interval Training: Conditioning for Sports and General Fitness. Philadelphia, Pa: WB Saunders Co; 1974; and McArdle WD, Katch FI, Katch VL. Exercise Physiology: Energy, Nutrition and Human Performance. 3rd ed. Philadelphia, PA: Lea & Febiger; 1991.

b. Exercise or work interval
c. Relief interval—rest or work relief[91]

Fartlek Training

Mode of Training
Figure 12–7 illustrates a sample method of fartlek training.

Intensity, Frequency, and Duration of Training
Fartlek training provides an anaerobic component within the context of aerobic activity. For example, the runner starts off at a steady pace and, from time to time, incorporates intense bursts of speed over a varied terrain. This type of training may eliminate boredom and delay the onset of fatigue; however, it prevents the runner from acquiring pace judgment due to the use of alternate fast and slow pace variations.[11] The use of a heart rate monitor may provide for a more structured program.[22]

In general, fartlek training programs may be designed by adjusting the following variables:

1. Varying the intensity according to how the runner feels during the training. The runner alternates slow and fast running but does not consider a specific pace during the training
2. Varying the frequency of the following:
   a. Number of days per week the fartlek training is performed
   b. Number of slow versus fast intervals
3. Varying the duration of the following:
   a. Total training program
   b. Slow versus fast intervals
4. Varying the terrain (eg, flat versus hilly, grassy versus rocky, snow, sand)

STRENGTH

Modes of Training
The following are sample methods of sport-specific strength training:

1. Single set system[54]
2. Multiple set system[54]
3. Triangle programs[54]
4. Super set system[54]
5. Tri-set system[54]
6. Multipoundage system[54]
7. Cheat system[54]
8. Split routine system[54]

START
warm-up
↓
stretch
↓

slow run   →   fast run
no specific intensity   no specific intensity
flat and grassy terrain   flat and grassy terrain
                                                 ↓
fast run   ←   slow run
no specific intensity   no specific intensity
hilly and rocky terrain   hilly and rocky terrain
↓
cool-down
↓
stretch

END

Figure 12–7. Sample fartlek training program.

9. Isolated exercise system[54]
10. Forced repetition system[54]
11. Super pump system[54]
12. Circuit weight training[96]
13. Interval weight training[115]
14. Functional isometrics[68,116,117]
15. Eccentric training[44,70,151]

Intensity, Frequency, and Duration of Training

For specific exercise prescription variables (ie, mode, intensity, frequency, duration) of sport-specific strength training, the clinician should refer to established guidelines and sources.[1,12,25,41,50,60,68,82,106,107,116,117,122,125,129,130,137,149,150,152,164,169] Tables 12–2 to 12–4 outline guidelines for determining weight percentages and standards for developing sport-specific strength conditioning programs.

SPEED

Modes of Training

The following are sample methods of speed training:

GENERAL TRAINING

1. Acceleration sprints
2. Interval sprints
3. Overdistance sprints

SPRINT-RESISTED TRAINING

1. Running uphill (eg, natural terrain, treadmill)
2. Running in sand[36,119]
3. Running in snow[36]
4. Running in water[36]
5. Running against the wind[36]
6. Running with a weighted vest
7. Running with ankle or wrist weights or both
8. Running while pulling a weighted sled[146]
9. Running against the restraint of a harness or belt (ie, pulling resistance is applied by a training partner)[10,146]
10. Running with a miniature parachute of varying sizes of small, medium, and large, providing approximate resistances of 9, 13, and 22 pounds, respectively[5,25,121]
11. Plyometric exercises (eg, hopping, horizontal jumping, vertical jumping, depth jumping)

SPRINT-ASSISTED TRAINING

1. Running downhill: natural terrain with the distance ranging from 30 to 75 yards and where the slope is approximately a 5% downhill grade, which means that for every 100 feet traveled forward the vertical drop is 5 feet.[76] Others have suggested a slope of 2.6 degrees or less[47]

TABLE 12–2. GUIDELINES FOR SPORT-SPECIFIC WEIGHT TRAINING

Training Variables	Percent of 1-RM	Repetition Range	Set Range
Power	> 90	1–3	1–2
Strength	70–90	5–10	2–3
Muscular endurance	60–70	8–12	3

Adapted with permission from Albert M, Lathrop J. Free weight training. In: Albert M. Eccentric Muscle Training in Sports and Orthopaedics. New York, NY: Churchill Livingstone; 1991:142.

TABLE 12–3. WEIGHT STANDARDS (BODY WEIGHT + LB)[a]

Level	Clean	Bench Press	Dead Lift	Front Squat	Back Squat
Very poor	−25	−50	BWT + 100	BWT + 100	BWT + 250
Poor	BWT	BWT	BWT + 125	BWT + 125	BWT + 275
Average	+25	+75	BWT + 150	BWT + 150	BWT + 300
Good	+50	+100	BWT + 200	BWT + 175	BWT + 325
Excellent	+75	+150	BWT + 275	BWT + 200	BWT + 350

[a]Totals expressed in body weight (BWT) ± additional weight.
Reprinted with permission from Albert M, Lathrop J. Free weight training. In: Albert M. Eccentric Muscle Training In Sports and Orthopaedics. New York, NY: Churchill Livingstone; 1991:149.

2. Overspeed running on a treadmill
3. Overspeed pedaling on a stationary bicycle
4. Running with the wind
5. Running into a motorized or elastic towline apparatus[36,47,146]
6. Performing a bicycling-type motion with the legs, either while lying supine

TABLE 12–4. WEIGHT PERCENTAGES

MAX	60%	70%	75%	80%	85%	90%	95%	100%	105%
500	300	350	375	400	425	450	475	500	525
490	295	345	370	390	415	440	465	490	515
480	290	335	360	385	410	430	455	480	505
470	280	330	350	375	400	425	445	470	495
460	275	320	345	365	390	415	435	460	485
450	270	315	335	360	380	405	425	450	475
440	265	310	330	350	375	395	420	440	460
430	260	300	320	345	365	385	410	430	450
420	250	295	315	335	355	380	400	420	440
410	245	285	305	330	350	370	390	410	430
400	240	280	300	320	340	360	380	400	420
390	235	275	290	310	330	350	370	390	410
380	230	265	285	305	325	340	360	380	400
370	220	260	275	295	315	330	350	370	390
360	215	250	270	290	305	325	340	360	380
350	210	245	260	280	295	315	330	350	370
340	205	240	255	270	290	305	325	340	355
330	200	230	245	265	280	295	315	330	345
320	190	225	240	255	270	290	305	320	335
310	185	215	230	250	265	280	295	310	325
300	180	210	225	240	255	270	285	300	315
290	175	205	215	230	245	260	275	290	305
280	170	195	210	225	240	250	265	280	295
270	160	190	200	215	230	245	255	270	285
260	155	180	195	210	220	235	245	260	275
250	150	175	185	200	210	225	235	250	265
240	145	170	180	190	205	215	230	240	250
230	140	160	170	185	195	205	220	230	240
220	130	155	165	175	185	200	210	220	230
210	125	145	155	170	180	190	200	210	220
200	120	140	150	160	170	180	190	200	210
190	115	135	140	150	160	170	180	190	200
180	110	125	135	145	155	160	170	180	190
170	100	120	130	135	145	155	160	170	180
160	95	110	120	130	135	145	150	160	170
150	90	105	110	120	130	135	145	150	160
140	85	100	105	110	120	125	135	140	145
130	80	90	100	105	110	115	125	130	135
120	70	85	90	95	100	110	115	120	125
110	65	75	80	90	95	100	105	110	115
100	60	70	75	80	85	90	95	100	105

Adapted with permission from Albert M, Lathrop J. Free weight training. In: Albert M. Eccentric Muscle Training in Sports and Orthopaedics. New York, NY: Churchill Livingstone; 1991:149–150. Data from Pasanella and Lathrop.[120]

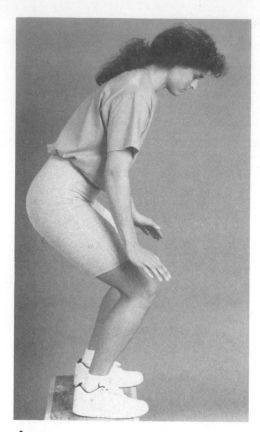

A

Figure 12–8. Depth jump exercise. (A) (Left) The client stands on an elevated surface (the height is chosen according to the client's strength level and sport-specific goal). **(B)** (Below) The client drops off (no jumping off the platform) from the elevated surface to the floor and lands with both feet together and knees bent to absorb the shock. **(C)** (Below) Upon landing, the client swings his or her arms upward and jumps as high vertically and as far horizontally as possible. The client then lands on both feet with the knees bent to absorb the shock, thus completing the exercise sequence.

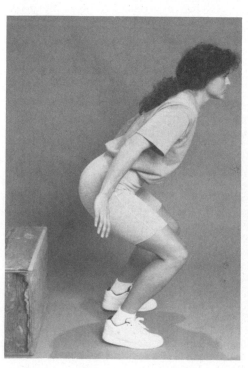

B

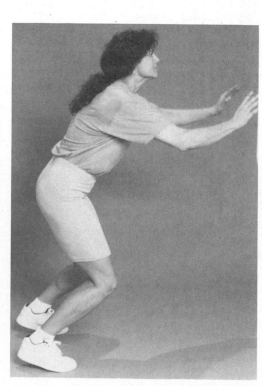

C

with the legs elevated, while holding onto a pull-up bar, or while suspended with a harness from a pull-up bar

7. Running behind a vehicle with either a shield for reducing wind resistance or with a towline for pulling the athlete (*Note:* these methods may be potentially dangerous)[47]

8. Plyometric exercises (eg, hopping, horizontal jumping, vertical jumping, depth jumping)

Intensity, Frequency, and Duration of Training

For specific exercise prescription variables (ie, mode, intensity, frequency, duration) of speed training, the clinician should refer to established guidelines and sources.[22,30,32,33,40,47,48,59,79,80,82,92,99,165]

POWER

Modes of Training

1. Plyometrics
   a. Upper body training
   b. Lower body training (see Figure 12–8)
2. Strength training
   a. Power cleans
   b. Olympic lifting—snatch lift
   c. Olympic lifting—clean and jerk lift
3. Functional activities
   a. Vertical jump
   b. Horizontal jump

Intensity, Frequency, and Duration of Training

For specific exercise prescription variables (ie, mode, intensity, frequency, duration) of power training, the clinician should refer to established guidelines and sources.[32,47-49,69,101,102,127,135,142-144,162]

BALANCE AND AGILITY

Modes, Intensity, Frequency, and Duration of Training

For specific exercise prescription variables (ie, mode, intensity, frequency, duration) of balance and agility training, the clinician should refer to the various references cited in Chapter seven for balance and agility testing.

SYSTEMS OF SPORT PERFORMANCE TRAINING

Periodization

Periodization is a concept that essentially divides the training process into yearly, monthly, and weekly cycles for the purpose of achieving a physical "peak" for either the competitive season (eg, football) or for the most important competition or meet (eg, Olympics). Table 12–5 outlines a hypothetical model of strength training using the concepts of periodization. Generally, periodization may be divided into the following three cycles:

1. Macrocycle: may range from 1 year (eg, football conditioning) to 4 years (eg, Olympic training)
2. Mesocycle: may range up to several months
3. Microcycle: may range up to several weeks

For specific exercise prescription variables (ie, mode, intensity, frequency, duration) of periodization training, the clinician should refer to established guidelines and sources.[18-20,22,46,58,66,103-105,153,154]

TABLE 12–5. HYPOTHETICAL MODEL OF STRENGTH TRAINING UTILIZING THE PRINCIPLES OF PERIODIZATION[a]

Variables	Preparation Period — Hypertrophy Phase	→	Transition 1 Period — Basic Strength Phase	→	Competition Period — Strength and Power Phase	→	Transition 2 Period — Peaking or Maintenance Phase[c]	→	Active Rest[b]
Sets	3–10		3–5		3–5		1–3		
Reps	8–12		4–6		2–3		1–3		
Days/week	3–4		3–5		3–5		1–5		
Times/day	1–3		1–3		1–2		1		
Intensity cycle (weeks)[d]	2–3/1		2–4/1		2–3/1		—		
Intensity	Low		High		High		Very high to low		
Volume	High		Moderate to high		Low		Very low		

[a]Associated with Matveyev's Periodization Model.[89,90]

[b]The athlete participates in his or her own sport or other sports at very low volumes and intensities as a transition between the Peaking and Hypertrophy Phases.[155]

[c]Peaking for sports with a definite climax or maintenance for sports with long seasons (eg, football).

[d]The ratio of the number of heavy training weeks to light training weeks.

Adapted with permission from the National Strength and Conditioning Association. Roundtable—Periodization (Part 1). Nat Strength Condit Assoc J. 1986;8(5):12–22. Lincoln, Neb: National Strength and Conditioning Association.

Cross Training

Cross training is a concept that combines two or more sports or activities into a single training session or cyclical program in order to provide variety to the various systems of the body (eg, cardiovascular, muscular, skeletal). An advantage of cross training is that the volume of training can be high without overtraining because the stresses imposed by training are spread throughout the various muscle groups.[148] Table 12–6 outlines a model of cross training for competitive runners (5000 to 10,000 meters), which may also serve as a model for designing other cross-training programs.

For specific exercise prescription variables (ie, mode, intensity, frequency, duration) of cross training, the clinician should refer to established guidelines and sources.[67,157,158]

DESIGNING TRAINING AND REHABILITATION PROGRAMS

When preparing exercise prescriptions for sports conditioning, the clinician may need to be familiar with the client's sport (ie, rules, regulations, equipment specifications, physical demands, etc). Therefore, the following list of sport-specific references will assist the clinician in understanding the physical, mental, and tactical dynamics of the sport:

1. Archery[93]
2. Badminton[16]
3. Baseball[123]
4. Basketball[138,166,167]
5. Bowling[88]
6. Cross-country skiing[15,136]
7. Cycling[27,28,94,139]
8. Dance[35,124]
9. Fencing[21]
10. Football[17,34,02]
11. Golf[9,98]
12. Gymnastics[131,159,163]
13. Hockey[86]
14. Jogging[53]
15. Marathon running[38]
16. Martial arts[75,110]
17. Olympic lifting[26,45,54,100]
18. Powerlifting[2,13,14,54,64,114]
19. Racquetball[4]
20. Running[84,85,112]
21. Scuba diving[141]
22. Soccer[126]
23. Softball[72,78]
24. Swimming/aquatics[81,140,160,161]
25. Tennis[65,71,111]
26. Track and field[22,23,30,31,37,39,55,56,59,87,128]
27. Triathlons[158]
28. Volleyball[51,52,77,132]
29. Walking[134]
30. Wrestling[7,74]

Figure 12–9 may be used for designing a 3- or 4-day (ie, weekly) advanced strength conditioning program for athletic conditioning.

TABLE 12–6. SAMPLE CROSS-TRAINING PROGRAM FOR COMPETITIVE RUNNERS (5000 TO 10,000 METERS)

	a.m.	p.m.
MONDAY	1. WT[a]—heavy intensity (45 minutes) 2. IT[c]—run (30 minutes)	1. LSDT[b]—cycle (60 minutes)
TUESDAY	1. LSDT—run (75 minutes) 2. Recovery—swim (15 minutes)	
WEDNESDAY	1. WT—light intensity (30 minutes)	1. IT—cycle (30 minutes)
THURSDAY	1. FT[d]—run on hills (60 minutes)	1. IT—swim (20 minutes)
FRIDAY	1. WT—medium intensity (45 minutes) 2. IT—run (30 minutes)	1. LSDT—bike (60 minutes)
SATURDAY	1. IT—run (40 minutes)	1. LSDT—bike (60 minutes)
SUNDAY	1. Recovery—swim (20 minutes)	

[a]WT = weight training
[b]LSDT = long, slow, distance training
[c]IT = interval training
[d]FT = fartlek training

Adapted with permission from O'Shea P. The science of cross-training: Theory and application for peak performance. Nat Strength Condit Assoc J. 1991;12(6):40–44. Lincoln, Neb: National Strength and Conditioning Association.

NAME: _____ AGE: _____ SEX: M F DATE: _____

WEIGHT: _____ lb _____ kg HEIGHT: _____ in _____ cm RESTING HR: _____ RESTING BP: _____ / _____

EXERCISES	SET 1 Reps / Intensity (#) (%) Weight / Rest (lb) (min)	SET 2 Reps / Intensity (#) (%) Weight / Rest (lb) (min)	SET 3 Reps / Intensity (#) (%) Weight / Rest (lb) (min)	SET 4 Reps / Intensity (#) (%) Weight / Rest (lb) (min)	SET 5 Reps / Intensity (#) (%) Weight / Rest (lb) (min)
DAY: _____					
1.	/ _____ /	/ _____ /	/ _____ /	/ _____ /	/ _____ /
2.	/ _____ /	/ _____ /	/ _____ /	/ _____ /	/ _____ /
3.	/ _____ /	/ _____ /	/ _____ /	/ _____ /	/ _____ /
4.	/ _____ /	/ _____ /	/ _____ /	/ _____ /	/ _____ /
5.	/ _____ /	/ _____ /	/ _____ /	/ _____ /	/ _____ /
6.	/ _____ /	/ _____ /	/ _____ /	/ _____ /	/ _____ /

Figure 12–9. Sample form for designing advanced resistance training programs.

REFERENCES

1. Albert M. *Eccentric Muscle Training in Sports and Orthopaedics*. New York, NY: Churchill Livingstone; 1991.
2. Algra B. An in-depth analysis of the bench press. *Nat Strength Condit Assoc J.* 1982;4(5):6.
3. Allen TE, Byrd RJ, Smith DP. Hemodynamic consequences of circuit weight training. *Res Q.* 1976;47:299–306.
4. Allsen PE, Witbeck P. *Racquetball*. 4th ed. Dubuque, Iowa: Wm C Brown Publishers; 1988.
5. All-Star Athletic Systems, Inc. *Speed Chute Training Device*. Memphis, Tenn: All-Star Athletic Systems, Inc; 1991.
6. Altuğ Z, Hoffman JL, Slane SM, et al. Work-circuit training. *Clin Management.* 1990;10(5):41–48.
7. American College of Sports Medicine. Position stand: Weight loss in wrestlers. *Med Sci Sports Exerc.* 1976;8(2):xi–xiii.
8. American College of Sports Medicine. Position stand: The recommended quantity and quality of exercise for developing and maintaining cardiorespiratory and muscular fitness in healthy adults. *Med Sci Sports Exerc.* 1990;22(2):265–274.
9. Amundson M. Golf. In: Mellion MB, Walsh WM, Shelton GL, eds. *The Team Physician's Handbook*. Philadelphia, Pa: Hanley & Belfus, Inc; 1990.
10. Armitage-Johnson S. Harness pull. *Nat Strength Condit Assoc J.* 1990;12(2):50–51.
11. Arnheim DD. *Modern Principles of Athletic Training*. 6th ed. St. Louis, Mo: Times Mirror/Mosby College Publishing; 1985.
12. Asmussen E. Positive and negative work. *Acta Physiol Scand.* 1953;28:364.
13. Baechle T, Kelso T, Barnes K. The bench press. *Nat Strength Condit Assoc J.* 1989;11(3):44–48.
14. Barnes K, Kelso T, Hill B, et al. The back squat. *Nat Strength Condit Assoc J.* 1989;11(2):18–24.
15. Bergh U. *Physiology of Cross-Country Skiing*. Champaign, Ill: Human Kinetics Publishers, Inc; 1982.
16. Bloss MV, Hales RS. *Badminton*. 6th ed. Dubuque, Iowa: Wm C Brown Publishers; 1990.
17. Bobo M. *Principles of Coaching Football*. Dubuque, Iowa: Wm C Brown Publishers; 1987.
18. Bompa TO. *Theory and Methodology of Training: The Key to Athletic Performance*. Dubuque, Iowa: Kendall Hunt; 1985.
19. Bompa TO. Physiological intensity values employed to plan endurance training. *Athl Train.* 1988;3(4):37–52.
20. Bompa TO. Periodization of strength: The most effective methodology of strength training. *Nat Strength Condit Assoc J.* 1990;12(5):49–52.
21. Bower M. *Foil Fencing*. 6th ed. Dubuque, Iowa: Wm C Brown Publishers; 1990.
22. Bowerman WJ, Freeman WH. *High-Performance Training for Track and Field*. 2nd ed. Champaign, Ill: Human Kinetics Publishers, Inc; 1991.
23. Brooks C. *Women's Hurdling*. Champaign, Ill: Human Kinetics Publishers, Inc; 1981.
24. Brownlie L, Brown S, Diewert G, et al. Cost-effective selection of fire fighter recruits. *Med Sci Sports Exerc.* 1985;17(6):661–666.
25. Brunner R, Tabachnik B. *Soviet Training and Recovery Methods*. Pleasant Hill, Calif: Sport Focus Publishing; 1990.
26. Burgener M, Bielick E, Huegli R. The power clean. *Nat Strength Condit Assoc J.* 1988;10(6):50–55.
27. Burke ER, ed. *Science of Cycling*. Champaign, Ill: Human Kinetics Publishers, Inc; 1986.
28. Burke ER, Newsom MM, eds. *Medical and Scientific Aspects of Cycling*. Champaign, Ill: Human Kinetics Publishers, Inc; 1988.
29. Cady LD, Bischoff DP, O'Connell ER, et al. Strength and fitness and subsequent back injuries in firefighters. *J Occup Med.* 1979;21(4):269–272.
30. Carr GA. *Fundamentals of Track and Field*. Champaign, Ill: Human Kinetics Publishers, Inc; 1991.
31. Cavanagh PR, ed. *Biomechanics of Distance Running*. Champaign, Ill: Human Kinetics Publishers, Inc; 1990.
32. Chu DA. *Jumping into Plyometrics*. Champaign, Ill: Leisure Press; 1992.

33. Chu D, Korchemny R. Sprinting stride actions: Analysis and evaluation. *Nat Strength Condit Assoc J.* 1989;11(6):6.

34. Clare PE. Football. In: Mellion MB, Walsh WM, Shelton GL, eds. *The Team Physician's Handbook.* Philadelphia, Pa: Hanley & Belfus, Inc; 1990.

35. Clarkson PM, Skrinar M, eds. *Science of Dance Training.* Champaign, Ill: Human Kinetics Publishers, Inc; 1988.

36. Costello F. Training for speed using resisted and assisted methods. *Nat Strength Condit Assoc J.* 1985;7(1):74–75.

37. Costill DL. *Inside Running: Basics of Sports Physiology.* Dubuque, Iowa: Brown & Benchmark; 1986.

38. Costill DL, Fox EL. Energetics of marathon running. *Med Sci Sports Exerc.* 1969;1:81–86.

39. Crawford T, Bertucci B, eds. *Winning Track and Field Drills for Women.* Champaign, Ill: Human Kinetics Publishers, Inc; 1985.

40. Cross T. Technique drills for speed development. *Nat Strength Condit Assoc J.* 1991;13(2):35–39.

41. Davies CTM, Barnes C. Negative (eccentric) work. Physiological responses to walking uphill and downhill on a motordriven treadmill. *Ergonomics.* 1972;15:121.

42. Davis PO, Biersner RJ, Barnard RJ, et al. Medical evaluation of fire fighters: How fit are they for duty? *Postgrad Med.* 1982;72(2):241–248.

43. Davis PO, Dotson CO, Maria DLS. Relationship between simulated fire fighting tasks and physical performance measures. *Med Sci Sports Exerc.* 1982;14(1):65–71.

44. Dean E. Physiology and therapeutic implications of negative work: A review. *Phys Ther.* 1988;68:233.

45. Derwin BP. The snatch: Technical description and periodization program. *Nat Strength Condit Assoc J.* 1990;12(2):6–15.

46. Dick F. *Training Theory.* 2nd ed. London, England: British Amateur Athletic Board; 1984.

47. Dintiman GB. *How to Run Faster.* West Point, NY: Leisure Press; 1984.

48. Dintiman GB, Ward RD. *Sport Speed.* Champaign, Ill: Human Kinetics Publishers, Inc; 1988.

49. Duda M. Plyometrics: A legitimate form of power training? *Physician Sportsmed.* 1988;16:213.

50. Duncan PW, Chandler JM, Cavanaugh DK, et al. Mode and speed specificity of eccentric and concentric exercise training. *J Orthop Sports Phys Ther.* 1989;11:70.

51. Egstrom GH, Schaafsma F. *Volleyball.* 3rd ed. Dubuque, Iowa: Wm C Brown Publishers; 1980.

52. Handel D, Mellion MB. Volleyball. In: Mellion MB, Walsh WM, Shelton GL, eds. *The Team Physician's Handbook.* Philadelphia, Pa: Hanley & Belfus, Inc; 1990.

53. Fisher AG, Allsen PE. *Jogging.* 2nd ed. Dubuque, Iowa: Wm C Brown Publishers; 1987.

54. Fleck SJ, Kraemer WJ. *Designing Resistance Training Programs.* Champaign, Ill: Human Kinetics Publishers, Inc; 1987.

55. Foreman K. *Coaching Track and Field Techniques.* 4th ed. Dubuque, Iowa: Wm C Brown Publishers; 1982.

56. Foreman K. *Track and Field.* 2nd ed. Dubuque, Iowa: Wm C Brown Publishers; 1983.

57. Fox EL, Mathews DK. *Interval Training: Conditioning for Sports and General Fitness.* Philadelphia, Pa: WB Saunders Co; 1974.

58. Freeman WH. *Peak When It Counts: Periodization for the American Coach.* Los Altos, Calif: Tafnews; 1988.

59. Gambetta V, ed. *The Athletics Congress's Track and Field Coaching Manual.* 2nd ed. Champaign, Ill: Human Kinetics Publishers, Inc; 1989.

60. Gamble JN. Strength and conditioning for the competitive athlete. In: Kulund DN, ed. *The Injured Athlete.* Philadelphia, Pa: JB Lippincott Co; 1988.

61. Gettman LR, Ayres JJ, Pollock ML, et al. The effect of circuit weight training on strength, cardiorespiratory function and body composition of adult men. *Med Sci Sports.* 1978;10:171–176.

62. Gettman LR, Pollock ML. Circuit weight training: A critical review of its physiological benefits. *Physician Sportsmed.* 1981;9(1):44–60.

63. Gill J. *A Guide to Building Fitness Trails.* Worthington, Ohio: Publishing Horizons, Inc; 1986.

64. Gotshalk L. Analysis of the deadlift. *Nat Strength Condit Assoc J.* 1985;6(6):4.

65. Groppel JL, Loehr JE, Melville DS, et al. *Science of Coaching Tennis*. Champaign, Ill: Human Kinetics Publishers, Inc; 1989.
66. Harre D. *Principles of Sport Training*. Berlin, Germany: Sportverlag; 1981.
67. Hickson RC. Interference of strength development by simultaneously training for strength and endurance. *Eur J Appl Physiol*. 1980;45(2–3):255–263.
68. Jackson A, Jackson T, Hnatek J, et al. Strength development: Using functional isometrics in an isotonic strength training program. *Res Q Exerc Sport*. 1985;56:234.
69. Javorek I. Plyometrics. *Nat Strength Condit Assoc J*. 1989;11(2):52–57.
70. Johnson BL. Eccentric versus concentric muscle training for strength development. *Med Sci Sports*. 1972;4:111.
71. Johnson JD, Xanthos PJ. *Tennis*. 5th ed. Dubuque, Iowa: Wm C Brown Publishers; 1988.
72. Jones BJ, Murray MJ. *Softball Concepts for Coaches and Teachers*. Dubuque, Iowa: Wm C Brown Publishers; 1978.
73. Kavanaugh T, Shephard RJ. Interval versus continuous training of post-coronary patients. *Med Sci Sports*. 1973;5:67.
74. Kelly TF. Wrestling. In: Mellion MB, Walsh WM, Shelton GL, eds. *The Team Physician's Handbook*. Philadelphia, Pa: Hanley & Belfus, Inc; 1990.
75. Kim D, Leland TW. *Karate*. 2nd ed. Dubuque, Iowa: Wm C Brown Publishers; 1978.
76. Klinzing J. Improving sprint speed for all athletes. *Nat Strength Condit Assoc J*. 1984;6(4):32–33.
77. Kluka DA, Dunn PJ. *Volleyball*. Dubuque, Iowa: Wm C Brown Publishers; 1988.
78. Kneer ME, McCord CL. *Softball: Slow and Fast Pitch*. 4th ed. Dubuque, Iowa: Wm C Brown Publishers; 1987.
79. Korchemny R. Training with the objective to improve stride length (Part 1). *Nat Strength Condit Assoc J*. 1988;10(2):21–25.
80. Korchemny R. Training with the objective to improve stride length (Part 2). *Nat Strength Condit Assoc J*. 1988;10(3):61–64.
81. Krasevec JA. *Y's Way to Water Exercise: Instructor's Guide*. Champaign, Ill: Human Kinetics Publishers, Inc; 1989.
82. Kroll WA. *Physical Conditioning for Winning Football*. 2nd ed. Dubuque, Iowa: Wm C Brown Publishers; 1991.
83. Lemon PWR, Hermiston RT. The human energy cost of fire fighting. *J Occup Med*. 1977;19(8):558–562.
84. Lüchtenberg D. Specific strength training for running (Part 1). *Nat Strength Condit Assoc J*. 1989;11(4):62–65.
85. Lüchtenberg D. Specific strength training for running (Part 2). *Nat Strength Condit Assoc J*. 1989;11(5):43–51.
86. MacAdam D, Reynolds G. *Hockey Fitness: Year-Round Conditioning, On and Off the Ice*. Champaign, Ill: Human Kinetics Publishers, Inc; 1988.
87. Martin D, Coe P. *Training Distance Runners*. Champaign, Ill: Human Kinetics Publishers, Inc; 1991.
88. Martin JL, Tandy RE, Agne-Traub C. *Bowling*. 6th ed. Dubuque, Iowa: Wm C Brown Publishers; 1990.
89. Matveyev L. *Periodisierang des sportlichen training*. Berlin, Germany: Berles and Wernitz; 1972.
90. Matveyev L. *Fundamentals of Sports Training*. Moscow, USSR: Progress; 1981.
91. McArdle WD, Katch FI, Katch VL. *Exercise Physiology: Energy, Nutrition and Human Performance*. 3rd ed. Philadelphia, Pa: Lea & Febiger; 1991.
92. McFarlane B. A look inside the biomechanics and dynamics of speed. *Nat Strength Condit Assoc J*. 1987;9(5):35–41.
93. McKinney WC, McKinney MW. *Archery*. 6th ed. Dubuque, Iowa: Wm C Brown Publishers; 1990.
94. Mellion MB, Hill JW. Bicycling. In: Mellion MB, Walsh WM, Shelton GL, eds. *The Team Physician's Handbook*. Philadelphia, Pa: Hanley & Belfus, Inc; 1990.
95. Meyer GC. The role of circuit interval and continuous conditioning in cardiac rehabilitation. In: Hall LK, Meyer GC, Hellerstein HK. *Cardiac Rehabilitation: Exercise Testing and Prescription*. Champaign, Ill: Human Kinetics Publishers, Inc; 1984.
96. Morgan RE, Adamson GT. *Circuit Weight Training*. London, England: G. Bell and Sons; 1961.
97. Mostardi RA, Urycki S. Entry level firefighter standards: Ergonomic assessment and

implementation. In: Mital A, ed. *Advances in Industrial Ergonomics and Safety I*. New York, NY: Taylor & Francis; 1989.

98. Nance VL, Davis EC. *Golf*. 6th ed. Dubuque, Iowa: Wm C Brown Publishers; 1990.

99. National Strength and Conditioning Association. Roundtable—Speed development. *Nat Strength Condit Assoc J*. 1984;5(6):12.

100. National Strength and Conditioning Association. Roundtable—Power clean. *Nat Strength Condit Assoc J*. 1985;6(6):10.

101. National Strength and Conditioning Association. Roundtable—Practical considerations for utilizing plyometrics (Part 1). *Nat Strength Condit Assoc J*. 1986;8(3):14–22.

102. National Strength and Conditioning Association. Roundtable—Practical considerations for utilizing plyometrics (Part 2). *Nat Strength Condit Assoc J*. 1986;8(4):14–24.

103. National Strength and Conditioning Association. Roundtable—Periodization (Part 1). *Nat Strength Condit Assoc J*. 1986;8(5):12–22.

104. National Strength and Conditioning Association. Roundtable—Periodization (Part 2). *Nat Strength Condit Assoc J*. 1987;8(6):17–24.

105. National Strength and Conditioning Association. Roundtable—Periodization (Part 3). *Nat Strength Condit Assoc J*. 1987;9(1):16–26.

106. National Strength and Conditioning Association. Roundtable—Sport-specific strength requirements (Part 1). *Nat Strength Condit Assoc J*. 1987;9(6):14–27.

107. National Strength and Conditioning Association. Roundtable—Sport-specific strength requirements (Part 2). *Nat Strength Condit Assoc J*. 1988;10(1):16–25.

108. National Strength and Conditioning Association. Roundtable—Circuit training (Part 1). *Nat Strength Condit Assoc J*. 1990;12(2):16–27.

109. National Strength and Conditioning Association. Roundtable—Circuit training (Part 2). *Nat Strength Condit Assoc J*. 1990;12(3):10–21.

110. Nelson JM. *Self-defense: Steps to Success*. Champaign, Ill: Human Kinetics Publishers, Inc; 1991.

111. Nichola TL. Tennis. In: Mellion MB, Walsh WM, Shelton GL, eds. *The Team Physician's Handbook*. Philadelphia, Pa: Hanley & Belfus, Inc; 1990.

112. Noakes T. *Lore of Running: Discover the Science and Spirit of Running*. 3rd ed. Champaign, Ill: Human Kinetics Publishers, Inc; 1991.

113. O'Connell ER, Thomas PC, Cady LD, et al. Energy costs of simulated stair climbing as a job-related task in fire fighting. *J Occup Med*. 1986;28(4):282–284.

114. O'Shea P. The parallel squat. *Nat Strength Condit Assoc J*. 1985;7(1):4.

115. O'Shea P. Interval weight training: A scientific approach to cross-training for athletic strength fitness. *Nat Strength Condit Assoc J*. 1987;9(2):53–57.

116. O'Shea P. Functional isometric lifting: Theory (Part 1). *Nat Strength Condit Assoc J*. 1987;9(6):44–46.

117. O'Shea P. Functional isometric lifting: Application (Part 2). *Nat Strength Condit Assoc J*. 1988;10(1):60–62.

118. O'Shea P, Nomak C, Garland F. Bicycle interval training for cardiovascular fitness. *Physician Sportsmed*. 1982;10(10):156–162.

119. Oviatt R, Hemba G. Oregon State: Sandblasting through the PAC. *Nat Strength Condit Assoc J*. 1991;13(4):40–46.

120. Pasanella D, Lathrop J. *Freshman Football Manual on Strength and Conditioning*. Atlanta, Ga: Georgia Tech Athletic Association; 1988.

121. Pauletto B. The speed chute. *Nat Strength Condit Assoc J*. 1991;13(4):47–48.

122. Pauletto B. *Strength Training for Coaches*. Champaign, Ill: Human Kinetics Publishers, Inc; 1991.

123. Pecci S. *Building a Better Hitter*. Dubuque, Iowa: Wm C Brown Publishers; 1990.

124. Peterson DR, Taylor AW, Lapenskie GP. *Medical Aspects of Dance*. Longmeadow, Mass: Mouvement Publications, Inc; 1986.

125. Poliquin C. Five steps to increasing the effectiveness of your strength training program. *Nat Strength Condit Assoc J*. 1988;10(3):34–39.

126. Puddu G, Caruso I, Cerullo G, et al. Soccer. In: Mellion MB, Walsh WM, Shelton GL, eds. *The Team Physician's Handbook*. Philadelphia, Pa: Hanley & Belfus, Inc; 1990.

127. Radcliffe JC, Farentinos RC. *Plyometrics: Explosive Power Training*. 2nd ed. Champaign, Ill: Human Kinetics Publishers, Inc; 1985.

128. Randolph J, ed. *Championship Track and Field* (Volume 2: *Field Events*). Champaign, Ill: Human Kinetics Publishers, Inc; 1982.

129. Rasch PJ. *Weight Training*. 5th ed. Dubuque, Iowa: Wm C Brown Publishers; 1990.

130. Robarge MB, Runzheimer K. *S.E.T.S.—The Strength and Endurance Training System.* Dubuque, Iowa: Brown & Benchmark; 1985.

131. Ryser O, Brown J. *A Manual for Tumbling and Apparatus Stunts.* 8th ed. Dubuque, Iowa: Wm C Brown Publishers; 1990.

132. Schaafsma F, Heck A, Sarver CT. *Volleyball for Coaches and Teachers.* 2nd ed. Dubuque, Iowa: Wm C Brown Publishers; 1985.

133. Schonfeld BR, Doerr DF, Convertino VA. An occupational performance test validation program for fire fighters at the Kennedy Space Center. *J Occup Med.* 1990;32(7):638–643.

134. Seiger LH, Hesson J. *Walking for Fitness.* Dubuque, Iowa: Wm C Brown Publishers; 1990.

135. Semenick DM, Adams KO. The vertical jump: A kinesiological analysis with recommendations for strength and conditioning programming. *Nat Strength Condit Assoc J.* 1987;9(3):5–9.

136. Sharkey BJ. *Training for Cross-Country Ski Racing: A Physiological Guide for Athletes and Coaches.* Champaign, Ill: Human Kinetics Publishers, Inc; 1984.

137. Sienna PA. *One Rep Max: A Guide to Beginning Weight Training.* Dubuque, Iowa: Brown & Benchmark; 1989.

138. Sitorius MA, Kwikkel M. Basketball. In: Mellion MB, Walsh WM, Shelton GL, eds. *The Team Physician's Handbook.* Philadelphia, Pa: Hanley & Belfus, Inc; 1990.

139. Sjogaard G, Nielsen B, Mikkelsen F, et al. *Physiology of Bicycling.* Longmeadow, Mass: Mouvement Publications, Inc; 1985.

140. Skinner AT, Thomson AM. *Duffield's Exercise in Water.* 3rd ed. Philadelphia, Pa: WB Saunders Co; 1983.

141. Smith RW, ed. *The New Science of Skin and Scuba Diving.* 6th ed. Champaign, Ill: Human Kinetics Publishers, Inc; 1985.

142. Smythe R. *Plyometrics: An Illustrated Guide.* Portland, Ore: Speed City, Inc; 1987.

143. Smythe R. *Acceleration: An Illustrated Guide.* Portland, Ore: Speed City, Inc; 1988.

144. Smythe R. *Jumping Higher: A Technique for Improved Jumping.* Portland, Ore: Speed City, Inc; 1988.

145. Sorani R. *Circuit Training.* Dubuque, Iowa: Wm C Brown Publishers; 1966.

146. Speed City. *Catalog.* Portland, Ore: Speed City, Inc; 1991.

147. Stamford B. What is interval training? *Physician Sportsmed.* 1989;17(9):193.

148. Stamford B. Task-specific training versus cross training. *Physician Sportsmed.* 1991;19(7):113–114.

149. Stanish WD, Rubinovich RM, Curwin S. Eccentric exercise in chronic tendinitis. *Clin Orthop.* 1986;208:65–68.

150. Stanton P, Purdam C. Hamstring injuries in sprinting: The role of eccentric exercise. *J Orthop Sports Phys Ther.* 1989;10(9):343–349.

151. Stauber WT. Eccentric action of muscles: Physiology, injury and adaptation. *Exerc Sports Sci Rev.* 1989;19:157.

152. Stone MH, Fleck SJ, Triplett NT, et al. Health- and performance-related potential of resistance training. *Sports Med.* 1991;11(4):210–231.

153. Stone MH, O'Bryant H. *Weight Training: A Scientific Approach.* Minneapolis, Minn: Burgess Publishing Co; 1984.

154. Stone MH, O'Bryant H, Garhammer J. A hypothetical model for strength training. *J Sports Med Phys Fit.* 1981;21(4):342–351.

155. Stone MH, O'Bryant H, Garhammer J, et al. A theoretical model of strength training. *Nat Strength Condit Assoc J.* 1982;4(4):36–39.

156. Stone MH, Wilson GD. Resistive training and selected effects. *Med Clin North Am.* 1985;69(1):109–122.

157. Stone WJ, Kroll WA. *Sports Conditioning and Weight Training: Programs for Athletic Competition.* 3rd ed. Dubuque, Iowa: Wm C Brown Publishers; 1991.

158. Town GP. *Science of Triathlon Training and Competition.* Champaign, Ill: Human Kinetics Publishers, Inc; 1985.

159. Turoff F. *Artistic Gymnastics: A Comprehensive Guide to Teaching and Performing Skills for Beginners and Advanced Beginners.* Dubuque, Iowa: Wm C Brown Publishers; 1991.

160. Ungerechts BE, Wilke K, Reischle K, eds. *Swimming Science V* (International Series on Sport Sciences). Champaign, Ill: Human Kinetics Publishers, Inc; 1988;8.

161. Vickers BJ, Vincent WJ. *Swimming.* 5th ed. Dubuque, Iowa: Wm C Brown Publishers; 1989.

162. Voight ML, Draovitch P. Plyometrics. In: Albert M. *Eccentric Muscle Training in Sports and Orthopaedics*. New York, NY: Churchill Livingstone; 1991.

163. Weber J. Gymnastics. In: Mellion MB, Walsh WM, Shelton GL, eds. *The Team Physician's Handbook*. Philadelphia, Pa: Hanley & Belfus, Inc; 1990.

164. Westcott WL. *Strength Fitness: Physiological Principles and Training Techniques*. 2nd ed. Dubuque, Iowa: Wm C Brown Publishers; 1987.

165. Whaley O. Improving foot quickness in the high school athlete. *Nat Strength Condit Assoc J*. 1987;9(1):47–49.

166. Wilkes GH. *Fundamentals of Coaching Basketball*. Dubuque, Iowa: Wm C Brown Publishers; 1982.

167. Wilkes GH. *Basketball*. 5th ed. Dubuque, Iowa: Wm C Brown Publishers; 1990.

168. Wilmore JH, Parr RB, Girandola RN, et al. Physiological alterations consequent to circuit weight training. *Med Sci Sports*. 1978;10:79–84.

169. Yessis M, Trubo R. *Secrets of Soviet Sports Fitness and Training*. New York, NY: Arbor House; 1987.

Suggested Readings

The suggested readings listed below may be used as supplemental references for those clinicians seeking additional information on special populations, special cases, exercise testing, exercise prescription, and rehabilitation.

The following are the individual sections in the suggested readings:

1. Anatomy
2. Arthritis
3. Asthma
4. Biomechanics and Kinesiology
5. Cardiovascular Disease
6. Cardiovascular Endurance—Exercise Prescription
7. Cardiovascular Endurance Testing
8. Children
9. Diabetes
10. Disabled
11. Elderly
12. Environment and Performance
13. Equipment and Performance
14. Ergogenic Aids and Drugs
15. Exercise Physiology
16. Exercise Safety and Liability
17. Exercise Testing
18. Facility Management
19. Flexibility and Range of Motion—Exercise Prescription
20. Flexibility and Range of Motion Testing
21. Health and Fitness
22. Kinanthropometric Testing
23. Low Back
24. Muscular Strength and Endurance—Exercise Prescription
25. Muscular Strength and Endurance Testing
26. Nutrition
27. Obesity and Weight Control
28. Osteoporosis
29. Physical Education
30. Physiologic Calculations
31. Pregnancy
32. Sport Performance—Exercise Prescription
33. Sport Performance Testing
34. Sport Psychology

35. Sports Medicine
36. Stress and Pain Management
37. Therapy and Rehabilitation
38. Women
39. Work Performance Testing

Anatomy

Donnelly JE. *Living Anatomy*. 2nd ed. Champaign, Ill: Human Kinetics Publishers, Inc; 1990.

Palastanga N, Field D, Soames R. *Anatomy and Human Movement: Structure and Function*. Stoneham, Mass: Butterworth-Heinemann; 1989.

Rasch PJ, Grabiner MD, Gregor RJ, et al. *Kinesiology and Applied Anatomy*. 7th ed. Philadelphia, Pa: Lea & Febiger; 1989.

Weineck J. *Functional Anatomy in Sports*. 2nd ed. St. Louis, Mo: Mosby-Year Book; 1990.

Wirhed R. *Athletic Ability and the Anatomy of Motion*. Boca Raton, Fla: CRC Press, Inc; 1988.

Arthritis

Clark AK, Allard L. *Rehabilitation Techniques in Rheumatology*. Baltimore, Md: Williams & Wilkins; 1987.

Ekblom B, Nordemar R. Rheumatoid arthritis. In: Skinner JS. *Exercise Testing and Exercise Prescription for Special Cases: Theoretical Basis and Clinical Application*. Philadelphia, Pa: Lea & Febiger; 1987.

Lane NE, Fries JF. Relationship of running to osteoarthritis and bone density. *Comp Ther*. 1988;14(2):7–15.

McCarty DJ. *Arthritis and Allied Conditions: A Textbook of Rheumatology*. 11th ed. Philadelphia, Pa: Lea & Febiger; 1989.

Moskowitz RW, Howell DS, Goldberg VM, et al. *Osteoarthritis: Diagnosis and Management*. Philadelphia, Pa: WB Saunders Co; 1984.

Nash HL. Sports activity and arthritis: Individually determined or preplanned? *Physician Sportsmed*. 1986;14(4):148.

Sayce V, Fraser I. *Exercise for Arthritis*. Fairfield, Ohio: Consumer Reports Books; 1989.

Sheon RP. A joint-protection guide for nonarticular rheumatic disorders. *Postgrad Med*. 1985;77(5):329.

Asthma

Fitch KD, Morton AR. Specificity of exercise in exercise-induced asthma. *Br Med J*. 1971;4:577–581.

Green MA. Exercise-induced asthma. *N Engl J Med*. 1980;302:522.

Morton AR, Fitch KD, Davis T. The effect of warm up on exercise-induced asthma. *Ann Allergy*. 1979;44:257–260.

Nickerson BG. Asthmatic patients and those with exercise-induced bronchospasm. In: Franklin BA, Gordon S, Timmis GC, eds. *Exercise in Modern Medicine*. Baltimore, Md: Williams & Wilkins; 1989.

Orenstein DM, Reed ME, Grogan FD, et al. Exercise conditioning in children with asthma. *J Pediatr*. 1985;106:555–560.

Szentagothai K, Gyene I, Szocska M, et al. Physical exercise program for children with bronchial asthma. *Pediatr Pulmonol*. 1987;3:166–172.

Biomechanics and Kinesiology

Adrian MJ, Cooper JM. *The Biomechanics of Human Movement*. Dubuque, Iowa: Brown & Benchmark; 1989.

Enoka RM. *Neuromechanical Basis of Kinesiology*. Champaign, Ill: Human Kinetics Publishers, Inc; 1988.

Goel VK, Weinstein JN. *Biomechanics of the Spine: Clinical and Surgical Perspective*. Boca Raton, Fla: CRC Press, Inc; 1989.

Groves R, Camaione DN. *Concepts in Kinesiology*. 2nd ed. Dubuque, Iowa: Wm C Brown Publishers; 1983.

Kirby RF, Roberts JA. *Introductory Biomechanics*. Longmeadow, Mass: Mouvement Publications, Inc; 1986.

Klein-Vogelbach S. *Functional Kinetics: Observing, Analyzing and Teaching Human Movement*. 4th ed. Berlin, Germany: Springer-Verlag; 1990.

Matsui H; Kobayashi K, ed. *Biomechanics VIII-A* (Congress at Nagoya, Japan). Champaign, Ill: Human Kinetics Publishers, Inc; 1983.

Matsui H; Kobayashi K, ed. *Biomechanics VIII-B* (Congress at Nagoya, Japan). Champaign, Ill: Human Kinetics Publishers, Inc; 1983.

Nordin M, Frankel VH, eds. *Basic Biomechanics of the Musculoskeletal System*. 2nd ed. Philadelphia, Pa: Lea & Febiger; 1989.

Northrip JW, Logan GA, McKinney WC. *Analysis of Sport Motion: Anatomic and Biomechanic Perspectives*. 3rd ed. Dubuque, Iowa: Wm C Brown Publishers; 1983.

Scheuchenzuber HJ. *Experiments in the Mechanics of Human Movement*. Longmeadow, Mass: Mouvement Publications, Inc; 1983.

Soderberg GL. *Kinesiology: Application to Pathological Motion*. Baltimore, Md: Williams and Wilkins; 1986.

Vaughan CL. *Biomechanics of Sport*. Boca Raton, Fla: CRC Press, Inc; 1988.

Vaughan CL, Murphy GN, du Toit LL. *Biomechanics of Human Gait: An Annotated Bibliography*. 2nd ed. Champaign, Ill. Human Kinetics Publishers, Inc; 1987.

Winter DA, Norman RW, Wells RP, et al, eds. *Biomechanics IX-A* (Congress at the University of Waterloo). Champaign, Ill: Human Kinetics Publishers, Inc; 1985.

Winter DA, Norman RW, Wells RP, et al, eds. *Biomechanics IX-B* (Congress at the University of Waterloo). Champaign, Ill: Human Kinetics Publishers, Inc; 1985.

Cardiovascular Disease

Barnard RJ, Hall JA. Patients with peripheral vascular disease. In: Franklin BA, Gordon S, Timmis GC, eds. *Exercise in Modern Medicine*. Baltimore, Md: Williams & Wilkins; 1989.

Franklin BA, Hellerstein HK, Gordon S, et al. Cardiac patients. In: Franklin BA, Gordon S, Timmis GC, eds. *Exercise in Modern Medicine*. Baltimore, Md: Williams & Wilkins; 1989.

Haskell WL. Coronary heart disease. In: Skinner JS. *Exercise Testing and Exercise Prescription for Special Cases: Theoretical Basis and Clinical Application*. Philadelphia, Pa: Lea & Febiger; 1987.

Jordon SC, Scott O. *Heart Disease in Pediatrics*. 3rd ed. Stoneham, Mass: Butterworth-Heinemann; 1989.

Moir TW. Nonischemic cardiovascular disease. In: Franklin BA, Gordon S, Timmis GC, eds. *Exercise in Modern Medicine*. Baltimore, Md: Williams & Wilkins; 1989.

Sannerstedt R. Hypertension. In: Skinner JS. *Exercise Testing and Exercise Prescription for Special Cases. Theoretical Basis and Clinical Application*. Philadelphia, Pa: Lea & Febiger; 1987.

Sharkey BJ. *New Dimensions in Aerobic Fitness (No 1, Current Issues in Exercise Science)*. Champaign, Ill: Human Kinetics Publishers, Inc; 1991.

Cardiovascular Endurance—Exercise Prescription

Amundsen LR. *Cardiac Rehabilitation*. New York, NY: Churchill Livingstone; 1981.

Amundsen LR. *Cardiac Rehabilitation: Outpatient Physical Training Methods*. Gaithersburg, Md: Aspen Publishers, Inc; 1987.

Brannon FJ, Geyer MJ, Foley NW. *Cardiac Rehabilitation*. Philadelphia, Pa: FA Davis Co; 1988.

Froelicher VF. Exercise testing and training: Clinical applications. *J Am Coll Cardiol*. 1983;1:114–125.

Frontera WR, Adams RP. Endurance exercise: Normal physiology and limitations imposed by pathological processes (Part 1). *Physician Sportsmed*. 1986;14(8):95–106.

Frontera WR, Adams RP. Endurance exercise: Normal physiology and limitations imposed by pathological processes (Part 2). *Physician Sportsmed*. 1986;14(9):109–120.

Hakki A, Hare TW, Iskandrian AS, et al. Prediction of maximal heart rates in men and women. *Cardiovasc Rev Rep*. 1983;4:997–999.

Harris KA, Holly RG. Physiological response to circuit weight training in borderline hypertensive subjects. *Med Sci Sports Exerc*. 1987;19:246–252.

Kelemen MH, Stewart KJ, Gillilan RE, et al. Circuit weight training in cardiac patients. *J Am Coll Cardiol*. 1986;7:38–42.

Klinger AK, Adrian MJ, Tyner-Wilson M. *Complete Encyclopedia of Aerobics: A Guide for the Aerobics Teacher*. Longmeadow, Mass: Mouvement Publications, Inc; 1986.

Léger L, Thivierge M. Heart rate monitors: Validity, stability and functionality. *Physician Sportsmed*. 1988;16 (5):143–151.

Mirwald RL, Bailey DA. *Maximal Aerobic Power: Longitudinal Analysis*. Longmeadow, Mass: Mouvement Publications, Inc; 1986.

Pashkow F, Pashkow P, Schafer M. *Successful Cardiac Rehabilitation*. Dubuque, Iowa: Brown & Benchmark; 1987.

Pechar GS, McArdle WD, Katch FI, et al. Specificity of cardiorespiratory adaptation to bicycle and treadmill training. *J Appl Physiol*. 1974;36:753–756.

Physician and Sportsmedicine. Roundtable—Walking for fitness. *Physician Sportsmed.* 1986;14(10):145–159.

Rippe JM, Ward A, Porcari JP, et al. Walking for health and fitness. *JAMA.* 1988;259:2720–2724.

Smith EL, Gilligan C. Physical activity prescription for the older adult. *Physician Sportsmed.* 1983;11:91.

Smith JJ. *Circulatory Response to the Upright Posture.* Boca Raton, Fla: CRC Press, Inc; 1990.

Stanford Alumni Association (Stanford Center for Research in Disease Prevention). *The Stanford Health and Exercise Handbook.* Champaign, Ill: Human Kinetics Publishers, Inc; 1987.

Stewart KJ, Mason M, Kelemen MH. Three-year participation in circuit weight training improves muscular strength and self-efficacy in cardiac patients. *J Cardiopul Rehabil.* 1988;8:292–296.

Cardiovascular Endurance Testing

American Heart Association. *Textbook of Advanced Cardiac Life Support.* Dallas, Tex: American Heart Association; 1987.

Cahalin LP, Blessey RL, Kummer D, et al. The safety of exercise testing performed independently by physical therapists. *J Cardiopul Rehabil.* 1987;7:269–276.

Detrano R, Froelicher VF. Exercise testing: Uses and limitations considering recent studies. *Prog Cardiovasc Dis.* 1988;31:173–204.

Doolittle TL. Aerobic testing for manual material handling jobs. In: Mital A, ed. *Advances in Industrial Ergonomics and Safety One.* Philadelphia, Pa: Taylor & Francis; 1989.

Fletcher GF, ed. *Exercise in the Practice of Medicine.* 2nd ed. Mount Kisco, NY: Futura Publishing; 1988.

Franz IW. *Ergometry in Hypertensive Patients: Implications for Diagnosis and Treatment.* New York, NY: Springer-Verlag; 1986.

Froelicher VF. *Exercise Testing and Training.* Chicago, Ill: Year Book Publishers, Inc; 1983.

Gibbons LW. Editorial: The safety of maximal exercise testing. *J Cardiopul Rehabil.* 1987;7:277.

Hall LK, Meyer GC, eds. *Cardiac Rehabilitation: Exercise Testing and Prescription.* Champaign, Ill: Human Kinetics Publishers, Inc; 1988;2.

Hall LK, Meyer GC, Hellerstein HK, eds. *Cardiac Rehabilitation: Exercise Testing and Prescription.* New York, NY: Spectrum Publications, Inc; 1984.

Holland GJ, Hoffmann JJ, Vincent W, et al. Treadmill vs steptreadmill ergometry. *Physician Sportsmed.* 1990;18(1):79.

Karam C. A *Practical Guide to Cardiac Rehabilitation.* Gaithersburg, Md: Aspen Publishers, Inc; 1989.

Leff AR, ed. *Cardiopulmonary Exercise Testing.* New York, NY: Grune & Stratton, Inc; 1986.

Löllgen H, Mellerowicz H, eds. *Progress in Ergometry: Quality Control and Test Criteria.* Berlin, Germany. Springer-Verlag; 1984.

Mellerowicz H, Smodlaka VN. *Ergometry: Basis of Medical Exercise Testing.* Baltimore, Md: Urban & Schwarzenberg; 1981.

Naughton J. *Exercise Testing: Physiological, Biomechanical and Clinical Principles.* Mt Kisco, NY: Futura Publishing; 1988.

Plyley MJ. Physiological principles of exercise testing. In: Torg JS, Welsh RP, Shephard RJ. *Current Therapy in Sports Medicine.* Philadelphia, Pa: ABC Decker, Inc; 1990;2.

Schauer JE, Hanson P. Usefulness of a branching treadmill protocol for evaluation of cardiac functional capacity. *Am J Cardiol.* 1987;60:1373–1377.

Shephard RJ. Tests of maximum oxygen intake: A critical review. *Sports Med.* 1984;1:99–124.

Wenger NK. *Exercise and the Heart.* 2nd ed. Philadelphia, Pa: FA Davis Co; 1985.

Wenger NK, Hellerstein HK. *Rehabilitation of the Coronary Patient.* New York, NY: John Wiley & Sons, Inc; 1978.

Wilson PK, Fardy PS, Froelicher OF. *Cardiac Rehabilitation, Adult Fitness and Exercise Testing.* Philadelphia, Pa: Lea & Febiger; 1981.

Winter EM. Cycle ergometry and maximal intensity exercise. *Sports Med.* 1991;11(6):351–357.

Children

American College of Sports Medicine. Opinion Statement: Physical fitness in children and youth. *Med Sci Sports Exerc.* 1988;20(4):422–423.

Avery ME, First LR. *Pediatric Medicine.* Baltimore, Md: Williams & Wilkins; 1988.

Bar-Or O. *Pediatric Sports Medicine for the Practitioner: From Physiologic Principles to Clinical Applications.* New York, NY: Springer-Verlag; 1983.

Bar-Or O, ed. *Advances in Pediatric Sport Sciences* (Vol 3: *Biological Issues*). Champaign, Ill: Human Kinetics Publishers, Inc; 1989.

Beunen GP, Malina RM, Van't Hof MA, et al. *Adolescent Growth and Motor Performance* (Vol 1, *Sports Science Monograph Series*). Champaign, Ill: Human Kinetics Publishers, Inc; 1988.

Binkhorst RA, Kemper HCG, Saris WHM, eds. *Children and Exercise XI* (Vol 15, *International Series on Sport Sciences*). Champaign, Ill: Human Kinetics Publishers, Inc; 1985.

Boileau RA, ed. *Advances in Pediatric Sport Sciences* (Vol 1: *Biological Issues*). Champaign, Ill: Human Kinetics Publishers, Inc; 1984.

Brown EW, Branta CF, eds. *Competitive Sports for Children and Youth: An Overview of Research and Issues*. Champaign, Ill: Human Kinetics Publishers, Inc; 1988.

Fish HT, Fish RB, Golding LA. *Starting Out Well: A Parents' Approach to Physical Activity and Nutrition*. Champaign, Ill: Human Kinetics Publishers, Inc; 1989.

Franks BD. *YMCA Youth Fitness Test Manual*. Champaign, Ill: Human Kinetics Publishers, Inc; 1989.

Gallahue DL. *Understanding Motor Development: Infants, Children, Adolescents*. 2nd ed. Dubuque, Iowa: Brown & Benchmark; 1989.

Gisolfi CV, Lamb DR, eds. *Youth, Exercise and Sport* (Vol 2, *Perspectives in Exercise Science and Sports Medicine*). Dubuque, Iowa: Brown & Benchmark; 1989.

Kirchner G. *Physical Education for Elementary School Children*. 7th ed. Dubuque, Iowa: Wm C Brown Publishers; 1989.

Malina RA, ed. *Young Athletes: Biological, Psychological and Educational Perspectives*. Champaign, Ill: Human Kinetics Publishers, Inc; 1988.

Martens R, Christina RW, Harvey JS, et al. *Coaching Young Athletes*. Champaign, Ill: Human Kinetics Publishers, Inc; 1981.

Molnar GE. *Pediatric Rehabilitation*. Baltimore, Md: Williams & Wilkins; 1985.

Oseid S, Carlsen KH, eds. *Children and Exercise XIII* (Vol. 19, *International Series on Sport Sciences*). Champaign, Ill: Human Kinetics Publishers, Inc; 1989.

Pipes PL. *Nutrition in Infancy and Childhood*. 4th ed. St Louis, Mo: CV Mosby Co; 1988.

Rotella RJ, Bunker LK. *Parenting Your Superstar*. Champaign, Ill: Human Kinetics Publishers, Inc; 1987.

Rowland TW. *Exercise and Children's Health*. Champaign, Ill: Human Kinetics Publishers, Inc; 1990.

Rutenfranz J, Mocellin R, Klimt F, eds. *Children and Exercise XII* (International Series on Sport Sciences). Champaign, Ill: Human Kinetics Publishers, Inc; 1986;17.

Smoll FL, Magill RA, Ash M, eds. *Children in Sport*. 3rd ed. Champaign, Ill: Human Kinetics Publishers, Inc; 1988.

Stull GA, Eckert HM, eds. *Effects of Physical Activity on Children* (The American Academy of Physical Education). Champaign, Ill: Human Kinetics Publishers, Inc; 1986;(19).

Sullivan JA, Grana WA, eds. *The Pediatric Athlete*. Chicago, Ill: American Academy of Orthopaedic Surgeons; 1990.

Tecklin JS. *Pediatric Physical Therapy*. Philadelphia, Pa: JB Lippincott Co; 1989.

Thomas KT, Lee AM, Thomas JR. *YMCA Youth Fitness Program*. Champaign, Ill: Human Kinetics Publishers, Inc; 1990.

Tillman K, Rizzo P. *What Are We Doing in the Gym Today? New Games and Activities for the Elementary Physical Education Class*. Englewood Cliffs, NJ: Prentice-Hall; 1983.

Tsang RC, Nichols BL, eds. *Nutrition During Infancy*. Philadelphia, Pa: Hanley & Belfus, Inc; 1988.

Wall J, Murray N. *Children and Movement: Physical Education in the Elementary School*. Dubuque, Iowa: Wm C Brown Publishers; 1990.

Weiss MR, Gould D, eds. *Sport for Children and Youths* (1984 Olympic Scientific Congress Proceedings). Champaign, Ill: Human Kinetics Publishers, Inc; 1986;10.

Diabetes

Berg KE. *Diabetic's Guide to Health and Fitness*. Champaign, Ill: Human Kinetics Publishers, Inc; 1986.

Cantu RC. *Diabetes and Exercise*. Longmeadow, Mass: Mouvement Publications, Inc; 1982.

Leon AS. Diabetes. In: Skinner JS. *Exercise Testing and Exercise Prescription for Special Cases: Theoretical Basis and Clinical Application*. Philadelphia, Pa: Lea & Febiger; 1987.

Leon AS. Patients with diabetes mellitus. In: Franklin BA, Gordon S, Timmis GC, eds. *Exercise in Modern Medicine*. Baltimore, Md: Williams & Wilkins; 1989.

Powers MA. *Handbook of Diabetes Nutritional Management*. Gaithersburg, Md: Aspen Publishers, Inc; 1987.

Disabled

Adams RC, McCubbin JA. *Games, Sports, and Exercises for the Physically Disabled*. 4th ed. Philadelphia, Pa: Lea & Febiger; 1991.

Berridge ME, Ward GR, eds. *International Perspectives on Adapted Physical Activity*. Champaign, Ill: Human Kinetics Publishers, Inc; 1987.

Davis R, Byrnes D. The competitive wheelchair stroke. *Nat Strength Condit Assoc J*. 1988;10(3):4–10.

Dreisinger TE, Londeree BR. Wheelchair exercise: A review. *Paraplegia*. 1982;20:20–24.

Dunn J, Fait H. *Special Physical Education: Adapted, Individualized Developmental*. 6th ed. Dubuque, Iowa: Wm C Brown Publishers; 1989.

Eason RL, Smith TL, Caron F, eds. *Adapted Physical Activity: From Theory to Application*. Champaign, Ill: Human Kinetics Publishers, Inc; 1983.

Eckert HM. *Motor Development*. 3rd ed. Dubuque, Iowa: Brown & Benchmark; 1987.

Glaser RM, Davis GM. Wheelchair-dependent individuals. In: Franklin BA, Gordon S, Timmis GC, eds. *Exercise in Modern Medicine*. Baltimore, Md: Williams & Wilkins; 1989.

Glaser RM, Sawka MN, Brune MF. Physiological responses to maximal effort wheelchair and arm ergometry. *J Appl Physiol*. 1980;48:1060–1064.

Horvat M. *Physical Education and Sport for Exceptional Students*. Dubuque, Iowa: Wm C Brown Publishers; 1990.

Jones JA, ed. *Training Guide to Cerebral Palsy Sports*. 3rd ed. Champaign, Ill: Human Kinetics Publishers, Inc; 1988.

Kennedy DW, Austin DR, Smith RW. *Special Recreation: Opportunities for Persons with Disabilities*. Dubuque, Iowa: Wm C Brown Publishers; 1987.

Letts RM. *Principles of Seating the Disabled*. Boca Raton, Fla: CRC Press, Inc; 1991.

Morris LR, Schulz L. *Creative Play Activities for Children with Disabilities: A Resource Book for Teachers and Parents*. 2nd ed. Champaign, Ill: Human Kinetics Publishers, Inc; 1989.

Paciorek MJ, Jones J. *Sports and Recreation for the Disabled: A Resource Manual*. Dubuque, Iowa: Brown & Benchmark; 1989.

Robinson J, Fox AD. *Scuba Diving With Disabilities*. Champaign, Ill: Human Kinetics Publishers, Inc; 1987.

Shephard RJ. *Fitness in Special Populations*. Champaign, Ill: Human Kinetics Publishers, Inc; 1990.

Sherrill C. *Adapted Physical Education and Recreation: A Multidisciplinary Approach*. 3rd ed. Dubuque, Iowa: Wm C Brown Publishers; 1986.

Sherrill C, ed. *Sport and the Disabled Athlete* (1984 Olympic Scientific Congress Proceedings). Champaign, Ill: Human Kinetics Publishers, Inc; 1986;9.

Smith RV, Leslie JH. *Rehabilitation Engineering*. Boca Raton, Fla: CRC Press, Inc; 1990.

Sullivan JV. *Fitness for the Handicapped: An Instructional Approach*. Springfield, Ill: Charles C Thomas Publisher; 1984.

Winnick JP, ed. *Adapted Physical Education and Sport*. Champaign, Ill: Human Kinetics Publishers, Inc; 1990.

Winnick JP, Short FX. *Physical Fitness Testing of the Disabled*. Champaign, Ill: Human Kinetics Publishers, Inc; 1985.

YMCA of the USA. *Aquatics for Special Populations*. Champaign, Ill: Human Kinetics Publishers, Inc; 1987.

Elderly

American Dietetic Association. Position Paper: Nutrition, aging, and the continuum of health care. Chicago, Ill: American Dietetic Association; 1987.

Andrews K. *Rehabilitation of the Older Adult*. Baltimore, Md: Williams & Wilkins; 1987.

Delafuente JC, Stewart RB. *Therapeutics in the Elderly*. Baltimore, Md: Williams & Wilkins; 1988.

deVries HA. Healthy elderly patients. In: Franklin BA, Gordon S, Timmis GC, eds. *Exercise in Modern Medicine*. Baltimore, Md: Williams & Wilkins; 1989.

Dychtwald K. *Wellness and Health Promotion for the Elderly*. Gaithersburg, Md: Aspen Publishers, Inc; 1986.

Elia EA. Exercise and the elderly. In: DiNubile NA, ed. *The Exercise Prescription* [Clinics in Sports Medicine 10(1)]. Philadelphia, Pa: WB Saunders Co; 1991.

Ferrini AF, Ferrini RL. *Health in Later Years*. Dubuque, Iowa: Wm C Brown Publishers; 1989.

Goldstein TS. *Geriatric Orthopaedics Rehabilitative Management of Common Problems*. Rockville, Md: Aspen Publishers, Inc; 1990.

Haywood KM. *Life Span Motor Development*. Champaign, Ill: Human Kinetics Publishers, Inc; 1986.

Haywood KM. *Laboratory Activities for Life Span Motor Development*. Champaign, Ill: Human Kinetics Publishers, Inc; 1988.

Jackson OL, ed. *Therapeutic Considerations for the Elderly* (Vol 14, *Clinics in Physical Therapy*). New York, NY: Churchill Livingstone; 1987.

Jacobsen JJ, ed. *Help! I'm Parenting My Parents*. Dubuque, Iowa: Brown & Benchmark; 1988.

Kaplan M. *Leisure: Lifestyle and Lifespan, Perspectives for Gerontology*. Dubuque, Iowa: Wm C Brown Publishers; 1979.

Lavizzo-Mourey RJ, Day SC, Diserens DF, et al, eds. *Practicing Prevention for the Elderly*. Philadelphia, Pa: Hanley & Belfus, Inc; 1989.

McPherson BD, ed. Sport and Aging (1984 Olympic Scientific Congress Proceedings). Champaign, Ill: Human Kinetics Publishers, Inc; 1986;5.

Ostrow AC, ed. *Aging and Motor Behavior*. Dubuque, Iowa: Brown & Benchmark; 1989.

Reichel W. *Clinical Aspects of Aging*. 3rd ed. Baltimore, Md: Williams & Wilkins; 1988.

Rikkers R. *Seniors on the Move*. Champaign, Ill: Human Kinetics Publishers, Inc; 1986.

Rockwell RE, Osborne NE. *Fitness and Nutrition for Seniors*. Springfield, Ill: Charles C Thomas Publisher; 1984.

Shea EJ. *Swimming for Seniors*. Champaign, Ill: Human Kinetics Publishers, Inc; 1986.

Shephard RJ. Physical training for the elderly. *Clin Sports Med.* 1986;5:515.

Shephard RJ. *Physical Activity and Aging*. 2nd ed. Gaithersburg, Md: Aspen Publishers, Inc; 1987.

Teague ML. *Health Promotion Programs: Achieving High-Level Wellness in the Later Years*. Dubuque, Iowa: Brown & Benchmark; 1987.

Wagstaff P, Coakley D. *Physiotherapy and the Elderly Patient*. Gaithersburg, Md: Aspen Publishers, Inc; 1988.

Environment and Performance

American College of Sports Medicine. Position Stand: The prevention of thermal injuries during distance running. *Med Sci Sports Exerc.* 1987;19(5):529–533.

Armstrong LE. Acclimatization: Transporting athletes into unique environments. *Nat Strength Condit Assoc J.* 1988;10(5):61–64.

Armstrong LE. Desynchronization of biological rhythms in athletes: Jet lag. *Nat Strength Condit Assoc J.* 1988;10(6):68–70.

Auerbach PS, Geehr EC. *Management of Wilderness and Environmental Emergencies*. 2nd ed. St Louis, Mo: Mosby-Year Book; 1989.

Bove AA, Davis JC, eds. *Diving Medicine*. 2nd ed. Philadelphia, Pa: WB Saunders Co; 1990.

Bowman WD. Safe exercise in the cold and cold injuries. In: Mellion MB, Walsh WM, Shelton GL, eds. *The Team Physician's Handbook*. Philadelphia, Pa: Hanley & Belfus, Inc; 1990.

Brendel W, Zink RA, eds. *High Altitude Physiology and Medicine*. New York, NY: Springer-Verlag; 1982.

Chambers MJ. Exercise: A prescription for a good night's sleep? *Physician Sportsmed.* 1991;19(8):107–114.

Folk GE. *Textbook of Environmental Physiology*. 2nd ed. Philadelphia, Pa: Lea & Febiger; 1974.

Haymes EM, Wells CL. *Environment and Human Performance*. Champaign, Ill: Human Kinetics Publishers, Inc; 1986.

Kryger MH, Roth T, Dement W. *Principles and Practice of Sleep Medicine*. Philadelphia, Pa: WB Saunders Co; 1989.

Maudgal DP, ed. *Hypothermia*. Elmsford, NY: Pergamon Press, Inc; 1987.

McCafferty WB. *Air Pollution and Athletic Performance*. Springfield, Ill: Charles C Thomas Publisher; 1981.

Pandolf KB, Sawka MN, Gonzalez RR, eds. *Human Performance Physiology and Environmental Medicine at Terrestrial Extremes*. Dubuque, Iowa: Brown & Benchmark; 1988.

Shiraki K, Yousef MK, Wilber CG. *Man in Stressful Environments: Diving, Hyper and Hypobaric Physiology*. Springfield, Ill: Charles C Thomas Publisher; 1988.

Shiraki K, Yousef MK, Wilber CG. *Man in Stressful Environments: Thermal and Work Physiology*. Springfield, Ill: Charles C Thomas Publisher; 1988.

Sutton JR, Coates G, Houston CS, eds. *Hypoxia: The Tolerable Limits*. Dubuque, Iowa: Brown & Benchmark; 1988.

Vallotton J. *A Color Atlas of Mountain Medicine*. St Louis, Mo: Mosby–Year Book; 1991.

Equipment and Performance

Flynn RB. Sports surfaces. In: Mellion MB, Walsh WM, Shelton GL, eds. *The Team Physician's Handbook*. Philadelphia, Pa: Hanley and Belfus, Inc; 1990.

Frederick EC, ed. *Sport Shoes and Playing Surfaces: Biomechanical Properties*. Champaign, Ill: Human Kinetics Publishers, Inc; 1984.

Nigg BM, ed. *Biomechanics of Running Shoes*. Champaign, Ill: Human Kinetics Publishers, Inc; 1986.

Segesser B, Pförringer W. *The Shoe in Sport*. Chicago, Ill: Year Book Medical Publishers, Inc; 1989.

Ergogenic Aids and Drugs

American College of Sports Medicine. Position Stand: The use of alcohol in sports. *Med Sci Sports Exerc*. 1982;14(6):ix–xi.

American College of Sports Medicine. Position Stand: The use of anabolic–androgenic steroids in sports. *Med Sci Sports Exerc*. 1987;19(5):534–539.

American College of Sports Medicine. Position Stand: Blood doping as an ergogenic aid. *Med Sci Sports Exerc*. 1987;19(5):540–543.

American Medical Association (Council on Scientific Affairs). Health effects of smokeless tobacco. *JAMA*. 1986;255(8):1038–1044.

Aronson V. Vitamins and minerals as ergogenic aids. *Physician Sportsmed*. 1986;14(3):209–212.

Aronson V. Protein and miscellaneous ergogenic aids. *Physician Sportsmed*. 1986;14(5):199–202.

Avis H. *Drugs and Life*. Dubuque, Iowa: Wm C Brown Publishers; 1990.

Cantwell JD. Cocaine and cardiovascular events. *Physician Sportsmed*. 1986;14(11):77–82.

Carroll CR. *Drugs in Modern Society*. 2nd ed. Dubuque, Iowa: Wm C Brown Publishers; 1989.

Friedl KE, Moore RJ, Marchitelli LJ. Steroid replacers: Let the athlete beware. *Nat Strength Condit Assoc J*. 1992;14(1):14–19.

Haupt HA, Rovere GD. Anabolic steroids: A review of the literature. *Am J Sports Med*. 1984;12:469–484.

Lamb DR. Anabolic steroids in athletics: How well do they work and how dangerous are they? *Am J Sports Med*. 1984;12(1):31–38.

Lamb DR, Williams M, eds. *Ergogenics: Enhancement of Performance in Exercise and Sport* (Vol 4, *Perspectives in Exercise Science and Sports Medicine*). Dubuque, Iowa: Brown & Benchmark; 1991.

Morgan WP, ed. *Ergogenic Aids and Muscular Performance*. New York, NY: Academic Press; 1972.

Mottram DR, ed. *Drugs in Sport*. Champaign, Ill: Human Kinetics Publishers, Inc; 1988.

National Strength and Conditioning Association. Position statement: Use and abuse of anabolic steroids. *Nat Strength Condit Assoc J*. 1985;7(5):44–59.

National Strength and Conditioning Association. Roundtable—Popularized ergogenic aids. *Nat Strength Condit Assoc J*. 1989;11(1):10–14.

Puffer JC, Green GA. Drugs and doping in athletes. In: Mellion MB, Walsh WM, Shelton GL, eds. *The Team Physician's Handbook*. Philadelphia, Pa: Hanley & Belfus, Inc; 1990.

Redda KK, Walker CA, Barnett G. *Cocaine, Marijuana, Designer Drugs: Chemistry, Pharmacology and Behavior*. Boca Raton, Fla: CRC Press, Inc; 1989.

Rogozkin VA. *Metabolism of Anabolic–Androgenic Steroids*. Boca Raton, Fla: CRC Press, Inc; 1990.

Shipe JR, Savory J. *Drugs in Competitive Athletics*. Boca Raton, Fla: CRC Press, Inc; 1991.

Strauss RH, ed. *Drugs and Performance in Sports*. Philadelphia, Pa: WB Saunders Co; 1987.

Tricker R, Cook D, eds. *Athletes at Risk: Drugs and Sport*. Dubuque, Iowa: Brown & Benchmark; 1990.

Wadler GI, Hainline B. *Drugs and the Athlete*. Philadelphia, Pa: FA Davis Co; 1989;2.

Wagner JC. Enhancement of athletic performance with drugs. *Sports Med*. 1991;12(4):250–265.

Williams MH. *Drugs and Athletic Performance*. Springfield, Ill: Charles C Thomas Publisher; 1974.

Williams MH. Nutritional ergogenic aids and athletic performance. *Nutr Today*. 1989;24(1):7–14.

Wright JE, Cowart WS. *Anabolic Steroids: Altered States.* Dubuque, Iowa: Brown & Benchmark; 1990.

Exercise Physiology

Adams WC. *Foundations of Physical Education, Exercise and Sport Sciences.* Philadelphia, Pa: Lea & Febiger; 1991.

Banister EW, Brown SR. The relative energy requirements of physical activity. In: Falls HB, ed. *Exercise Physiology.* New York, NY: Academic Press; 1968.

Barrow HM, Brown JP. *Man and Movement: Principles of Physical Education.* 4th ed. Philadelphia, Pa: Lea & Febiger; 1988.

Berne RM, Levy MN, eds. *Cardiovascular Physiology.* 5th ed. St Louis, Mo: CV Mosby Co; 1986.

Borer KT, Edington DW, White TP, eds. *Frontiers of Exercise Biology* (Big Ten Body of Knowledge Symposium Series). Champaign, Ill: Human Kinetics Publishers, Inc; 1983;13.

Burke EJ, ed. *Toward an Understanding of Human Performance.* Longmeadow, Mass: Mouvement Publications, Inc; 1980.

Cavanagh PR, Kram R. The efficiency of human movement—A statement of the problem. *Med Sci Sports Exerc.* 1985;17(3):304–308.

Cavanagh PR, Kram R. Mechanical and muscular factors affecting the efficiency of human movement. *Med Sci Sports Exerc.* 1985;17(3):326–331.

deVries HA. *Physiology of Exercise for Physical Education and Athletics.* 4th ed. Dubuque, Iowa: Wm C Brown Publishers; 1986.

Fox EL. *Sports Physiology.* 2nd ed. Dubuque, Iowa: Wm C Brown Publishers; 1984.

Fox EL, Bowers RW, Foss ML. *The Physiological Basis of Physical Education and Athletics.* 4th ed. Dubuque, Iowa: Wm C Brown Publishers; 1989.

Guyton AC. *Human Physiology and Mechanisms of Disease.* 4th ed. Philadelphia, Pa: WB Saunders Co; 1987.

Jones NL, McCartney N, McComas AJ, eds. *Human Muscle Power.* Champaign, Ill: Human Kinetics Publishers, Inc; 1986.

Karpman VL. *Cardiovascular System and Physical Exercise.* Boca Raton, Fla: CRC Press, Inc; 1987.

Kausen K, Hemmingsen I, Rasmussen B. *Basic Sport Science.* Longmeadow, Mass: Mouvement Publications, Inc; 1982.

Knuttgen HG, Vogel JA, Poortmans J, eds. *Biochemistry of Exercise* (Vol 13, International Series on Sport Sciences). Champaign, Ill: Human Kinetics Publishers, Inc; 1983.

Lamb DR, Murray R, eds. *Prolonged Exercise* (Vol 1, *Perspectives in Exercise Science and Sports Medicine*). Dubuque, Iowa: Brown & Benchmark; 1988.

Mackinnon LT. *Exercise and Immunology (No 2, Current Issues in Exercise Science).* Champaign, Ill: Human Kinetics Publishers, Inc; 1992.

Malina RM, Bouchard C, eds. *Sport and Human Genetics* (1984 Olympic Scientific Congress Proceedings). Champaign, Ill: Human Kinetics Publishers, Inc; 1986;4.

Malina RM, Eckert HM, eds. *Physical Activity in Early and Modern Populations* (The American Academy of Physical Education). Champaign, Ill: Human Kinetics Publishers, Inc; 1988;(21).

Michael ED, Burke EJ, Avakian EV. *Laboratory Experiences in Exercise Physiology.* 2nd ed. Longmeadow, Mass: Mouvement Publications, Inc; 1987.

Morrow JR, Pivarnik JM. *Simulated Exercise Physiology Laboratories* (software package). Champaign, Ill: Human Kinetics Publishers, Inc; 1989.

Nazar K, Terjung RL, Kaciuba-Uscilko H, et al, eds. *International Perspectives in Exercise Physiology.* Champaign, Ill: Human Kinetics Publishers, Inc; 1990.

Pandolf KB. *Exercise and Sport Sciences Reviews* (American College of Sports Medicine Series). Baltimore, Md: Williams & Wilkins; 1989;17.

Saltin B, ed. *Biochemistry of Exercise VI: Metabolic Regulation and Its Practical Significance* (International Series on Sport Sciences). Champaign, Ill: Human Kinetics Publishers, Inc; 1986;16.

Sharkey BJ. *Coaches Guide to Sport Physiology.* Champaign, Ill: Human Kinetics Publishers, Inc; 1986.

Shephard RJ. *Biochemistry of Physical Activity.* Springfield, Ill: Charles C Thomas Publisher; 1984.

Singer RN. *Peak Performance . . . and More*. Longmeadow, Mass: Mouvement Publications Inc; 1986.

Squire JM. *Molecular Mechanisms in Muscular Contraction*. Boca Raton, Fla: CRC Press, Inc; 1989.

Stone MH, Keith RE, Kearney JT, et al. Overtraining: A review of the signs, symptoms and possible causes. *J Appl Sport Sci Res*. 1991;5(1):35–50.

Sykes MK, Vickers MD, Hull CJ. *Principles of Clinical Measurement*. 2nd ed. Boston, Mass: Blackwell Scientific Publications; 1981.

Taylor AW, Gollnick PD, Green HJ, et al, eds. *Biochemistry of Exercise VII* (International Series on Sport Science). Champaign, Ill: Human Kinetics Publishers, Inc; 1990;21.

Tietz NW, ed. *Clinical Guide to Laboratory Tests*. 2nd ed. Philadelphia, Pa: WB Saunders Co; 1990.

Viru A. *Hormones in Muscular Activity*. Boca Raton, Fla: CRC Press, Inc; 1985;1,2.

Williams RS, Wallace A, eds. *Biological Effects of Physical Activity* (Sport Science Monograph Series). Champaign, Ill: Human Kinetics Publishers, Inc; 1989;2.

Exercise Safety and Liability

Bailey JA, Matthews DL. *Law and Liability in Athletics, Physical Education and Recreation*. 2nd ed. Dubuque, Iowa: Wm C Brown Publishers; 1989.

Clement A. *Law in Sport and Physical Activity*. Dubuque, Iowa: Brown & Benchmark; 1988.

Exercise Testing

Canadian Standards Association. *Canadian Metric Practice Guide*. Rexdale, Ontario: Canadian Standards Association; 1976.

Corbin CB, Lindsey R. *Concepts of Physical Fitness with Laboratories*. 6th ed. Dubuque, Iowa: Wm C Brown Publishers; 1988.

Kirkendall DR, Gruber JJ, Johnson RE. *Measurement and Evaluation for Physical Educators*. 2nd ed. Champaign, Ill: Human Kinetics Publishers, Inc; 1987.

Rothstein JM, ed. *Measurement in Physical Therapy* (Vol 7, *Clinics in Physical Therapy*). New York, NY: Churchill Livingstone; 1986.

Safrit MJ, Wood TM, eds. *Measurement Concepts in Physical Education and Exercise Science*. Champaign, Ill: Human Kinetics Publishers, Inc; 1989.

Shephard RJ, Lavallee H. *Physical Fitness Assessment: Principles, Practice and Application*. Springfield, Ill: Charles C Thomas Publisher; 1978.

Thomas JR, Nelson JK. *Research Methods in Physical Activity*. 2nd ed. Champaign, Ill: Human Kinetics Publishers, Inc; 1990.

Facility Management

American College of Sports Medicine. *ACSM's Health/Fitness Facility Standards and Guidelines*. Champaign, Ill: Human Kinetics Publishers, Inc; 1992.

Association for Fitness in Business. *Guidelines for Employee Health Promotion Programs*. Champaign, Ill: Human Kinetics Publishers, Inc; 1992.

Chenoweth DH. *Planning Health Promotion at the Worksite*. Dubuque, Iowa: Brown & Benchmark; 1987.

Dignan MB, Carr PA. *Program Planning for Health Education and Health Promotion*. Philadelphia, Pa: Lea & Febiger; 1987.

Gerson RF. *Marketing Health/Fitness Services*. Champaign, Ill: Human Kinetics Publishers, Inc; 1989.

Parks JB, Zanger BRK, eds. *Sport and Fitness Management: Career Strategies and Professional Content*. Champaign, Ill: Human Kinetics Publishers, Inc; 1990.

Patton RW, Grantham WC, Gerson RF, et al. *Developing and Managing Health/Fitness Facilities*. Champaign, Ill: Human Kinetics Publishers, Inc; 1986.

Shephard RJ. *Economic Benefits of Enhanced Fitness*. Champaign, Ill: Human Kinetics Publishers, Inc; 1986.

Sol N, Wilson PK, eds. *Hospital Health Promotion*. Champaign, Ill: Human Kinetics Publishers, Inc; 1989.

Flexibility and Range of Motion—Exercise Prescription

Alter MJ. *Science of Stretching*. Champaign, Ill: Human Kinetics Publishers, Inc; 1988.

Anderson B, Burke ER. Scientific, medical and practical aspects of stretching. In: DiNubile

NA, ed. *The Exercise Prescription* [Clinics in Sports Medicine 10(1)]. Philadelphia, Pa: WB Saunders Co; 1991.

Buroker KX, Schwane JA. Does postexercise static stretching alleviate delayed muscle soreness? *Physician Sportsmed*. 1989;17:83.

Cornelius WL. PNF ankle stretching: Partner/no-partner procedures. *Nat Strength Condit Assoc J*. 1991;13(1):59–63.

deVries HA. Flexibility. In: deVries HA, ed. *Physiology of Exercise for Physical Education and Athletics*. 3rd ed. Dubuque, Iowa: Wm C Brown Publishers; 1980.

Etnyre BR, Lee EJ. Comments on proprioceptive neuromuscular facilitation stretching techniques. *Res Q Exerc Sport*. 1987;58:184–188.

Gose JC, Schweizer P. Iliotibial band tightness. *J Orthop Sports Phys Ther*. 1989;10(10):399–407.

Madding SW, Wong JG, Hallum A, et al. Effects of duration or passive stretching on hip abduction range of motion. *J Orthop Sports Phys Ther*. 1987;8:409–416.

Moore MA, Hutton RS. Electromyographic investigation of muscle stretching techniques. *Med Sci Sports Exerc*. 1980;12:322–329.

Sady SP, Wortman M, Blanke D. Flexibility training: Ballistic, static or proprioceptive neuromuscular facilitation? *Arch Phys Med Rehabil*. 1982;63:261–263.

Siff MC. Modified PNF as a system of physical conditioning. *Nat Strength Condit Assoc J*. 1991;13(4):73–77.

Trombly CA, ed. *Occupational Therapy for Physical Dysfunction*. 2nd ed. Baltimore, Md: Williams & Wilkins; 1983.

Voss DE, Ionta MK, Myers BJ. *Proprioceptive Neuromuscular Facilitation*. Philadelphia, Pa: Harper & Row; 1985.

Wiktorsson-Möller M, Öberg B, Ekstrand J, et al. Effects of warming up, massage and stretching on range of motion and muscle strength in the lower extremity. *Am J Sports Med*. 1983;11(4):249–252.

Zachazewski JE. Flexibility. In: Scully R, Barnes ML, eds. *Physical Therapy*. Philadelphia, Pa: JB Lippincott Co; 1989.

Zachazewski JE, Reischl SR. Flexibility for the runner: Specific program considerations. *Top Acute Care Trauma Rehabil*. 1986;1:9-27.

Flexibility and Range of Motion Testing

Boone DC, Azen SP, Lin CM, et al. Reliability of goniometric measurements. *Phys Ther*. 1978;58:1355–1360.

Cooper DL, Fair J. Developing and testing flexibility. *Physician Sportsmed*. 1978;6:137–138.

Corbin C. Flexibility. *Clin Sports Med*. 1984;3:101–117.

Kapandji IA. *Physiology of the Joints*. 2nd ed. Baltimore, Md: Williams & Wilkins; 1970;2.

Micheli LJ. Overuse injuries in children's sports: The growth factor. *Orthop Clin North Am*. 1983;14:337–360.

Moll J, Wright V. Measurement of spinal movement. In: Jayson J. *The Lumbar Spine in the Back Pain Patient*. New York, NY: Grune & Stratton, Inc; 1976.

Moore MA, Hutton RS. Electromyographic investigation of muscle stretching techniques. *Med Sci Sports Exerc*. 1980;12:322–329.

Pearcy M, Portek I, Shepherd J. The effect of low back pain on lumbar spinal movements measured by three-dimensional x-ray analysis. *Spine*. 1985;10:150–153.

Reynolds P. Measurement of spinal mobility: A comparison of three methods. *Rheum and Rehab*. 1975;14:180–185.

Tibrewal S, Pearcy J, Portek I, et al. A perspective study of lumbar spinal movements before and after discectomy using bi-planar radiography. *Spine*. 1985;10:455–460.

Health and Fitness

Allsen PE, Harrison JM, Vance B. *Fitness for Life: An Individualized Approach*. 4th ed. Dubuque, Iowa: Wm C Brown Publishers; 1989.

American College of Sports Medicine. *ACSM Fitness Book*. Champaign, Ill: Human Kinetics Publishers, Inc; 1992.

Baloh RW. *Dizziness, Hearing Loss and Tinnitus: The Essentials of Neurotology*. Philadelphia, Pa: FA Davis Co; 1984.

Bouchard C, Shephard RJ, Stephens T, et al, eds. *Exercise, Fitness and Health: A Consensus of Current Knowledge*. Champaign, Ill: Human Kinetics Publishers, Inc; 1990.

Carey MI. *Lifestyle Workshops*. Champaign, Ill: Human Kinetics Publishers, Inc; 1989.

Corbin CB, Lindsey R. *The Ultimate Fitness Book*. Champaign, Ill: Human Kinetics Publishers, Inc; 1984.

Decker JI, Orcutt G, Sammann P. *Y's Way to Fitness Walking: Leader's Guide*. Champaign, Ill: Human Kinetics Publishers, Inc; 1989.

Dickman SR. *Pathways to Wellness*. Champaign, Ill: Human Kinetics Publishers, Inc; 1988.

Dishman RK, ed. *Exercise Adherence: Its Impact on Public Health*. Champaign, Ill: Human Kinetics Publishers, Inc; 1988.

Dossey BM, Keegan L, Kolkmeier LG, et al. *Holistic Health Promotion: A Guide for Practice*. Gaithersburg, Md: Aspen Publishers, Inc; 1989.

Emmett A. *The Bare Facts: The Effect of Sun on Skin*. Philadelphia, Pa: FA Davis Co; 1989.

Franks BD, Howley ET. *Fitness Facts: The Healthy Living Handbook*. Champaign, Ill: Human Kinetics Publishers, Inc; 1989.

Franks BD, Howley ET. *Fitness Leader's Handbook*. Champaign, Ill: Human Kinetics Publishers, Inc; 1989.

Gavin J. *The Exercise Habit*. Champaign, Ill: Human Kinetics Publishers, Inc; 1992.

Gavrilov LA, Gavrilova NS. *The Biology of Life Span: A Quantitative Approach*. New York, NY: Harwood Academic Publishers; 1991.

Getchell B. *The Fitness Book* (The National Institute for Fitness and Sport). Dubuque, Iowa: Brown & Benchmark; 1987.

Howley ET, Franks BD. *Health/Fitness Instructor's Handbook*. Champaign, Ill: Human Kinetics Publishers, Inc; 1986.

Katz J. *FitnessWorks*. Champaign, Ill: Human Kinetics Publishers, Inc; 1988.

Knudsen JF. Noise-induced hearing loss. *Resident Staff Phys*. 1986;32(11):92.

Munnings F. Sun safety: Shedding light on the risks of exposure. *Physician Sportsmed*. 1991;19(7):100–107.

Patton RW, Corry JM, Gettman LR, et al. *Implementing Health/Fitness Programs*. Champaign, Ill: Human Kinetics Publishers, Inc; 1986.

Rejeski WJ, Kenny EA. *Fitness Motivation: Preventing Participant Dropout*. Champaign, Ill: Human Kinetics Publishers, Inc; 1988.

Solis KM. *Ropics: The Next Jump Forward in Fitness*. Champaign, Ill: Human Kinetics Publishers, Inc; 1992.

Sweeting RL. *A Values Approach to Health Behavior*. Champaign, Ill: Human Kinetics Publishers, Inc; 1990.

Vanderschmidt HF, Koch-Weser D, Woodbury PA, eds. *Handbook of Clinical Prevention*. Baltimore, Md: Williams & Wilkins; 1987.

Kinanthropometric Testing

Himes JH, Bouchard C. Do the new Metropolitan Life Insurance weight-height tables correctly assess body frame and body fat relationships? *American Journal of Public Health*. 1985;75:1076–1079.

Houmard JA, Israel RG, McCammon MR, et al. Validity of a near-infrared device for estimating body composition in a college football team. *J Appl Sport Sci Res*. 1991;5(2):53–59.

Katch FI, Katch VL. Measurement and prediction errors in body composition assessment and the search for a perfect prediction equation. *Res Q Exerc Sport*. 1980;51:249–260.

Lohman TG. Research progress in validation of laboratory methods of assessing body composition. *Med Sci Sports Exerc*. 1984;16:596–603.

Lohman TG. *Advances in Body Composition Assessment (No 3, Current Issues in Exercise Science)*. Champaign, Ill: Human Kinetics Publishers, Inc; 1992.

Lohman TG. Assessment of body composition in children. *Pediatr Exerc Sci*. 1989;1:19–30.

Lukaski HC. Methods for the assessment of human body composition: Traditional and new. *Am J Clin Nutr*. 1987;46:537–556.

Malina RM. Bioelectric methods for estimating body composition: An overview and discussion. *Hum Biol*. 1987;59:329–335.

Martin AD, Drinkwater DT. Variability in the measures of body fat: Assumptions or technique. *Sports Med*. 1991;11(5):277–288.

National Strength and Conditioning Association. Roundtable—Body composition: Scientific considerations (Part 1). *Nat Strength Condit Assoc J*. 1987;9(3):12–26.

National Strength and Conditioning Association. Roundtable—Body composition: Practical considerations (Part 2). *Nat Strength Condit Assoc J*. 1987;9(4):10–20.

Ostyn M, Beunen G, Simons J. Kinanthropometry II (*International Series on Sport Sciences*). Baltimore, Md: University Park Press; 1980;9.

Pett LB, Ogilvie GF. The report on Canadian average weights, heights and skinfolds. *Canadian Bulletin of Nutrition*. 1957;5:1–81.

Pollock ML, Schmidt DH, Jackson AS. Measurement of cardiorespiratory fitness and body composition in the clinical setting. *Comprehensive Ther*. 1980;6:12–27.

Low Back

Borenstein DG, Wiesel SW. *Low Back Pain: Medical Diagnosis and Comprehensive Management*. Philadelphia, Pa: WB Saunders Co; 1989.

Bureau of Labor Statistics. Back injuries associated with lifting. Washington, DC: US Government Printing Office. Bulletin 2144; August, 1982.

Cailliet R. *Understand Your Backache: A Guide to Prevention, Treatment and Relief*. Philadelphia, Pa: FA Davis Co; 1984.

Cailliet R. *Low Back Pain Syndrome*. 4th ed. Philadelphia, Pa: FA Davis Co; 1988.

Cailliet R. *Soft Tissue Pain and Disability*. 2nd ed. Philadelphia, Pa: FA Davis Co; 1988.

Cox JM. *Low Back Pain: Mechanism, Diagnosis and Treatment*. 5th ed. Baltimore, Md: Williams & Wilkins; 1990.

Floman Y., ed. *Disorders of the Lumbar Spine*. Gaithersburg, Md: Aspen Publishers, Inc; 1990.

Giles LGF. *Anatomical Basis of Low Back Pain*. Baltimore, Md: Williams & Wilkins; 1989.

Ghosh P. *The Biology of the Intervertebral Disc*. Boca Raton, Fla: CRC Press, Inc; 1988;1.

Ghosh P. *The Biology of the Intervertebral Disc*. Boca Raton, Fla: CRC Press, Inc; 1988;2.

Griffiths HJ. *Imaging Strategies for Low Back Pain*. Gaithersburg, Md: Aspen Publishers, Inc; 1990.

Gustilo RB. *The Fracture Classification Manual*. St Louis, Mo: Mosby-Year Book; 1991.

Haldeman S. *Principles and Practice of Chiropractic*. 2nd ed. Norwalk, Conn: Appleton & Lange; 1992.

Hebert LA. *Sex and Back Pain*. Bangor, Me: IMPACC, Inc; 1987.

Ishmael WK, Shorbe HB. *Care of the Back*. 3rd ed. Philadelphia, Pa: JB Lippincott Co; 1985.

Jayson M. *The Lumbar Spine and Back Pain*. New York, NY: Churchill Livingstone; 1989.

Junghanns H; Hager HJ, ed. *Clinical Implications of Normal Biomechanical Stresses on Spinal Function*. Gaithersburg, Md: Aspen Publishers, Inc; 1990.

Kenna CJ, Murtagh JE. *Back Pain and Spinal Manipulation: A Practical Guide*. Stoneham, Mass: Butterworth-Heinemann; 1989.

Liemohn W, Snodgrass LB, Sharpe GL. Unresolved controversies in back management: A review. *J Orthop Sports Phys Ther*. 1988;9(7):239–244.

Macnab I, McCulloch JA. *Backache*. 2nd ed. Baltimore, Md: Williams & Wilkins; 1990.

Mandell P, Lipton MH, Burnstein J, et al. *Low Back Pain: An Historical and Contemporary Overview of the Occupational, Medical and Psychosocial Issues of Chronic Back Pain*. Thorofare, NJ: SLACK, Inc; 1989.

Mayer TG, Mooney V, Gatchel RJ, eds. *Contemporary Conservative Care for Painful Spinal Disorders*. Philadelphia, Pa: Lea & Febiger; 1991.

McKenzie R. *The Lumbar Spine: Mechanical Diagnosis and Therapy*. Lower Hutt, New Zealand: Spinal Publications Ltd; 1981.

McKenzie R. *Treat Your Own Neck*. Lower Hutt, New Zealand: Spinal Publications Ltd; 1983.

McKenzie R. *Treat Your Own Back*. Lower Hutt, New Zealand: Spinal Publications Ltd; 1985.

McKenzie R. *The Cervical and Thoracic Spine: Mechanical Diagnosis and Therapy*. Lower Hutt, New Zealand: Spinal Publications Ltd; 1991.

Ponte DJ, Jensen GJ, Kent BE. A preliminary report on the use of the McKenzie protocol versus Williams protocol in the treatment of low back pain. *J Orthop Sports Phys Ther*. 1984;6(2):130–139.

Porterfield JA, DeRosa C. *Mechanical Low Back Pain: Perspectives in Functional Anatomy*. Philadelphia, Pa: WB Saunders Co; 1991.

Saudek CE, Palmer KA. Back pain revisited. *J Orthop Sports Phys Ther*. 1987;8:556.

Sullivan MS. Back support mechanisms during manual lifting. *Phys Ther*. 1989;96(1):38–45.

Thomas JE. *Chiropractic Manual of Low Back and Leg Pain*. Norwalk, Conn: Appleton & Lange; 1991.

Tollison CD, Kriegel ML, eds. *Interdisciplinary Rehabilitation of Low Back Pain*. Baltimore, Md: Williams & Wilkins; 1989.

Twomey LT, Taylor JR, eds. *Physical Therapy of the Low Back* (Vol 13, *Clinics in Physical Therapy*). New York, NY: Churchill Livingstone; 1987.

Waddell G. A new clinical model for the treatment of low-back pain. *Spine*. 1987;12:632–644.

White AH, Anderson R, eds. *The Conservative Care of Low Back Pain*. Baltimore, Md: Williams & Wilkins; 1991.

YMCA of the USA. *Y's Way to a Healthy Back*. Champaign, Ill: Human Kinetics Publishers, Inc; 1991.

Zacharkow D. *The Healthy Lower Back: Laying the Foundation Through Proper Lifting, Sitting and Exercise*. Springfield, Ill: Charles C Thomas Publisher; 1984.

Zacharkow D. *Posture: Sitting, Standing, Chair Design and Exercise*. Springfield, Ill: Charles C Thomas Publisher; 1988.

Muscular Strength and Endurance—Exercise Prescription

Abraham WM. Exercise-induced muscle soreness. *Physician Sportsmed*. 1979;7(10):57.

Arendt EA. Strength development: A comparison of resistive exercise techniques. *Contemp Orthop*. 1984;9:67–72.

Armstrong RB. Mechanisms of exercise-induced delayed onset muscular soreness: A brief review. *Med Sci Sports Exerc*. 1984;16:529.

Auble TE, Schwartz L, Robertson RJ. Aerobic requirements for moving handweights through various ranges of motion while walking. *Physician Sportsmed*. 1987;15:133–140.

Byrnes WC, Clarkson PM, White JS, et al. Delayed onset muscle soreness following repeated bouts of downhill running. *J Appl Physiol*. 1985;59:710.

Dudley GA, Djamil R. Incompatibility of endurance and strength training modes of exercise. *J Appl Physiol, Respiratory, Environmental and Exerc Physiol*. 1985;59:1336–1451.

Dvir Z. Clinical applicability of isokinetics: A review. *Clin Biomech*. 1991;6(3):133–144.

Enoka RM. Muscle strength and its development: New perspectives. *Sports Med*. 1988;6:146–168.

Falkel JE, Sawka MN, Levine L, et al. Upper to lower body muscular strength and endurance ratios for women and men. *Ergonomics*. 1985;28:1661–1670.

Fleck SJ, Falkel JE. Value of resistance training for the reduction of sports injuries. *Sports Med*. 1986;3:61–68.

Fleck SJ, Kraemer WJ. Resistance training: Basic principles (Part 1 of 4). *Physician Sportsmed*. 1988;16(3):160.

Fleck SJ, Kraemer WJ. Resistance training: Physiological responses and adaptations (Part 2 of 4). *Physician Sportsmed*. 1988;16(4):108.

Fleck SJ, Kraemer WJ. Resistance training: Physiological responses and adaptations (Part 3 of 4). *Physician Sportsmed*. 1988;16(5):63.

Fleck SJ, Kraemer WJ. Resistance training: Exercise prescription (Part 4 of 4). *Physician Sportsmed*. 1988;16(6):69.

Fleck SJ, Schutt R. Types of strength training. *Clin Sports Med*. 1985;4:159–168.

Foran B. Advantages and disadvantages of isokinetics, variable resistance and free weights. *Nat Strength Condit Assoc J*. 1985;7(1):24–25.

Francis KT. Delayed muscle soreness: A review. *J Orthop Sports Phys Ther*. 1983;5:10.

Fry AC. The effect of weight training on the heart. *Nat Strength Condit Assoc J*. 1986;8(4):38–41.

Graves JE, Martin AD, Miltenberger LA, et al. Physiological responses to walking with hand weights, wrist weights and ankle weights. *Med Sci Sports Exerc*. 1988;20:265–271.

Graves JE, Pollock ML, Leggett SH, et al. Effect of reduced training frequency on muscular strength. *Int J Sports Med*. 1988;9:316–319.

Graves JE, Pollock ML, Montain SJ, et al. The effect of hand-held weights on the physiological responses to walking exercise. *Med Sci Sports Exerc*. 1987;19:260–265.

Graves JE, Sagiv ME, Pollock ML, et al. Effects of hand-held weights and wrist weights on metabolic and hemodynamic responses to submaximal exercise in hypertensive responders. *J Cardiopul Rehabil*. 1988;8:134–140.

Harman EA, Rosenstein RM, Frykman PN, et al. Effects of a belt on intra-abdominal pressure during weight lifting. *Med Sci Sports Exerc*. 1989;21:186–190.

Haslam DR, McCartney N, McKelvie RS, et al. Direct measurements of arterial blood pressure during formal weight lifting in cardiac patients. *J Cardiopul Rehabil*. 1988;8:213–225.

Hettinger T. *Physiology of Strength*. Springfield, Ill: Charles C Thomas Publisher; 1961.

Jacobson BH, Kulling FA. Effect of resistive weight training in prepubescents. *J Orthop Sports Phys Ther*. 1989;11(3):96–99.

Karpovich PV. *Physiology of Muscular Activity*. Philadelphia, Pa: WB Saunders Co; 1959.

Kraemer WJ, Deschenes M, Fleck SJ. Physiological adaptations to resistance exercise: Implications for athletic conditioning. *Sports Med.* 1988;6:246–256.

Kraemer WJ, Fleck SJ, Deschenes M. A review: Factors in exercise prescription of resistance training. *Nat Strength Condit Assoc J.* 1988;10(5):36–41.

Lander JE, Simonton RL, Giacobbe JKF. The effectiveness of weight-belts during the squat exercise. *Med Sci Sports Exerc.* 1990;22(1):117–126.

MacDougall JD, Tuxen D, Sale DG, et al. Arterial blood pressure responses to heavy resistance exercise. *J Appl Physiol.* 1985;58:785–790.

McGlynn G. *Dynamics of Fitness: A Practical Approach.* 2nd ed. Dubuque, Iowa: Wm C Brown Publishers; 1990.

Moffroid MT, Whipple RH. Specificity of speed of exercise. *Phys Ther.* 1970;50:1699–1704.

Moran G, McGlynn G. *Dynamics of Strength Training.* Dubuque, Iowa: Wm C Brown Publishers; 1990.

Müller EA. Influence of training and of inactivity on muscle strength. *Arch Phys Med Rehabil.* 1970;51:449–462.

National Strength and Conditioning Association. Roundtable—Determining factors of strength (Part 1). *Nat Strength Condit Assoc J.* 1985;7(1):10.

National Strength and Conditioning Association. Roundtable—Determining factors of strength (Part 2). *Nat Strength Condit Assoc J.* 1985;7(2):10.

National Strength and Conditioning Association. Roundtable—Cardiovascular effects of weight training. *Nat Strength Condit Assoc J.* 1987;9(2):10.

National Strength and Conditioning Association. Roundtable—Breathing during weight training. *Nat Strength Condit Assoc J.* 1987;9(5):17–25.

National Strength and Conditioning Association. Position paper: Strength training for female athletes (Part 1). *Nat Strength Condit Assoc J.* 1989;11(4):43–55.

National Strength and Conditioning Association. Position paper: Strength training for female athletes (Part 2). *Nat Strength Condit Assoc J.* 1989;11(5):29–36.

O'Shea P. *Scientific Principles and Methods of Strength and Fitness.* 2nd ed. Reading, Mass: Addison-Wesley Publishing Co; 1976.

Palmieri GA. Weight training and repetition speed. *J Appl Sport Sci Res.* 1987;1(2):36–38.

Panariello RA. The closed kinetic chain in strength training. *Nat Strength Condit Assoc J.* 1991;13(1):29–33.

Petrofsky JS. *Isometric Exercise and its Clinical Implications.* Springfield, Ill: Charles C Thomas Publisher; 1982.

Riley DP. *Strength Training by the Experts.* 2nd ed. Champaign, Ill: Human Kinetics Publishers, Inc; 1982.

Rutherford OM, Jones DA. The role of learning and coordination in strength training. *Eur J Appl Physiol.* 1986;55:100.

Sale DG. Neural adaptation to resistance training. *Med Sci Sports Exerc.* 1988;20:S135–S145.

Sapega AA. Current concepts review: Muscle performance evaluation in orthopaedic practice. *J Bone Joint Surg (Am).* 1990;72-A(10):1562–1574.

Sawka MN. Physiology of upper body exercise. In: Pandolf KB, ed. *Exercise and Sport Sciences Reviews.* New York, NY: Macmillan Publishing Co; 1986;14.

Seliger V, Dolejs L, Kares V. A dynamometric comparison of maximum eccentric, concentric and isometric contractions using emg and energy expenditure measurements. *Eur J Appl Physiol.* 1980;45:235.

Smith MJ, Melton P. Isokinetic versus isotonic variable-resistance training. *Am J Sports Med.* 1981;9:275–279.

Talag TS. Residual muscular soreness influenced by concentric, eccentric and static contractions. *Res Q.* 1973;44:458.

Temkin LP. Isometric exercise: A danger or a benefit? *Ariz Med.* 1986;6:380–383.

Thorstensson A. Observations on strength training and detraining. *Acta Physiol Scand.* 1977;100:491.

Zarandora JE, Nelson AG, Conlee RK, et al. Physiological responses to hand-carried weights. *Physician Sportsmed.* 1986;14:113–120.

Muscular Strength and Endurance Testing

Anderson T, Kearney JT. Muscular strength and absolute and relative endurance. *Res Q Exerc Sport.* 1982;53:1–7.

Andrews AW. Hand-held dynamometry for measuring muscle strength. *J Hum Muscle Perform.* 1991;1(1):35–50.

Baltzopoulos V, Brodie DA. Isokinetic dynamometry: Applications and limitations. *Sports Med.* 1989;8:101–116.

Bohannon RW. The clinical measurement of strength. *Clin Rehabil.* 1987;1:5–16.

Bohannon RW. Make tests and break tests of elbow flexor muscle strength. *Phys Ther.* 1988;68:193–194.

Bohannon RW, Smith MB. Differentiation of maximal and submaximal knee extension efforts by isokinetic testing. *Clin Biomech.* 1988;3:215–218.

Bosco C, Mognoni P, Luhtanen P. Relationship between isokinetic performance and ballistic movement. *Eur J Appl Physiol.* 1983;51:357–364.

Burnie J, Brodie DA. Isokinetics in the assessment of rehabilitation: A case report. *Clin Biomech.* 1986;1:140–145.

Delitto A. Isokinetic dynamometry. *Muscle Nerve.* 1990;13:S53–S57.

Fess E. The effects of Jamar dynamometer handle position and test protocol on normal grip strength. *J Hand Surg.* 1982;7:308.

Fess E. A method for checking Jamar dynamometer calibration. *J Hand Ther.* 1987;1:28.

Gilbert JC, Knowlton RG. Simple method to determine the sincerity of effort during a maximal isometric test of grip strength. *Am J Phys Med.* 1983;62:135–144.

Hildreth DH, Briendenback WC, Lister GD, et al. Detection of submaximal effort by use of rapid exchange grip. *J Hand Surg.* 1989;14A:742–745.

Hinson MN, Smith WC, Funk S. Isokinetics: A clarification. *Res Q.* 1979;50:30–35.

Knapik JJ, Right JE, Mawdsley RH, et al. Isokinetic, isometric and isotonic strength relationships. *Arch Phys Med Rehabil.* 1983;64:77–80.

Kroemer KHE, Howard JM. Towards standardization of muscle strength testing. *Med Sci Sports.* 1970;2:224–230.

Mendell JR, Florence J. Manual muscle testing. *Muscle Nerve.* 1990;13:S16–S20.

Osternig LR. Isokinetic dynamometry: Implications for muscle testing and rehabilitation. In: Pandolf KB, ed. *Exercise and Sport Sciences Reviews.* New York, NY: Macmillan Publishing Co; 1986;14.

Patterson R. Muscle testing and therapeutic exercise in rehabilitation. In: Webster JG, ed. *Encyclopedia of Medical Devices and Instrumentation.* New York, NY: John Wiley & Sons; 1988.

Patterson R, Amundsen L, Baxter T, et al. A system for testing isometric muscle strength, endurance and response time. In: *Physical Medicine and Rehabilitation: State of the Art Reviews.* Philadelphia, Pa: Hanley & Belfus; 1989;3(2).

Petrofsky JS. *Isometric Exercise and Its Clinical Implications.* Springfield, Ill: Charles C Thomas Publisher; 1982.

Pytel LJ, Kamon E. Dynamic strength testing as a predictor for maximal lifting. *Ergonomics.* 1981;24:663–672.

Saunders NE, Bohannon RW. Can feigned maximal efforts be distinguished from maximal efforts? *J Hum Muscle Perform.* 1991;1(1):16–24.

Simonson E, ed. *Physiology of Work Capacity and Fatigue.* Springfield, Ill: Charles C Thomas Publisher; 1971.

Smith GA, Nelson RC, Sadoff SJ, et al. Assessing sincerity of effort in maximal grip strength tests. *Am J Phys Med Rehabil.* 1989;68:73–80.

Solgaard S, Kristiansen B, Jensen JS. Evaluation of instruments for measuring grip strength. *Acta Orthop Scand.* 1984;55:569.

Thorngren KG, Werner CO. Normal grip strength. *Acta Orthop Scand.* 1979;50:255.

Tornvall G. Assessment of physical capabilities. *Acta Physiol Scand.* 1963;58(Suppl 201).

Watkins MP, Harris BA. Evaluation of isokinetic muscle performance. *Clin Sports Med.* 1983;2:37–53.

Winter DA, Wells RP, Orr GW. Errors in the use of isokinetic dynamometers. *Eur J Appl Physiol.* 1981;46:397–408.

Nutrition

American Dietetic Association. Position Paper: Sports nutrition. Chicago, Ill: American Dietetic Association; 1986.

American Dietetic Association. Position Paper: Nutrition for physical fitness and athletic performance for adults. Chicago, Ill: American Dietetic Association; 1987.

American Dietetic Association. Position Paper: Vegetarian diet. Chicago, Ill: American Dietetic Association; 1988.

Belko AZ. Vitamins and exercise—An update. *Med Sci Sports Exerc.* 1987;19(Suppl):S191–S196.

Berning J, Steen SN. *Sports Nutrition: The Health Professional's Handbook*. Gaithersburg, Md: Aspen Publishers, Inc; 1991.

Bursztein S, Elwyn DH, Askanazi J, et al. *Energy Metabolism, Indirect Calorimetry and Nutrition*. Baltimore, Md: Williams & Wilkins; 1989.

Clark N. *Nancy Clark's Sports Nutrition Guidebook*. Champaign, Ill: Human Kinetics Publishers, Inc; 1990.

Coleman E. *Eating for Endurance*. Palo Alto, Calif: Bull Publishing Co; 1988.

Ellis D, Gabel K. Weight gain guidelines for athletes. *Nat Strength Condit Assoc J*. 1991;13(3):20–23.

Feldman EB. *Essentials of Clinical Nutrition*. Philadelphia, Pa: FA Davis Co; 1988.

Forbes GB. *Human Body Composition: Growth, Aging, Nutrition and Activity*. New York, NY: Springer-Verlag; 1987.

Garner DM, Rosen LW. Eating disorders among athletes: Research and recommendations. *J Appl Sport Sci Res*. 1991;5(2):100–107.

Gines DJ. *Nutrition Management in Rehabilitation*. Gaithersburg, Md: Aspen Publishers, Inc; 1990.

Grandjean AC. The vegetarian athlete. *Physician Sportsmed*. 1987;15(5):191–194.

Grandjean AC. Sports nutrition. In: Mellion MB, Walsh WM, Shelton GL, eds. *The Team Physician's Handbook*. Philadelphia, Pa: Hanley & Belfus, Inc; 1990.

Hafen BQ. *Nutrition, Food and Weight Control*. Dubuque, Iowa: Wm C Brown Publishers; 1981.

Haskell W, Scala J, Whittam J. *Nutrition and Athletic Performance*. Palo Alto, Calif: Bull Publishing Co; 1982.

Hickson JF, Wolinsky I. *Nutrition in Exercise and Sport*. Boca Raton, Fla: CRC Press, Inc; 1989.

Hodgson P. Review of popular diets. In: Storlie J, Jordon HA, eds. *Nutrition and Exercise in Obesity Management*. New York, NY: Spectrum Publications; 1984.

Kris-Etherton PM, ed. *Cardiovascular Disease: Nutrition for Prevention and Treatment*. Chicago, Ill: American Dietetic Association; 1990.

Leaf DA. *Exercise and Nutrition in Preventive Cardiology*. Dubuque, Iowa: Brown & Benchmark; 1991.

Marderosian AD, Liberti L. *Natural Product Medicine: A Scientific Guide to Foods, Drugs, Cosmetics*. Philadelphia, Pa: JB Lippincott Co; 1988.

Pennington JAT. *Bowes and Church's Food Values of Portions Commonly Used*, 15th ed. Philadelphia, Pa: JB Lippincott Co; 1989.

Perkin JE. *Food Allergies and Adverse Reactions*. Gaithersburg, Md: Aspen Publishers, Inc; 1990.

Roe DA. *Handbook on Drug and Nutrient Interactions: A Problem-Oriented Reference Guide*. 4th ed. Chicago, Ill: American Dietetic Association; 1989.

Shils ME, Young VR. *Modern Nutrition in Health and Disease*. 7th ed. Philadelphia, Pa: Lea & Febiger; 1988.

Simko MD, Cowell C, Hreha MS. *Practical Nutrition: A Quick Reference for the Health Care Practitioner*. Gaithersburg, Md: Aspen Publishers, Inc; 1989.

Smith NJ, Worthington-Roberts BS. *Food for Sport*. Palo Alto, Calif: Bull Publishing Co; 1989.

Snetselaar LG. *Nutrition Counseling Skills: Assessment, Treatment and Evaluation*. 2nd ed. Gaithersburg, Md: Aspen Publishers, Inc; 1988.

Tribole E. *Eating on the Run*. 2nd ed. Champaign, Ill: Human Kinetics Publishers, Inc; 1992.

Van Der Leeden F, Troise FL, Todd DK. *The Water Encyclopedia*. 2nd ed. Boca Raton, Fla: CRC Press, Inc; 1990.

Williams MH. *Nutrition Aspects of Human Physical and Athletic Performance*. 2nd ed. Springfield, Ill: Charles C Thomas Publisher; 1985.

Williams MH. *Nutrition for Fitness and Sport*. 2nd ed. Dubuque, Iowa: Wm C Brown Publishers; 1988.

Wilmore JH, Freund BJ. Nutritional enhancement of athletic performance. *Nutr Ab Rev*. 1984;54(1):1–16.

Obesity and Weight Control

Bjorntorp P, Brodoff B. *Obesity*. Philadelphia, Pa: JB Lippincott Co; 1991.

Brownell KD, Rodin J, Wilmore J, eds. *Eating, Body Weight and Performance in Athletes: Disorders of Modern Society*. Baltimore, Md: Williams & Wilkins; 1992.

Buskirk ER. Obesity. In: Skinner JS. *Exercise Testing and Exercise Prescription for Special Cases: Theoretical Basis and Clinical Application*. Philadelphia, Pa: Lea & Febiger; 1987.

Clark KL, Parr RB, Castelli WP, eds. *Evaluation and Management of Eating Disorders: Anorexia, Bulimia and Obesity*. Champaign, Ill: Human Kinetics Publishers, Inc; 1988.

Cotterman SK. *Y's Way to Weight Management*. Champaign, Ill: Human Kinetics Publishers, Inc; 1985.

Edwards TL, Lau B. *Weight Loss to Super Wellness*. 2nd ed. Champaign, Ill: Human Kinetics Publishers, Inc; 1988.

Eisenman PA, Johnson SC, Benson JE. *Coaches Guide to Nutrition and Weight Control*. 2nd ed. Champaign, Ill: Human Kinetics Publishers, Inc; 1990.

Ferguson JM. *Habits Not Diets: The Secret to Lifetime Weight Control*. Palo Alto, Calif: Bull Publishing Co; 1988.

Frankle RT, Yang MU. *Obesity and Weight Control: The Health Professional's Guide to Understanding and Treatment*. Gaithersburg, Md: Aspen Publishers, Inc; 1988.

Ikeda J. *Winning Weight Loss for Teens*. Palo Alto, Calif: Bull Publishing Co; 1987.

Kingsbury BD. *Full Figure Fitness: A Program for Teaching Overweight Adults*. Champaign, Ill: Human Kinetics Publishers, Inc; 1988.

Krasnegor NA, Grave GD, Kretchmer N. *Childhood Obesity: A Biobehavioral Perspective*. Boca Raton, Fla: CRC Press, Inc; 1990.

Lampman RM, Schteingart DE. Moderate and extreme obesity. In: Franklin BA, Gordon S, Timmis GC, eds. *Exercise in Modern Medicine*. Baltimore, Md: Williams & Wilkins; 1989.

LeBow MD. *The Thin Plan*. Champaign, Ill: Human Kinetics Publishers, Inc; 1988.

Lyons P, Burgard D. *Great Shape: The First Fitness Guide for Large Women*. Palo Alto, Calif: Bull Publishing Co; 1990.

Powers PS. *Obesity: The Regulation of Weight*. Baltimore, Md: Williams & Wilkins; 1980.

Rotatori AF, Fox RA. *Obesity in Children and Youth: Measurement, Characteristics, Causes and Treatment*. Springfield, Ill: Charles C Thomas Publisher; 1989.

Storlie J, Jordan HA, eds. *Evaluation and Treatment of Obesity*. Champaign, Ill: Human Kinetics Publishers, Inc; 1984.

Storlie J, Jordan HA, eds. *Nutrition and Exercise in Obesity Management*. Champaign, Ill: Human Kinetics Publishers, Inc; 1984.

Storlie J, Jordan HA, eds. *Behavioral Management of Obesity*. Champaign, Ill: Human Kinetics Publishers, Inc; 1988.

Osteoporosis

Aloia JF. *Osteoporosis: A Guide to Prevention and Treatment*. Champaign, Ill: Human Kinetics Publishers, Inc; 1989.

Sinaki M, Dale DA, Hurley DL. *Living with Osteoporosis: Guidelines for Women Before and After Diagnosis*. Philadelphia, Pa: BC Decker, Inc; 1988.

Smith EL, Gilligan C. Effects of inactivity and exercise on bone. *Physician Sportsmed*. 1987;15(11):91.

Physical Education

Christina RW, Corcos DM. *Coaches Guide to Teaching Sports Skills*. Champaign, Ill: Human Kinetics Publishers, Inc; 1988.

Clegg R, Thompson WA. *Modern Sports Officiating: A Practical Guide*. 4th ed. Dubuque, Iowa: Wm C Brown Publishers; 1989.

Cylkowski GJ. *Developing a Career in Sports and Athletics*. Longmeadow, Mass: Mouvement Publications Inc; 1987.

Jones BJ, Wells LJ, Peters RE, et al. *Guide to Effective Coaching: Principles and Practice*. 2nd ed. Dubuque, Iowa: Wm C Brown Publishers; 1988.

Knuttgen HG, Qiwei M, Zhongyuan W, eds. *Sport in China*. Champaign, Ill: Human Kinetics Publishers, Inc; 1990.

Martens R. *Successful Coaching*. 2nd ed. Champaign, Ill: Human Kinetics Publishers, Inc; 1990.

Pate RR, McClenaghan B, Rotella, R. *Scientific Foundations of Coaching*. Dubuque, Iowa: Wm C Brown Publishers; 1984.

Seidel BL, Biles FR, Figley GE, et al. *Sports Skills: A Conceptual Approach to Meaningful Movement*. 2nd ed. Dubuque, Iowa: Wm C Brown Publishers; 1980.

Spears B, Swanson RA. *History of Sport and Physical Education in the United States*. 3rd ed. Dubuque, Iowa: Wm C Brown Publishers; 1989.

Voy R. *Drugs, Sport and Politics*. Champaign, Ill: Human Kinetics Publishers, Inc; 1991.

White JR, ed. *Sports Rules Encyclopedia*. Champaign, Ill: Human Kinetics Publishers, Inc; 1990.

Physiologic Calculations

Adams WC. Influence of age, sex and body weight on energy expenditure in bicycle riding. *J Appl Physiol.* 1967;22: 539–545.

Claremont A, Reddan WG, Smith EL. Metabolic costs and feasibility of water support exercises for the elderly. In: Nagle FJ, Montoye HJ, eds. *Exercise in Health and Disease.* Springfield, Ill: Charles C Thomas Publisher; 1981.

Dill DB. Oxygen use in horizontal and grade walking and running on the treadmill. *J Appl Physiol.* 1965;20:19–22.

Katch VL, Villanacci JF, Sady SP. Energy costs of rebound-running. *Res Q Exerc Sport.* 1981;52:269–272.

Knuttgen HG. Force, work, power and exercise. *Med Sci Sports.* 1978;10:227–228.

Souci SW. *Food Composition and Nutrition Tables.* 4th ed. Boca Raton, Fla: CRC Press, Inc; 1990.

Pregnancy

American College of Obstetricians and Gynecologists. Exercise during pregnancy and the postnatal period (ACOG Home Exercise Programs). Washington, DC: American College of Obstetricians and Gynecologists; 1985.

Artal LR, Masaki DI, Khodiguian N, et al. Exercise prescription in pregnancy: Weight-bearing versus non-weight-bearing exercise. *Am J Obstet Gynecol.* 1989;161:1464–1469.

Clapp JF. Pregnancy. In: Franklin BA, Gordon S, Timmis GC, eds. *Exercise in Modern Medicine.* Baltimore, Md: Williams & Wilkins; 1989.

Egbert BJ. *A Handbook of Physical Conditioning for Pregnant Women.* Worthington, Ohio: Publishing Horizons, Inc; 1985.

Freyder SC. Exercising while pregnant. *J Orthop Sports Phys Ther.* 1989;10(9):358–365.

Holstein BB. *Shaping Up for a Healthy Pregnancy.* Champaign, Ill: Human Kinetics Publishers, Inc; 1988.

Knuttgen HG. Pregnancy. In: Skinner JS. *Exercise Testing and Exercise Prescription for Special Cases: Theoretical Basis and Clinical Application.* Philadelphia, Pa: Lea & Febiger; 1987.

Mittelmark RA, Wiswell RA, Drinkwater BL, eds. *Exercise in Pregnancy.* 2nd ed. Baltimore, Md: Williams & Wilkins; 1991.

Winick M. *Nutrition, Pregnancy and Early Infancy.* Baltimore, Md: Williams & Wilkins; 1989.

Worthington-Roberts BS, Williams SR. *Nutrition in Pregnancy and Lactation.* 4th ed. St Louis, Mo: CV Mosby Co; 1989.

Sport Performance—Exercise Prescription

Baechle TR, Groves BR. *Weight Training: Steps to Success.* Champaign, Ill: Human Kinetics Publishers, Inc; 1992.

Behm DG. Surgical tubing for sport and velocity specific training. *Nat Strength Condit Assoc J.* 1988;10(4):66–70.

Benyo R. *The Exercise Fix.* Champaign, Ill: Human Kinetics Publishers, Inc; 1990.

Blackmore C, Hawkes N, Burton E. *Drill to Skill: Teacher Tactics in Physical Education.* Dubuque, Iowa: Wm C Brown Publishers; 1991.

Chu DA. *Jumping into Plyometrics.* Champaign, Ill: Human Kinetics Publishers, Inc; 1992.

Colwin CM. *Swimming into the 21st Century.* Champaign, Ill: Human Kinetics Publishers, Inc; 1992.

Costill DL, Maglischo EW, Richardson AB. *Swimming (Handbook of Sports Medicine and Science).* Champaign, Ill: Human Kinetics Publishers, Inc; 1992.

Dintiman G. The effects of various training programs on running speed. *Res Q.* 1964;35:456–463.

Dintiman G. *Sprinting Speed: Its Improvement for Major Sports Competition.* Springfield, Ill: Charles C Thomas Publisher; 1970.

Garhammer J. Power production by Olympic lifters. *Med Sci Sports Exerc.* 1980;12:54.

Komi PV, ed. *Strength and Power in Sport (The Encyclopedia of Sports Medicine).* Boston, Mass: Blackwell Scientific Publications; 1992.

Leighton JR. *Fitness, Body Development and Sports Conditioning Through Weight Training.* 2nd ed. Springfield, Ill: Charles C Thomas Publisher; 1983.

Leonard J. *Science of Coaching Swimming.* Champaign, Ill: Human Kinetics Publishers, Inc; 1992.

McFarlane B. Warm-up pattern design. *Nat Strength Condit Assoc J.* 1987;9(4):22–29.

McIntosh M. *Lifetime Aerobics.* Dubuque, Iowa: Wm C Brown Publishers; 1990.

Mullen KD, Gold RS, Belcastro PA, et al. *Connections for Health*. 2nd ed. Dubuque, Iowa: Wm C Brown Publishers; 1990.

Shephard RJ, Åstrand P-O, eds. *Endurance in Sport (The Encyclopedia of Sports Medicine)*. Champaign, Ill: Human Kinetics Publishers, Inc; 1992.

Simon HB, Levisohn SR. *The Athlete Within: A Personal Guide to Total Fitness*. Boston, Mass: Little, Brown and Company; 1987.

Sleamaker R. *Serious Training for Serious Athletes*. Champaign, Ill: Human Kinetics Publishers, Inc; 1989.

Timmer CAW. Cycling biomechanics: A literature review. *J Orthop Sports Phys Ther*. 1991;14(3):106–113.

Yacenda J. *Alpine Skiing: Steps to Success*. Champaign, Ill: Human Kinetics Publishers, Inc; 1992.

Sport Performance Testing

Altuğ Z, Altuğ T, Altuğ A. A test selection guide for assessing and evaluating athletes. *Nat Strength Condit Assoc J*. 1987;9(3):62–66.

Dainty DA, Norman RW, eds. *Standardizing Biomechanical Testing in Sport*. Champaign, Ill: Human Kinetics Publishers, Inc; 1987.

Hastad DN, Lacy AC. *Measurement and Evaluation in Contemporary Physical Education*. Scottsdale, Ariz: Gorsuch Scarisbrick; 1989.

Sport Psychology

Bunker LK, Rotella RJ. *Sports Psychology: Psychological Considerations in Maximizing Sport Performance*. Longmeadow, Mass: Mouvement Publications, Inc; 1984.

Cox RH. *Sport Psychology: Concepts and Applications*. 2nd ed. Dubuque, Iowa: Wm C Brown Publishers; 1990.

Hendrickson TP, Rowe SJ. The role of sports psychology/psychiatry. In: Mellion MB, Walsh WM, and Shelton GL, eds. *The Team Physician's Handbook*. Philadelphia, Pa: Hanley & Belfus, Inc; 1990.

Martens R, Vealey RS, Burton D. *Competitive Anxiety in Sport*. Champaign, Ill: Human Kinetics Publishers, Inc; 1990.

Orlick T. *In Pursuit of Excellence: How to Win in Sport and Life Through Mental Training*. Champaign, Ill: Human Kinetics Publishers, Inc; 1990.

Ostrow AC, ed. *Directory of Psychological Tests in the Sport and Exercise Sciences*. Morgantown, WVa: Fitness Information Technology, Inc; 1990.

Roberts GC. *Motivation in Sport and Exercise*. Champaign, Ill: Human Kinetics Publishers, Inc; 1992.

Sports Medicine

Adams S, Adrian M, Bayless MA, eds. *Catastrophic Injuries in Sports: Avoidance Strategies*. 2nd ed. Dubuque, Iowa: Brown & Benchmark; 1987.

American Academy of Orthopaedic Surgeons. *Athletic Training and Sports Medicine*. 2nd ed. Park Ridge, Ill: American Academy of Orthopaedic Surgeons; 1991.

Andrews JR, Harrelson GL. *Physical Rehabilitation of the Injured Athlete*. Philadelphia, Pa: WB Saunders Co; 1991.

Arnheim D. *Essentials of Athletic Training*. 2nd ed. St Louis, Mo: Mosby-Year Book; 1991.

Bergeron JD, Greene H. *Coaches Guide to Sport Injuries*. Champaign, Ill: Human Kinetics Publishers, Inc; 1989.

Bernhardt DB, ed. *Sports Physical Therapy (Clinics in Physical Therapy)*. New York, NY: Churchill Livingstone; 1986;10.

Bloomfield J, Fricker PA, Fitch KD, eds. *Textbook of Science and Medicine in Sport*. Champaign, Ill: Human Kinetics Publishers, Inc; 1992.

Booher JM, Thibodeau GA. *Athletic Injury Assessment*. 2nd ed. St Louis, Mo: Mosby-Year Book; 1989.

Bunker TD, Wallace WA. *Shoulder Arthroscopy*. St Louis, Mo: Mosby-Year Book; 1991.

Cantu RC, Micheli LJ, eds. *ACSM Guidelines for the Team Physician*. Philadelphia, Pa: Lea & Febiger; 1991.

Casey MJ, Foster C, Hixson EG, eds. *Winter Sports Medicine*. Philadelphia, Pa: FA Davis Co; 1990;3.

Croce P. *The Baseball Player's Guide to Sports Medicine*. Champaign, Ill: Human Kinetics Publishers, Inc; 1987.

Cross MJ, Crichton KJ. *Clinical Examination of the Injured Knee*. Baltimore, Md: Williams & Wilkins; 1987.

D'Ambrosia RD, Drez D, eds. *Prevention and Treatment of Running Injuries*. 2nd ed. Thorofare, NJ: SLACK, Inc; 1989.

Dirix A, Knuttgen HG, Tittel K, eds. *The Olympic Book of Sports Medicine (Encyclopedia of Sports Medicine)*. Champaign, Ill: Human Kinetics Publishers, Inc; 1988;1.

Firooznia H, Golimbu CN, Rafii M, et al. *MRI and CT of the Musculoskeletal System*. St Louis, Mo: Mosby-Year Book; 1992.

Flegel MJ. *Sport First Aid*. Champaign, Ill: Human Kinetics Publishers, Inc; 1992.

Garrick JG, Webb DR. *Sports Injuries: Diagnosis and Management*. Philadelphia, Pa: WB Saunders Co; 1990.

Gates SJ, Mooar PA, eds. *Orthopaedics and Sports Medicine for Nurses*. Baltimore, Md: Williams & Wilkins; 1989.

Grana WA, Lomardo JA, Sharkey BJ, et al, eds. *Advances in Sports Medicine and Fitness*. Chicago, Ill: Year Book Medical Publishers, Inc; 1988;1.

Grana WA, Lomardo JA, Sharkey BJ, et al, eds. *Advances in Sports Medicine and Fitness*. Chicago, Ill: Year Book Medical Publishers, Inc; 1990;3.

Griffith HW. *Complete Guide to Sports Injuries*. Philadelphia, Pa: Lea & Febiger; 1986.

Grisogono V, ed. *Sports Injuries (International Perspectives in Physical Trauma)*. New York, NY: Churchill Livingstone; 1989.

Hochschuler SH. *The Spine in Sports*. St Louis, Mo: Mosby–Year Book; 1990.

Hossler P. *Handbook of Athletic Training*. Longmeadow, Mass: Mouvement Publications, Inc; 1984.

Jokl E. *Sudden Death of Athletes*. Springfield, Ill: Charles C Thomas Publisher; 1985.

Jordon BD, Tsairis P, Warren RF. *Sports Neurology*. Gaithersburg, Md: Aspen Publishers, Inc; 1989.

Kuprian W, ed. *Physical Therapy for Sports*. Philadelphia, Pa: WB Saunders Co; 1982.

McLatchie GR, ed. *Essentials of Sports Medicine*. New York, NY: Churchill Livingstone; 1986.

Mellion MB. *Office Management of Sports Injuries and Athletic Problems*. Philadelphia, Pa: Hanley and Belfus, Inc; 1987.

Mercier LR, Pettid FJ, Tamisiea DF, et al. *Practical Orthopedics*. 3rd ed. St Louis, Mo: Mosby–Year Book; 1991.

Millar AP. *Sports Injuries and Their Management*. Philadelphia, Pa: FA Davis Co; 1987.

Moore JR, Wade G. Prevention of anterior cruciate ligament injuries. *Nat Strength Condit Assoc J*. 1989;11(3):35–40.

Morris AF. *Sports Medicine: Prevention of Athletic Injuries*. Dubuque, Iowa: Wm C Brown Publishers; 1984.

Moseley JB, Jobe FW, Pink M, et al. EMG analysis of the scapular muscles during a shoulder rehabilitation program. *Am J Sports Med*. 1992;20(2):128–134.

Mueller FO, Ryan AJ, eds. *Prevention of Athletic Injuries: The Role of the Sports Medicine Team*. Philadelphia, Pa: FA Davis Co; 1991;4.

National Collegiate Athletic Association. *NCAA Sports Medicine Handbook*. Overland Park, Kan; National Collegiate Athletic Association; 1992.

Nicholas JA, Hershman EB, eds. *The Lower Extremity and Spine in Sports Medicine*. St Louis, Mo: Mosby–Year Book; 1986;1,2.

Nicholas JA, Hershman EB, Posner MA, eds. *The Upper Extremity in Sports Medicine*. St Louis, Mo: Mosby–Year Book; 1990.

Nieman DC. *Fitness and Sports Medicine: An Introduction*. 2nd ed. Palo Alto, Calif: Bull Publishing Co; 1990.

O'Donoghue DH. *Treatment of Injuries to Athletes*. 4th ed. Philadelphia, Pa: WB Saunders Co; 1984.

Peterson L, Renstrom P. *Sports Injuries: Their Prevention and Treatment*. St Louis, Mo: Mosby–Year Book; 1986.

Philipp JA, Wilkerson JD. *Teaching Team Sports: A Coeducational Approach*. Champaign, Ill: Human Kinetics Publishers, Inc; 1990.

Prentice WE, ed. *Rehabilitation Techniques in Sports Medicine*. St Louis, Mo: Mosby–Year Book; 1990.

Prentice WE. *Therapeutic Modalities in Sports Medicine*. 2nd ed. St Louis, Mo: Mosby–Year Book; 1990.

Reid DC. *Sports Injury Assessment and Rehabilitation*. New York, NY: Churchill Livingstone; 1992.

Reider B, ed. *Sports Medicine: The School-Age Athlete*. Philadelphia, Pa: WB Saunders Co; 1991.

Ritter MA, Albohm MJ. *Your Injury: A Common Sense Guide to Sports Injuries*. Dubuque, Iowa: Brown & Benchmark; 1987.

Roy S, Irvin R. *Sports Medicine Prevention, Evaluation, Management and Rehabilitation*. Englewood Cliffs, NJ: Prentice-Hall; 1983.

Sataloff RT, Brandfonbrener AG, Lederman RJ, eds. *Textbook of Performing Arts*. New York, NY: Raven Press; 1990.

Schneider RC, Kennedy JC, Plant ML. *Sports Injuries: Mechanisms, Prevention and Treatment*. Baltimore, Md: Williams & Wilkins; 1985.

Scott WN. *Ligament and Extensor Mechanism Injuries of the Knee: Diagnosis and Treatment*. St Louis, Mo: Mosby–Year Book; 1991.

Scott WN, Nisonson B, Nicholas JA. *Principles of Sports Medicine*. Baltimore, Md: Williams & Wilkins; 1984.

Scriber K, Burke E, ed. *Relevant Topics in Athletic Training*. Longmeadow, Mass: Mouvement Publications, Inc; 1978.

Shields CL, ed. *Manual of Sports Surgery*. New York, NY: Springer-Verlag; 1987.

Smith NJ. *Common Problems in Pediatric Sports Medicine*. St Louis, Mo: Mosby–Year Book; 1988.

Smith NJ, Stanitski CL. *Sports Medicine: A Practical Guide*. Philadelphia, Pa: WB Saunders Co; 1987.

Strauss RH. *Sports Medicine*. Philadelphia, Pa: WB Saunders Co; 1984.

Subotnick SI. *Sports Medicine of the Lower Extremity*. New York, NY: Churchill Livingstone; 1988.

Sutton G. Hamstrung by hamstring strains: A review of the literature. *J Orthop Sports Phys Ther*. 1984;5(4):184–195.

Sutton JR, Brock RM, eds. *Sports Medicine for the Mature Athlete*. Dubuque, Iowa: Brown & Benchmark; 1986.

Taylor PM, Taylor DK. *Conquering Athletic Injuries*. Champaign, Ill: Human Kinetics Publishers, Inc; 1988.

Teitz CC. *Scientific Foundations of Sports Medicine*. Philadelphia, Pa: BC Decker, Inc; 1989.

Tippett SR. *Coaches Guide to Sport Rehabilitation*. Champaign, Ill: Human Kinetics Publishers, Inc; 1990.

Torg JS. *Athletic Injuries to the Head, Neck and Face*. 2nd ed. St Louis, Mo: Mosby–Year Book; 1991.

Torg JS, Vegso JJ, Torg E. *Rehabilitation of Athletic Injuries: An Atlas of Therapeutic Exercise*. Chicago, Ill: Year Book Medical Publishers, Inc; 1987.

Townsend H, Jobe FW, Pink M, et al. Electromyographic analysis of the glenohumeral muscles during a baseball rehabilitation program. *Am J Sports Med*. 1991;19(3):264–272.

Wilk KE, Keirns MA, Andrews JR, et al. Anterior cruciate ligament reconstruction rehabilitation: A six-month follow-up of isokinetic testing in recreational athletes. *Isokinetics and Exercise Science*. 1991;1(1):36–43.

Williams JGP. *Diagnostic Picture Tests in Injury in Sport*. St Louis, Mo: Mosby–Year Book; 1988.

Williams LA, Evans RC, Shirley PD. *Imaging of Sports Injuries*. Philadelphia, Pa: WB Saunders Co; 1989.

Wolpa ME. *The Sports Medicine Guide: Treating and Preventing Common Athletic Injuries*. Champaign, Ill: Human Kinetics Publishers, Inc; 1982.

Zarins B, Andrews JR, Carson WG. *Injuries to the Throwing Arm*. Philadelphia, Pa: WB Saunders Co; 1985.

Stress and Pain Management

Bonica JJ. *Management of Pain*. 2nd ed. Philadelphia, Pa: Lea & Febiger; 1989.

Greenberg JS. *Comprehensive Stress Management*. 3rd ed. Dubuque, Iowa: Wm C Brown Publishers; 1990.

Muse M, LeFew B, Shafiei M, et al. *Exercise for the Chronic Pain Patient*. Longmeadow, Mass: Mouvement Publications, Inc; 1984.

Travell JG. *Myofascial Pain and Dysfunction: The Trigger Point Manual (Vol 2)*. Baltimore, Md: Williams & Wilkins; 1991.

Wells PE, Frampton V, Bowsher D. *Pain Management in Physical Therapy*. Norwalk, Conn: Appleton & Lange; 1988.

Therapy and Rehabilitation

Basmajian JV. *Manipulation, Traction and Massage*. 3rd ed. Baltimore, Md: Williams & Wilkins; 1985.

Basmajian JV, Kirby RL. *Medical Rehabilitation*. Baltimore, Md: Williams & Wilkins; 1984.

Bauer D. *Foundations of Physical Rehabilitation: A Management Approach*. New York, NY: Churchill Livingstone; 1989.

Bordelon LR. *Surgical and Conservative Foot Care*. Thorofare, NJ: SLACK, Inc; 1988.

Bunch WH. *Scoliosis: Making Clinical Decisions*. St Louis, Mo: Mosby–Year Book; 1989.

Campion MR. *Adult Hydrotherapy: A Practical Approach*. Stoneham, Mass: Butterworth-Heinemann; 1990.

Cohen J, Bonfiglio M, Campbell CJ. *Orthopedic Pathophysiology in Diagnosis and Treatment*. New York, NY: Churchill Livingstone; 1990.

Colson JHC, Collison FW. *Progressive Exercise Therapy in Rehabilitation and Physical Education*. 4th ed. Bristol, England: John Wright and Sons; 1983.

Corrigan B, Maitland GD. *Practical Orthopaedic Medicine*. Stoneham, Mass: Butterworth-Heinemann; 1983.

Cyriax J, Coldham M. *Textbook of Orthopaedic Medicine, Vol 2, Treatment by Manipulation, Massage and Injection*. 11th ed. Philadelphia, Pa: WB Saunders Co; 1984.

Cyriax J, Cyriax P. *Illustrated Manual of Orthopaedic Medicine*. Stoneham, Mass: Butterworth-Heinemann; 1983.

Daniels L, Worthingham C. *Therapeutic Exercise for Body Alignment and Function*. 2nd ed. Philadelphia, Pa: WB Saunders Co; 1977.

DiGiovanna EL, Schiowitz S, eds. *An Osteopathic Approach to Diagnosis and Treatment*. Philadelphia, Pa: JB Lippincott Co; 1991.

Donatelli R, ed. *The Biomechanics of the Foot and Ankle*. Philadelphia, Pa: FA Davis Co; 1990;3.

Donatelli RA, ed. *Physical Therapy of the Shoulder*. 2nd ed. New York, NY: Churchill Livingstone; 1991.

Echternach JL, ed. *Physical Therapy of the Hip*. New York, NY: Churchill Livingstone; 1990.

Eder M, Tilscher H, Gengenbach M, ed. *Chiropractic Therapy: Diagnosis and Treatment*. Rockville, Md: Aspen Publishers, Inc; 1990.

Goodman CC, Snyder TEK. *Differential Diagnosis in Physical Therapy: Musculoskeletal and Systemic Conditions*. Philadelphia, Pa: WB Saunders Co; 1990.

Granger CV, Gresham GE. *Functional Assessment in Rehabilitation Medicine*. Baltimore, Md: Williams & Wilkins; 1984.

Greenman PE. *Principles of Manual Medicine*. Baltimore, Md: Williams & Wilkins; 1989.

Hartley A. *Practical Joint Assessment: A Sports Medicine Approach*. St Louis, Mo: Mosby-Year Book; 1990.

Hammer WI. *Functional Soft Tissue Examination and Treatment by Manual Methods. The Extremities*. Gaithersburg, Md: Aspen Publishers, Inc; 1990.

Hollis M. *Practical Exercise Therapy*. 3rd ed. Boston, Mass: Blackwell Scientific Publications; 1989.

Kannus P, Alosa D, Cook L, et al. Effect of one-legged exercise on the strength, power and endurance of the contralateral leg: A randomized, controlled study using isometric and concentric isokinetic training. *Eur J Appl Physiol*. 1992;64:117–126.

Kottke FJ, Lehmann JF. *Krusen's Handbook of Physical Medicine and Rehabilitation*. 4th ed. Philadelphia, Pa: WB Saunders Co; 1990.

Leek J, Gershwin ME, Fowler WM, eds. *Principles of Physical Medicine and Rehabilitation in the Musculoskeletal Diseases*. Philadelphia, Pa: WB Saunders Co; 1986.

Lewit K. *Manipulative Therapy in Rehabilitation of the Motor System*. Stoneham, Mass: Butterworth-Heinemann; 1985.

Low J, Reed A. *Electrotherapy Explained: Principles and Practice*. Stoneham, Mass: Butterworth-Heinemann; 1990.

Maitland GD. *Vertebral Manipulation*. 5th ed. Stoneham, Mass: Butterworth-Heinemann; 1986.

Maitland GD. *Peripheral Manipulation*. 3rd ed. Stoneham, Mass: Butterworth-Heinemann; 1990.

Michlovitz SL. *Thermal Agents in Rehabilitation*. 2nd ed. Philadelphia, Pa: FA Davis Co; 1991.

Okamoto GA, Phillips TJ. *Physical Medicine and Rehabilitation*. Philadelphia, Pa: WB Saunders Co; 1984.

O'Sullivan SB, Schmitz TJ. *Physical Rehabilitation: Assessment and Treatment*. 2nd ed. Philadelphia, Pa: FA Davis Co; 1988.

Palmer ML, Epler ME. *Clinical Assessment Procedures in Physical Therapy*. Philadelphia, Pa: JB Lippincott Co; 1990.

Palmer ML, Toms JE. *Manual for Functional Training*. 3rd ed. Philadelphia, Pa: FA Davis Co; 1992.

Pecina M, Krmpotic-Nemanic J, Markiewitz AD. *Tunnel Syndromes*. Boca Raton, Fla: CRC Press, Inc; 1991.

Perry J. *Gait Analysis: Normal and Pathological Function*. Thorofare, NJ: SLACK, Inc; 1992.

Phillips CA. *Functional Electrical Rehabilitation: Technological Restoration After Spinal Cord Injury*. New York, NY: Springer-Verlag; 1991.

Rothman J, Levine R. *Prevention Practice: Strategies for Physical Therapy and Occupational Therapy*. Philadelphia, Pa: WB Saunders Co; 1992.

Rothstein JM, Roy SH, Wolf SL. *The Rehabilitation Specialist's Handbook*. Philadelphia, Pa: FA Davis Co; 1991.

Ruskin AP, ed. *Current Therapy in Physiatry: Physical Medicine and Rehabilitation*. Philadelphia, Pa: WB Saunders Co; 1984.

Scully R, ed, Barnes MR, Canfield J, et al, *Physical Therapy*. Philadelphia, Pa: JB Lippincott Co; 1989.

Shurr DG, Cook TM. *Prosthetics and Orthotics*. Norwalk, Conn: Appleton & Lange; 1990.

Smidt GL, ed. *Gait in Rehabilitation*. New York, NY: Churchill Livingstone; 1990.

Somers MF. *Spinal Cord Injury: Functional Rehabilitation*. Norwalk, Conn: Appleton & Lange; 1992.

Szabo RM, ed. *Nerve Compression Syndromes: Diagnosis and Treatment*. Thorofare, NJ: SLACK, Inc; 1989.

Tappan FM. *Healing Massage Techniques: Holistic, Classic and Emerging Methods*. 2nd ed. Norwalk, Conn: Appleton & Lange; 1988.

Whittle M. *Gait Analysis: An Introduction*. Stoneham, Mass: Butterworth-Heinemann; 1991.

Women

American College of Sports Medicine. Opinion statement: The participation of the female athlete in long-distance running. *Med Sci Sports Exerc*. 1979;11(4):ix–xi.

Drinkwater BL, ed. *Female Endurance Athletes*. Champaign, Ill: Human Kinetics Publishers, Inc; 1986.

Polden M, Mantle J. *Physiotherapy in Obstetrics and Gynaecology*. Stoneham, Mass: Butterworth-Heinemann; 1990.

Puhl JL, Brown CH, eds. *The Menstrual Cycle and Physical Activity*. Champaign, Ill: Human Kinetics Publishers, Inc; 1986.

Puhl JL, Brown CH, Voy RO, eds. *Sport Science Perspectives for Women*. Champaign, Ill: Human Kinetics Publishers, Inc; 1988.

Shangold MM, Mirkin G, eds. *Women and Exercise: Physiology and Sports Medicine*. Philadelphia, Pa: FA Davis Co; 1988;1.

Wells CL. *Women, Sport and Performance: A Physiological Perspective*. 2nd ed. Champaign, Ill: Human Kinetics Publishers, Inc; 1991.

Work Performance Testing

Aquilano NJ. A physiological evaluation of time standards for strenuous work as set by stopwatch time study and two predetermined motion time data systems. *J Ind Eng*. 1968;19:425.

Ayoub MM, Mital A. *Manual Materials Handling Design and Injury Control Through Ergonomics*. Philadelphia, Pa: Taylor & Francis; 1989.

Ayoub M, Mital A, Bakken L, et al. Development of strength and capacity norms for manual materials handling activities: The state-of-the-art. *Hum Factors*. 1980;22:271–283.

Bezold C, Carlson RJ, Peck JC. *The Future of Work and Health*. Dover, Mass: Auburn House; 1986.

Brouha L. *Physiology in Industry*. New York, NY: Pergamon Press; 1960.

Buckle P, ed. *Musculoskeletal Disorders at Work*. New York, NY: Taylor & Francis; 1987.

Bullock MI. *Ergonomics: The Physiotherapist in the Workplace*. New York, NY: Churchill Livingstone; 1990;6.

Damos D, ed. *Multiple Task Performance*. Philadelphia, Pa: Taylor & Francis; 1991.

Demers LM. *Work Hardening: A Practical Guide*. Boston, Mass: Andover Medical Publishers; 1992.

Fraser TM. *Fitness for Work: The Role of Physical Demands Analysis and Physical Capacity Assessment*. Philadelphia, Pa: Taylor & Francis; 1992.

Garg A, Chaffin DB, Herrin GD. Prediction of metabolic rates for manual materials handling jobs. *Am Ind Hyg Assoc J*. 1978;39:661–674.

Grandjean E. *Fitting the Task to the Man*. 4th ed. Philadelphia, Pa: Taylor & Francis; 1988.

Himmelstein JS, Pransky GS. *Worker Fitness and Risk Evaluations*. Philadelphia, Pa: Hanley & Belfus, Inc; 1988.

Hoffman JL, Altuğ Z. Cardiovascular exercise testing in work hardening. In: Slane SM. *Functional Capacities Assessment in Work Hardening*. Thorofare, NJ: SLACK, Inc; in prep.

Hopkins HL, Smith HD. *Willard and Spackman's Occupational Therapy*. 7th ed. Philadelphia, Pa: JB Lippincott Co; 1988.

Kaneko M, ed. *Fitness for the Aged, Disabled and Industrial Worker* (International Series on Sport Science). Champaign, Ill: Human Kinetics Publishers, Inc; 1990;20.

Key GL. Industrial physical therapy: An introduction. In: Gould JA, ed. *Orthopaedic and Sports Physical Therapy*. 2nd ed. St Louis, Mo: CV Mosby Co; 1990.

Keyserling W, Herrin G, Chaffin D. Isometric strength testing as a means of controlling medical incidents on strenuous jobs. *J Occup Med*. 1980;22:332–336.

Kishino N, Mayer T, Gatchel R, et al. Quantification of lumbar function. Part 4: Isometric and isokinetic simulation in normal subjects and low-back dysfunction patients. *Spine*. 1985;10:921–927.

Landau K, Rohmert W, eds. *Recent Development in Job Analysis*. New York, NY: Taylor & Francis; 1989.

Mayer TG, Gatchel RJ, Kishino N. Objective assessment of spine function following industrial injury. *Spine*. 1985;10:482–493.

Ogden-Niemeyer L, Jacobs K. *Work Hardening: State of the Art*. Thorofare, NJ: SLACK, Inc; 1989.

Passmore R, Durnin JVGA. Human energy expenditure. *Physiol Rev*. 1955;35:801.

Pheasant S. *Bodyspace Anthropometry, Ergonomics and Design*. Philadelphia, Pa: Taylor & Francis; 1986.

Pheasant S. *Ergonomics Work and Health*. Gaithersburg, Md: Aspen Publishers, Inc; 1991.

Pope MH, Andersson GBJ, Frymoyer JW, et al. *Occupational Low Back Pain: Assessment, Treatment and Prevention*. St Louis, Mo: Mosby-Year Book; 1991.

Putz-Anderson V, ed. *Cumulative Trauma Disorders: A Manual for Musculoskeletal Diseases of the Upper Limbs*. Philadelphia, Pa: Taylor & Francis; 1988.

Ridley J, ed. *Safety at Work*. 3rd ed. Stoneham, Mass: Butterworth-Heinemann; 1990.

Rodahl K. *The Physiology of Work*. Philadelphia, Pa: Taylor & Francis; 1989.

Rodgers SH, Eggleton EM, eds. *Ergonomic Design for People at Work*. New York, NY: Van Nostrand Reinhold Co; 1983;1.

Scheer SJ, ed. *Medical Perspectives in Vocational Assessment of Impaired Workers*. Gaithersburg, Md: Aspen Publishers, Inc; 1990.

Scheer SJ. *Multidisciplinary Perspectives in Vocational Assessment of Impaired Workers*. Gaithersburg, Md: Aspen Publishers, Inc; 1990.

Tichauer ER. *The Biomechanical Basis of Ergonomics: Anatomy Applied to the Design of Work Situations*. New York, NY: John Wiley & Sons, Inc; 1978.

Williams TA. *Computers, Work and Health*. Philadelphia, PA: Taylor & Francis; 1989.

Wilson JR, Corlett EN, eds. *Evaluation of Human Work: A Practical Ergonomics Methodology*. Philadelphia, Pa: Taylor & Francis; 1990.

Appendices

Appendix A

Abbreviations, Symbols, and Conversion Factors*

The abbreviations, symbols, and conversion factors in Tables A-1 to A-6 have generally been represented as they appear in the original source and may be used by clinicians seeking specific conversion factors used in exercise testing and prescription.

Units in symbolic form may be represented as: $mL \cdot kg^{-1} \cdot min^{-1}$, $mL/kg \cdot min$ or $mL \cdot kg^{-1}/min$ (not mL/kg/min) [40] Therefore, the superscript "$^{-1}$" can be read as "per," as in milliliters per kilogram per minute. Also, for example, the notation W/t can be read as work divided by time.[3]

For further information regarding terminology and units of measurement, one should consult the American College of Sports Medicine Guidelines.[4]

TABLE A-1. LIST OF ABBREVIATIONS AND SYMBOLS[20,41,43]

1. Conversion abbreviations

atm = atmosphere	kg · m = kilogram-meter
Btu = British thermal unit	kJ = kilojoule
C = Celsius	km = kilometer
cal = calorie	kp = kilopond
cc = cubic centimeter	kPa = kilopascal
cm = centimeter	kp · m = kilopond-meter
dyn = dyne	kW = kilowatt
F = Fahrenheit	L = liter
fl = fluid	lb = pound (mass) or pound-force (lbf)
ft = foot	m = meter
g = gram	MET = metabolic equivalent
gal = gallon	mi = mile
hp = horsepower	min = minute
hr = hour	mL = milliliter
in = inch	mm = millimeter
J = joule	N = newton
K = Kelvin	oz = ounce
kcal = kilocalorie	Pa = pascal
kg = kilogram or kilogram-force (kgf)	psi = pounds per square inch
	pt = pint

(continued)

---

*Prepared by Aykut Altuğ, BS

229

TABLE A–1. (Continued)

qt = quart	≠ is not equal to
rev = revolution	≡ is identical to, is defined as
rev/min (rpm) = revolutions per minute	> is greater than
s = second	< is less than
t = ton	+ plus
Tbsp = tablespoon	− minus
tsp = teaspoon	± plus or minus
US = United States	× multiplied by; magnification
W = watt	∝ is proportional to
yd = yard	% percent
2. Mathematical Signs and Symbols	° degree
= equals	# number; pounds
≈ equals approximately	

TABLE A–2. STANDARD SI (SYSTÈME INTERNATIONAL D'UNITÉS) PREFIXES

Name	Symbol	Factor		
tera	T	1 000 000 000 000	=	10^{12}
giga	G	1 000 000 000	=	10^{9}
mega	M	1 000 000	=	10^{6}
kilo	k	1 000	=	10^{3}
hecto	h	100	=	10^{2}
deka	da	10	=	10^{1}
deci	d	0.1	=	10^{-1}
centi	c	0.01	=	10^{-2}
milli	m	0.001	=	10^{-3}
micro	μ	0.000 001	=	10^{-6}
nano	n	0.000 000 001	=	10^{-9}
pico	p	0.000 000 000 001	=	10^{-12}

Adapted with permission from Shigley JE, Mischke CR. Mechanical Engineering Design. 5th ed. Copyright 1989, New York, NY: McGraw-Hill Book Co; p 727.

TABLE A–3. SI BASE UNITS

Quantity	Name	Symbol
Length	meter	m
Mass	kilogram	kg
Time	second	s
Electric current	ampere	A
Temperature	kelvin	K
Amount of a substance	mole	mol

Adapted with permission from Halliday D, Resnick R. Fundamentals of Physics. 2nd ed. Copyright 1986, New York, NY: John Wiley & Sons; p A1.

TABLE A–4. SI DERIVED UNITS WITH SPECIAL NAMES[48]

Quantity	Name	Symbol	Equivalent in Other Units	Expressed in Base Units
Force	newton	N	—	$m \cdot kg \cdot s^{-2}$
Frequency	hertz	Hz	—	s^{-1}
Power	watt	W	$J \cdot s^{-1}$	$m^{2} \cdot kg \cdot s^{-3}$
Pressure	pascal	Pa	$N \cdot m^{-2}$	$m^{-1} \cdot kg \cdot s^{-2}$
Work, energy, quantity of heat	joule	J	$N \cdot m$	$m^{2} \cdot kg \cdot s^{-2}$

TABLE A–5. SOME SI DERIVED UNITS

Quantity	Name of Unit	Symbol
Area	square meter	m^2
Volume	cubic meter	m^3
Mass density	kilogram per cubic meter	$kg \cdot m^{-3}$
Speed, velocity	meter per second	$m \cdot s^{-1}$
Angular velocity	radian per second	$rad \cdot s^{-1}$
Acceleration	meter per second squared	$m \cdot s^{-2}$
Angular acceleration	radian per second squared	$rad \cdot s^{-2}$

Adapted with permission from Halliday D, Resnick R. Fundamentals of Physics, 2nd ed. Copyright 1986, New York, NY: John Wiley & Sons; p A2.

TABLE A–6. CONVERSION FACTORS[1,3,6,8,9,14,17,30,33,34,36,38,40,43,46]

1. ACCELERATION
$1 ft \cdot s^{-2} = 0.3048 m \cdot s^{-2}$
$1 m \cdot s^{-2} = 3.2808 ft \cdot s^{-2}$
acceleration of gravity $= 9.81 m \cdot s^{-2}$

2. AREA
$1 ft^2 = 929 cm^2$
$1 ft^2 = 0.0929 m^2$
$1 in^2 = 6.4516 cm^2$
$1 in^2 = 6.4516 \times 10^{-4} m^2$
$1 m^2 = 10.764 ft^2$

3. DENSITY
$1 kg \cdot m^{-3} = 0.06243 lb \cdot ft^{-3}$
$1 lb \cdot ft^{-3} = 16.019 kg \cdot m^{-3}$
$1 lb \cdot in^{-3} = 27.680 g \cdot cm^{-3}$
$1 lb \cdot in^{-3} = 27.680 \times 10^3 kg \cdot m^{-3}$

4. FORCE
$1 dyn = 2.248 \times 10^{-6} lb$
$1 kg = 1 kp = 9.80665 N$
$1 lb = 32.174 ft \cdot lb \cdot s^{-2}$
$1 lb = 4.4482 N$
$1 lb = 4.4482 kg \cdot m \cdot s^{-2}$
$1 N = 1 kg \cdot m \cdot s^{-2}$
$1 N = 0.102 kg$
$1 N = 10^5 dyn$
$1 N = 0.22481 lb$

5. LENGTH
$1 cm = 0.3937 in$
$1 cm = 10 mm$
$1 cm = 10^{-2} m$
$1 ft = 30.48 cm$
$1 ft = 0.3048 m$
$1 ft = 12 in$
$1 in = 25.4 mm$
$1 in = 2.54 cm$
$1 in = 2.54 \times 10^{-2} m$
$1 km = 1000 m$
$1 km = 0.62137 mi$
$1 m = 39.37 in$
$1 m = 3.2808 ft$
$1 m = 1.0936 yd$
$1 m = 100 cm = 1000 mm = 0.001 km$
$100 m = 109 yd = 328 ft$
$200 m = 219 yd = 656 ft$
$400 m = 437 yd = 1312 ft$
$800 m = 875 yd = 2624 ft$
$1500 m = 1640 yd = 4920 ft$
$1 mi = 1609.34 m$

$1 mi = 1.60934 km$
$1 mi = 5280 ft$
$1 mm = 10^{-3} m = 0.001 m$
1 rev = 3 m for a Tunturi bicycle ergometer
1 rev = 6 m for a Monark bicycle ergometer
$1 yd = 3 ft$
$1 yd = 91.44 cm$
$1 yd = 0.9144 m$
$100 yd = 300 ft$

6. MASS
$1 g = 1000 mg$
$1 kg = 2.2046 lb$
$1 kg = 1000 g$
$1 lb = 16 oz$
$1 lb = 453.6 g$
$1 lb = 0.4536 kg$
$1 oz = 28.3495 g$
$1 t (metric) = 1000 kg$
$1 t (metric) = 2205 lb$
$1 ton (short) = 2000 lb$
$1 ton (long) = 2240 lb$

7. MEASURES AND WEIGHTS
$1 cup = 8 fl oz$
$1 cup = 12 Tbsp (dry)$
$1 cup = 16 Tbsp (liquid)$
$1 fl oz = 30 g = 30 cc$
$1 fl oz = 2 Tbsp$
$1 g = 1 cm^3 (1 cc) = 1 mL$
$1 gal (US) = 4 qt$
$1 gal (US) = 8 pt$
$1 gal (US) \approx 8 lb$
$1 gal (US) = 128 fl oz$
$1 L = 1.0567 qt$
$1 L = 33.8 fl oz$
$1 lb \approx 2 cups$
1 lb = 12 oz (Apothecaries' and Troy weight)
1 lb = 16 oz (avoirdupois weight)
$1 pt = 2 cups$
$1 pt = 16 fl oz$
$1 qt = 4 cups$
1 qt = 2 pt (dry and liquid)
$1 qt = 0.9464 L$
$1 Tbsp = ½ fluid ounce$
$1 Tbsp = 15 g$
$1 Tbsp = 3 tsp$
$1 tsp fluid = 5 g$
$1 tsp dry = 4 g$

(continued)

TABLE A–6. (Continued)

8. *NUTRITION*

1 g carbohydrate = 4 cal
1 g protein = 4 cal
1 g fat = 9 cal
1 g alcohol = 7 cal

9. *POWER*

$1 \text{ Btu} \cdot \text{h}^{-1} = 0.2931 \text{ W}$
$1 \text{ Btu} \cdot \text{h}^{-1} = 3.93 \times 10^{-4} \text{ hp}$
$1 \text{ hp} = 2545 \text{ Btu} \cdot \text{h}^{-1}$
$1 \text{ hp} = 550 \text{ ft} \cdot \text{lb} \cdot \text{s}^{-1}$
$1 \text{ hp} = 745.7 \text{ W} = 745.7 \text{ J} \cdot \text{s}^{-1}$
$1 \text{ hp} = 75 \text{ kg} \cdot \text{m} \cdot \text{s}^{-1}$
$1 \text{ hp} = 4562 \text{ kg} \cdot \text{m} \cdot \text{min}^{-1}$
$1 \text{ hp} = 10.69 \text{ kcal} \cdot \text{min}^{-1}$
$1 \text{ kcal} \cdot \text{min}^{-1} = 69.767 \text{ W}$
$1 \text{ kg} \cdot \text{m} \cdot \text{min}^{-1} = 1 \text{ kp} \cdot \text{m} \cdot \text{min}^{-1}$
$1 \text{ kg} \cdot \text{m} \cdot \text{min}^{-1} = 0.1635 \text{ W}$
$1 \text{ kg} \cdot \text{m} \cdot \text{min}^{-1} = 0.000219 \text{ hp}$
$1 \text{ kp (or 1 kg)} \approx 50 \text{ W} \approx 300 \text{ kg} \cdot \text{m} \cdot \text{min}^{-1}$
$1 \text{ kW} = 1000 \text{ W}$
$1 \text{ kW} = 1.34 \text{ hp}$
$1 \text{ MET} = 3.5 \text{ mL} \cdot \text{kg}^{-1} \cdot \text{min}^{-1}$
$1 \text{ MET} \approx 1 \text{ kcal} \cdot \text{kg}^{-1} \cdot \text{hr}^{-1}$
$1 \text{ MET} \approx 1.6 \text{ km} \cdot \text{hr}^{-1}$ (running on a horizontal surface)
$1 \text{ MET} \approx 1.0 \text{ mi} \cdot \text{hr}^{-1}$ (running on a horizontal surface)
$1 \text{ W} = 6.12 \text{ kg} \cdot \text{m} \cdot \text{min}^{-1} \approx 6 \text{ kg} \cdot \text{m} \cdot \text{min}^{-1}$ (or $\text{kp} \cdot \text{m} \cdot \text{min}^{-1}$)
$1 \text{ W} = 0.1019 \text{ kg} \cdot \text{m} \cdot \text{s}^{-1}$
$1 \text{ W} = 1 \text{ J} \cdot \text{s}^{-1} = 1 \text{ N} \cdot \text{m} \cdot \text{s}^{-1}$
$1 \text{ W} = 60 \text{ J} \cdot \text{min}^{-1} = 0.060 \text{ kJ} \cdot \text{min}^{-1}$
$1 \text{ W} = 60 \text{ N} \cdot \text{m} \cdot \text{min}^{-1}$
$1 \text{ W} = 0.001 \text{ kW}$
$1 \text{ W} = 0.73756 \text{ ft} \cdot \text{lb} \cdot \text{s}^{-1}$
$1 \text{ W} = 0.01433 \text{ kcal} \cdot \text{min}^{-1}$
$1 \text{ W} = 0.00134 \text{ hp}$
$20 \text{ W} = 120 \text{ kg} \cdot \text{m} \cdot \text{min}^{-1}$ (pedaling frequency of 40 rpm)
$40 \text{ W} = 240 \text{ kg} \cdot \text{m} \cdot \text{min}^{-1}$ (pedaling frequency of 40 rpm)
$60 \text{ W} = 360 \text{ kg} \cdot \text{m} \cdot \text{min}^{-1}$ (pedaling frequency of 40 rpm)
$80 \text{ W} = 480 \text{ kg} \cdot \text{m} \cdot \text{min}^{-1}$ (pedaling frequency of 40 rpm)
$100 \text{ W} = 600 \text{ kg} \cdot \text{m} \cdot \text{min}^{-1}$ (pedaling frequency of 40 rpm)
$120 \text{ W} = 720 \text{ kg} \cdot \text{m} \cdot \text{min}^{-1}$ (pedaling frequency of 40 rpm)
$25 \text{ W} = 150 \text{ kg} \cdot \text{m} \cdot \text{min}^{-1} = 0.5 \text{ kp}$ (pedaling frequency of 50 rpm)
$50 \text{ W} = 300 \text{ kg} \cdot \text{m} \cdot \text{min}^{-1} = 1.0 \text{ kp}$ (pedaling frequency of 50 rpm)
$75 \text{ W} = 450 \text{ kg} \cdot \text{m} \cdot \text{min}^{-1} = 1.5 \text{ kp}$ (pedaling frequency of 50 rpm)
$100 \text{ W} = 600 \text{ kg} \cdot \text{m} \cdot \text{min}^{-1} = 2.0 \text{ kp}$ (pedaling frequency of 50 rpm)
$125 \text{ W} = 750 \text{ kg} \cdot \text{m} \cdot \text{min}^{-1} = 2.5 \text{ kp}$ (pedaling frequency of 50 rpm)
$150 \text{ W} = 900 \text{ kg} \cdot \text{m} \cdot \text{min}^{-1} = 3.0 \text{ kp}$ (pedaling frequency of 50 rpm)
$30 \text{ W} = 180 \text{ kg} \cdot \text{m} \cdot \text{min}^{-1}$ (pedaling frequency of 60 rpm)
$60 \text{ W} = 360 \text{ kg} \cdot \text{m} \cdot \text{min}^{-1}$ (pedaling frequency of 60 rpm)
$90 \text{ W} = 540 \text{ kg} \cdot \text{m} \cdot \text{min}^{-1}$ (pedaling frequency of 60 rpm)
$120 \text{ W} = 720 \text{ kg} \cdot \text{m} \cdot \text{min}^{-1}$ (pedaling frequency of 60 rpm)
$150 \text{ W} = 900 \text{ kg} \cdot \text{m} \cdot \text{min}^{-1}$ (pedaling frequency of 60 rpm)
$180 \text{ W} = 1080 \text{ kg} \cdot \text{m} \cdot \text{min}^{-1}$ (pedaling frequency of 60 rpm)
$35 \text{ W} = 210 \text{ kg} \cdot \text{m} \cdot \text{min}^{-1}$ (pedaling frequency of 70 rpm)
$70 \text{ W} = 420 \text{ kg} \cdot \text{m} \cdot \text{min}^{-1}$ (pedaling frequency of 70 rpm)
$105 \text{ W} = 630 \text{ kg} \cdot \text{m} \cdot \text{min}^{-1}$ (pedaling frequency of 70 rpm)
$140 \text{ W} = 840 \text{ kg} \cdot \text{m} \cdot \text{min}^{-1}$ (pedaling frequency of 70 rpm)
$175 \text{ W} = 1050 \text{ kg} \cdot \text{m} \cdot \text{min}^{-1}$ (pedaling frequency of 70 rpm)
$210 \text{ W} = 1260 \text{ kg} \cdot \text{m} \cdot \text{min}^{-1}$ (pedaling frequency of 70 rpm)

(continued)

TABLE A–6. (Continued)

10. *PRESSURE*

1 atm = 760 torr
1 atm = 760 mm Hg at 0°C
1 atm = 14.696 lb · in^{-2}
1 atm = 2116.2 lb · ft^{-2}
1 atm = 1.01325 × 10^5 N · m^{-2}
1 atm = 1.01325 bar
1 bar = 10^5 N · m^{-2} = 10^5 Pa
1 in = 25.4 torr
29.92 in Hg = 760 torr
1 kPa = 7.5 mm Hg
1 lb · in^{-2} ≡ 1 psi = 6894.76 N · m^{-2}
1 lb · ft^{-2} = 47.880 N · m^{-2}
1 Pa = 1 N · m^{-2} = 1 kg · m^{-1} · s^{-2}
1 Pa = 0.0075 mm Hg
1 torr = 1 mm Hg at 0°C
1 torr = 133.322 Pa

11. *SPEED (VELOCITY if both magnitude and direction are specified)*

1 ft · s^{-1} = 0.3048 m · s^{-1}
1 ft · s^{-1} = 0.6818 mi · hr^{-1}
1 km · hr^{-1} (or kph) = 0.62137 mi · hr^{-1}
1 km · hr^{-1} = 0.9113 ft · s^{-1}
1 m · min^{-1} = 0.03728 mi · hr^{-1}
1 m · s^{-1} = 3.2808 ft · s^{-1}
1 m · s^{-1} = 2.2371 mi · hr^{-1}
1 mi · hr^{-1} (or mph) = 1.4667 ft · s^{-1}
1 mi · hr^{-1} = 0.4470 m · s^{-1}
1 mi · hr^{-1} = 26.822 m · min^{-1}
1 mi · hr^{-1} = 1.6093 km · hr^{-1}
1 mi · min^{-1} = 88.00 ft · s^{-1} = 60.00 mi · hr^{-1}

12. *TEMPERATURE*

°C = K − 273.15
°C = (°F − 32)/1.8
°F = (1.8 × °C) + 32
K = °C + 273.15
Boiling point of H$_2$O = 212°F and 100°C
Freezing point of H$_2$O = 32°F and 0°C

13. *VOLUME*

1 cm^3 = 0.06102 in^3
1 ft^3 = 0.0283168 m^3
1 ft^3 = 28.3168 L
1 ft^3 = 7.4805 gal (US)
1 gal (US) = 3.7854 L
1 gal (US) = 3.7854 × 10^{-3} m^3

1 gal (US) = 0.13368 ft^3
1 gal (US) = 231 in^3
1 in^3 = 16.387 cm^3
1 L = 1000 mL
1 L = 0.001 m^3
1 L = 0.035315 ft^3
1 L = 1 kg = 1000 cm^3 = 1000 mL (of water at 4°C)
1 m^3 = 35.315 ft^3
1 oz (US fluid) = 29.573 cm^3

14. *WORK, ENERGY, AND HEAT*

1 Btu = 107.56 kp · m
1 Btu = 1055.04 J
1 Btu = 251.98 cal
1 Btu = 0.25198 kcal
1 Btu = 778.161 ft · lb
1 cal = 4.186 J
1 cal = 3.968 × 10^{-3} Btu
1 erg = 1.0197 × 10^{-8} kp · m
1 erg = 2.3889 × 10^{-11} kcal
1 ft · lb = 3.2389 × 10^{-4} kcal
1 ft · lb = 1.35582 J
1 ft · lb = 0.13825 kp · m
1 ft · lb = 1.3560 N · m
1 J = 1 W · s = 1 N · m
1 J = 10^7 erg
1 J = 0.73756 ft · lb
1 J = 2.3889 × 10^{-4} kcal
1 J = 0.10197 kp · m
1 kcal = 3.968 Btu
1 kcal = 3087 ft · lb
1 kcal = 4186 J
1 kcal = 4.186 kJ
1 kcal = 426.85 kp · m at 100% efficiency
1 kg · m = 1 kp · m
1 kg · m = 9.80665 J
1 kg · m ≈ 1.8 mL O$_2$
1 kg · m = 7.2330 ft · lb
1 kg · m = 3.6529 × 10^{-6} hp · hr^{-1}
1 kg · m = 2.3427 × 10^{-3} kcal
1 kJ = 1000 J
1 kJ = 1000 N · m
1 kJ = 0.234 kcal
1 kp · m = 9.80665 J
1 L O$_2$ ≈ 5 kcal
1 N · m = 0.102 kg · m
1 N · m = 0.7375 ft · lb

Physical Science Formulas*

The symbols, units and formulas in Tables B–1 and B–2 have generally been represented as they appear in the original source and may be used by clinicians seeking specific physical science formulas used in exercise science.

TABLE B–1. LIST OF SYMBOLS AND UNITS[31,44]

1. Equation Symbols
   - α = alpha
   - ω = omega
   - ρ = rho
   - θ = theta

2. Units
   - α = $rad \cdot s^{-2}$
   - ω = $rad \cdot s^{-1}$
   - ρ = $kg \cdot m^{-3}$
   - θ = rad (radian)
   - I = $kg \cdot m^2$
   - L = $kg \cdot m \cdot s^{-2}$
   - m = g or kg
   - M = $kg \cdot m \cdot s^{-1}$
   - T = $N \cdot m$
   - V = L or mL
   - W = kg of weight

---

*Prepared by Aykut Altuğ, BS

TABLE B–2. PHYSICAL SCIENCE FORMULAS[31,44]

1. Linear Velocity or Speed[a] $= \dfrac{\text{Linear Displacement}}{\text{Time}}$

$$v = \frac{d}{t}$$

2. Angular Velocity or Speed[a] $= \dfrac{\text{Angular Displacement}}{\text{Time}}$

$$\omega = \frac{\theta}{t}$$

3. Linear Acceleration $= \dfrac{\text{Change in Linear Velocity}}{\text{Time}}$

$$a = \frac{v_2 - v_1}{t}$$

4. Angular Acceleration $= \dfrac{\text{Change in Angular Velocity}}{\text{Time}}$

$$\alpha = \frac{\omega_2 - \omega_1}{t}$$

5. Resultant Force $=$ Mass $\times$ Acceleration

$$F = ma$$

6. Torque $=$ Force $\times$ Perpendicular Distance

$$T = Fd_\perp$$

7. Power $= \dfrac{\text{Work}}{\text{Time}}$

$$P = \frac{w}{t}$$

8. Power $=$ Force $\times$ Velocity at Which Force Is Applied

$$P = Fv$$

9. Work $=$ Force $\times$ Distance the Force Is Applied

$$w = Fd$$

10. Linear Momentum $=$ Mass $\times$ Velocity

$$M = mv$$

11. Angular Momentum $=$ Rotational Inertia $\times$ Angular Velocity

$$L = I\omega$$

12. Density $= \dfrac{\text{Mass}}{\text{Volume}}$

$$\rho = \frac{m}{V}$$

13. Mass $= \dfrac{\text{Weight}}{\text{Gravitational Acceleration}}$

$$m = \frac{W}{g}$$

(Continued)

TABLE B–2. (Continued)

14. Weight = Mass × Gravitational Acceleration

$$W = mg$$

15. Volume = $\dfrac{\text{Mass}}{\text{Density}}$

$$V = \dfrac{m}{\rho}$$

16. Pressure = $\dfrac{\text{Force}}{\text{Area}}$

$$p = \dfrac{F}{A}$$

[a]When both the magnitude and direction (a vector quantity) are specified for a system, it is the velocity, not the speed (a scalar quantity designating by magnitude only), that is defined.

Sources of Testing and Prescription Calculations

The following list provides references for those clinicians seeking specific information regarding calculation formats for various formulas and conversion factors used in exercise testing and prescription.

CARDIOVASCULAR

A. Treadmill calculations[3,38,49]
B. Leg cycle ergometry calculations[3,9,38,49]
C. Arm cycle ergometry calculations[3,49]
D. Stepping calculations[3,9,38,49]
E. Field test calculations[3]
F. Oxygen consumption calculations[1,11,18,32,37,38,42,45,49]
G. Carbon dioxide production calculations[32]
H. Respiratory quotient/respiratory exchange ratio calculations[3,32]
I. Respiratory calculations (vital capacity, forced vital capacity, forced expiratory volumes, residual volume, total lung capacity, tidal volume, ventilatory equivalent)[1,45]
J. Electrocardiographic (ECG) analysis (resting and exercise)[1,11,15,16,19]
K. Exercise blood pressure calculations (mean blood pressure, rate pressure product)[1]

MUSCULAR STRENGTH AND ENDURANCE

A. Isokinetic calculations[1,40]
B. Isometric handgrip calculations[1]

ANTHROPOMETRIC AND BODY COMPOSITION

    A. Hydrostatic weighing calculations[1]
    B. Skinfold calculations[1]
    C. Girth calculations[1]
    D. Stature–weight index calculations[1]

NUTRITION[12,27,35,36,39,47]

    A. 24-hour recall
    B. Food frequency questionnaire
    C. Food diary
    D. Weighted food intake

Rehabilitation Evaluation Forms

Figures D–1 to D–4 outline various evaluation forms and a health screening questionnaire that may be used in a clinical setting.[10,24,25,28,32]

Specific informed consent formats have not been presented in this section because each facility may wish to consider consulting with legal counsel prior to the adoption of these forms.[21-23,29] Table D–1 provides sources of informed consent forms presented by various associations and researchers.

TABLE D–1. SOURCES OF INFORMED CONSENT FORMS

1. American Association of Cardiovascular and Pulmonary Rehabilitation[2]
2. American College of Sports Medicine[5]
3. American Heart Association[7]
4. Others[13,25,26,37]

Last Name: _____   First Name: _____   Date: _____

Age: _____ Sex: M   F Weight: _____ Height: _____

Address: _____

Phone: (Home) _____ (Work) _____

Employer: _____   Occupation: _____

Are you currently working? ( ) Yes ( ) No If no, since when ____ /____ /____

Referring Physician: _____

In case of emergency contact: _____   Phone: _____

PLEASE MARK (X) IF THE ANSWER IS YES:
Medical History

Do you have or have you ever had?

( ) Alcohol abuse problems
( ) Allergies
( ) Angina
( ) Arthritis
( ) Back injuries
( ) Cancer
( ) Circulatory problems
( ) Diabetes
( ) Dislocations (joints)
( ) Epilepsy
( ) Gastrointestinal problems
( ) Gout
( ) Hearing loss
( ) Heart attack(s)
( ) Heart disease
( ) Heart surgery
( ) High blood cholesterol
( ) High blood pressure
( ) Jaw injury
( ) Kidney disease
( ) Ligament injuries
( ) Lung disease
( ) Muscle/tendon injuries
( ) Neck injuries
( ) Nervous or emotional problems
( ) Paralysis
( ) Phlebitis
( ) Stroke(s)
( ) TMJ (temporomandibular disorders)
( ) Tumor(s)
( ) Varicose veins

Have you recently experienced?

( ) A wound that does not heal
( ) Blurred or double vision
( ) Calf pain with exercise
( ) Change in bowel or bladder habits
( ) Change in speech pattern (eg, slurring)
( ) Chest pain or pressure
( ) Clicking or locking of jaw
( ) Constant pain unrelieved by rest or movement
( ) Difficulty keeping balance
( ) Difficulty opening mouth
( ) Difficulty sleeping
( ) Difficulty swallowing
( ) Dizziness, fainting, or blackouts
( ) Falls
( ) Headaches
( ) Muscular pain at rest
( ) Muscular pain with exertion
( ) Ringing in ears
( ) Shortness of breath
( ) Swollen ankles or legs
( ) Swollen, stiff, or painful joints
( ) Tingling, numbness, or loss of feeling
( ) Tremors
( ) Unexplained weight loss
( ) Unusual skin coloration
( ) Unusual weakness or fatigue

Figure D–1. Sample medical screening questionnaire. (*Continued*)

Family History

Have any blood relatives (eg, parents, sister) had?

( )   Congenital heart disease

( )   Diabetes

( )   Heart attack(s)

( )   Heart operations

( )   High blood cholesterol

( )   High blood pressure

Lifestyle History

Do you smoke? ( ) Yes ( ) No ( ) Quit

Smoke how many years? _____

Smoke how much? _____

Gained weight? ( ) Yes   ( ) No

Gained how much? _____

Lost weight? ( ) Yes   ( ) No

Lost how much? _____

Do you exercise? ( ) Yes   ( ) No

Type of exercise? _____

_____

Exercise how often? _____

Please comment here on any additional problems or symptoms mentioned above:

_____

_____

Are you pregnant? ( ) Yes   ( ) No

Identify any allergies (eg, pollens, food, medications): _____

_____

Please describe any surgery and/or hospitalizations: _____

_____

Please list all current diagnostic tests (location and date):

X-rays _____

MRI _____

CAI scan _____

_____

_____

Please list all the medications you are taking: _____

_____

Please list all the supplements you are currently using (eg, vitamins, minerals, protein): _____

_____

Identify any assistive devices you are currently using (eg, cane, knee brace, back brace): _____

_____

Please identify any past treatments by a physician, physical therapist, or chiropractor. _____

_____

I, the undersigned, state that I have answered this questionnaire to the best of my knowledge.

_____   _____

Patient's Signature   Date

THANK YOU FOR TAKING TIME TO PROVIDE US WITH THIS NEEDED INFORMATION.

Figure D-1.

I. INTAKE INTERVIEW

DATE OF EXAM: _____

NAME: _____

AGE: _____ SEX: M   F   WEIGHT: _____ HEIGHT: _____

ADDRESS: _____

OCCUPATION: _____

JOB DUTIES: _____

_____

PRESENTLY WORKING: Y   N   DATE LAST WORKED: _____

REFERRING PHYSICIAN: _____ DATE OF M.D. EXAM: _____

DIAGNOSIS: _____

DATE OF INJURY: _____

HISTORY: _____

_____

_____

_____

HOSPITALIZATIONS: _____

PREVIOUS INJURIES: _____

_____

PREVIOUS TREATMENT: _____

_____

DIAGNOSTIC TESTS: _____

_____

_____

PREVIOUS SURGERY: Y   N   _____

MEDICATIONS: _____

DURATION ON MEDICATIONS: _____

IS THERE LITIGATION PENDING? Y   N

II. ORTHOPEDIC ASSESSMENT

A. Subjective Reports

PAIN SCALE: 0–10 (1 = min, 5 = mod, 10 = max) _____

WHAT INCREASES SYMPTOMS: _____

_____

WHAT EASES SYMPTOMS: _____

_____

_____

B. Observation/Inspection

ASSISTIVE DEVICES: Y   N   _____

STANDING POSTURE: GOOD   FAIR   POOR   SITTING POSTURE: GOOD   FAIR   POOR

GAIT: EVEN or UNEVEN   COMFORTABLE or ANTALGIC   BALANCED or UNBALANCED

C. Postural Analysis

HEAD: normal _____ forward _____ retracted _____ sidebent: R L rotated: R L

SHOULDERS: normal _____ rounded _____ elevated: B R L depressed: B R L
          protracted: B R L retracted: B R L

ARMS: normal _____   IR: B R L   ER: B R L

THORACIC SPINE: normal _____ flat _____ kyphotic _____ lordotic _____

LUMBAR SPINE: normal _____ flat _____ kyphotic _____ lordotic _____

ROTOSCOLIOSIS: thoracic: R L lumbar: R L

SCOLIOSIS: Y N convex: R L

Figure D–2. Sample physical assessment form. (*Continued*)

HIPS: iliac crest: = R L   PSIS: = R L   ASIS: = R L   GT: = R L
      sacral position: = R_____ L_____
LEGS: normal _____   IR: B R L   ER: B R L
KNEES: normal _____   varus: B R L   valgus: B R L   recurvatum: B R L
      flexion deformity: B R L
POPLITEAL: = R L
FEET: normal _____   supinated: B R L   pronated: B R L
SAGITTAL PLANE ANALYSIS: _____
_____
FRONTAL PLANE ANALYSIS: _____
_____

D. Range of Motion Testing

Cervical Range of Motion

Flexion: _____   Extension: _____
Sidebending L: _____ R: _____
Rotation L: _____ R: _____

Extremity _____ Range of Motion
_____ L: _____ R: _____
_____ L: _____ R: _____
_____ L: _____ R: _____
_____ L: _____ R: _____

Lumbar Range of Motion

Flexion: _____   Extension: _____
Sidebending L: _____ R: _____
Rotation L: _____ R: _____

Extremity _____ Range of Motion
_____ L: _____ R: _____
_____ L: _____ R: _____
_____ L: _____ R: _____
_____ L: _____ R: _____

E. Manual Muscle Testing

Upper Quarter

	L	R
SCM	_____	_____
Scalenes	_____	_____
Trapezius	_____	_____
Middle Delt	_____	_____
Shoulder IR	_____	_____
Shoulder ER	_____	_____
Serratus Ant	_____	_____
Middle Trap	_____	_____
Lower Trap	_____	_____
Biceps	_____	_____
Triceps	_____	_____
Brach Rad	_____	_____
Wrist Flex	_____	_____
Wrist Ext	_____	_____
Thumb Ext	_____	_____
Intrinsics	_____	_____

Lower Quarter

	L	R
Rectus Abdominus	_____	
Oblique Abdominus	_____	
Ilio Psoas	_____	_____
Psoas	_____	_____
Hip IR	_____	_____
Hip ER	_____	_____
Quads	_____	_____
Tib Ant	_____	_____
EHL	_____	_____
Peroneals	_____	_____
Erector Spinae	_____	_____
Gluteus Maximus	_____	_____
Gluteus Medius	_____	_____
Adductors	_____	_____
Hamstrings	_____	_____
Gastroc/Soleus	_____	_____

F. Flexibility Testing

Upper Quarter

	L	R
Pect Major ST	_____	_____
Pect Major CL	_____	_____
Pect Minor	_____	_____
Latissimus/Teres	_____	_____
Shoulder Flex	_____	_____
Shoulder Ext	_____	_____
Shoulder Abd	_____	_____
Shoulder ER	_____	_____
Shoulder IR	_____	_____

Lower Quarter

	L	R
SLR	_____	_____
Thomas Test	_____	_____
Long Sit	_____	_____
Ober's Test	_____	_____
Gastroc/Soleus	_____	_____
Rectus Femoris	_____	_____
Hip Abduction	_____	_____
Hip Adduction	_____	_____
Piriformis	_____	_____
Supine Leg Length	_____	_____
Supine ASIS	_____	_____
Prone Leg Length	_____	_____
Hamstrings	_____	_____
Hip ER	_____	_____
Hip IR	_____	_____

Figure D–2. (Continued)

G. Reflex Testing

Cervical   Lumbar

	L	R
C5		
C6		
C7		
Hoffman		

	L	R
L 3-4		
S 1-2		
Babinski		
Clonus		

H. Sensation Testing

_____
_____

I. Coordination/Balance Testing

_____
_____

J. Palpation Testing

_____
_____

K. Joint Stability Testing

_____
_____

L. Cardiovascular Testing

Resting Blood Pressure: _____/_____   Resting Heart Rate: _____

M. Special Tests

_____

III. ASSESSMENT

_____
_____
_____
_____

IV. GOALS

_____
_____
_____
_____
_____

V. PLAN OF CARE AND RECOMMENDATIONS

_____
_____
_____
_____

_____   _____
Evaluator   Date

KEY: B = bilateral   R = right   L = left
       ER = external rotation   IR = internal rotation
       GT = greater trochanter

Figure D–2.

I. INTAKE INTERVIEW

DATE OF EXAM: _____

NAME: _____

AGE: _____ SEX: M   F   WEIGHT: _____ HEIGHT: _____

ADDRESS: _____

OCCUPATION: _____

JOB DUTIES: _____

_____

PRESENTLY WORKING: Y   N   DATE LAST WORKED: _____

REFERRING PHYSICIAN: _____ DATE OF MD EXAM: _____

DIAGNOSIS: _____

DATE OF INJURY: _____

HISTORY: _____

_____

_____

_____

_____

HOSPITALIZATIONS: _____

PREVIOUS INJURIES: _____

_____

PREVIOUS TREATMENT: _____

_____

DIAGNOSTIC TESTS: _____

_____

_____

PREVIOUS SURGERY: Y   N _____

MEDICATIONS: _____

DURATION ON MEDICATIONS: _____

II. DIETARY ASSESSMENT

A. What is your desired weight? _____

What is the most you have ever weighed? _____ Date: _____

What is the least you have ever weighed? _____ Date: _____

B. What are your five favorite foods? _____

What are your five least favorite foods? _____

What are your favorite snacks? _____

What are your favorite beverages? _____

What are your favorite sports or activities? _____

What are your favorite hobbies? _____

C. Describe a typical breakfast: _____

Describe a typical lunch: _____

Figure D–3. Sample nutrition assessment form. *Adapted from Heyward VH. Advanced Fitness Assessment and Exercise Prescription. 2nd ed. Champaign, Ill: Human Kinetics Publishers, Inc; 1991; and Peterson M, Peterson K. Eat to Compete: A Guide to Sports Nutrition. Chicago, Ill: Year Book Medical Publishers, Inc; 1988. (Continued)*

Describe a typical dinner: _____

Describe typical snacks and frequency: _____

Describe the amount of water consumed per day: _____
Describe all supplements you are using: _____

D. Describe in detail any food-related allergies or intolerances: _____

E. Describe your current exercise program: _____

Describe your typical weekday activities: _____

Describe your typical weekend activities: _____

Describe your typical work-related activities: _____

F. Describe foods or drinks commonly consumed before exercise or competition: _____

G. Do you normally eat your meals at home or in restaurants? _____

H. What specific questions or concerns do you have regarding nutrition? _____

III. ASSESSMENT
General Impressions:
_____
_____

IV. GOALS
_____
_____
_____
_____

V. PLAN OF CARE AND RECOMMENDATIONS
_____
_____
_____
_____

_____   _____
Evaluator   Date

Figure D–3.

NAME: _____ DATE: _____

AGE: _____ SEX: M   F

1. What exercise equipment do you have access to? (check those that apply)

_____ Stationary cycle		_____ Treadmill	
_____ Bicycle		_____ Cross-country ski simulator	
_____ Barbell/dumbbell weights		_____	
_____ VCR aerobic tape		_____	

2. What exercise facilities do you have access to? (check those that apply)

_____ Health/fitness club	_____ Swimming pool
_____ Aerobic exercise class	_____ Track
_____ Park	_____ Outdoor trail
_____ Bicycle path/route	_____

3. List the type of fitness equipment you would consider purchasing for your home.

_____

_____

4. Would you prefer indoor or outdoor fitness activities?

_____

_____

5. Would you prefer an individual (eg, swimming) or a group (eg, basketball) type of fitness activity?

_____

_____

6. Please list the sports and activities that you are skilled in:

_____ Basketball	_____ Cycling
_____ Volleyball	_____ Walking
_____ Hunting	Swimming
_____ Cross-country skiing	_____ Hiking

7. Please list the sports and activities that you would enjoy participating in:

_____ Basketball	_____ Cycling
_____ Volleyball	_____ Walking
_____ Hunting	_____ Swimming
_____ Cross-country skiing	_____ Hiking

8. What are your health and fitness goals?

_____ Weight loss   How much? _____

_____ Weight gain   How much? _____

_____ Body shaping/toning

9. Additional Comments: _____

_____

Figure D–4. Sample home exercise program questionnaire.

Appendix

Laboratory Tests Affected by Exercise or Related Conditions

Table E–1 may be used to compare values obtained from laboratory tests to normal values as well as to individual responses to exercise.

TABLE E-1. LABORATORY TESTS AND NORMAL RANGES FOR ADULTS AND CHILDREN AFFECTED BY EXERCISE OR RELATED CONDITIONS

Test	Normal Value		Response to Exercise	Rationale
Hemoglobin (inner core of the RBC[a] in a given volume)	Male:	13.5–18 g/dL (140–180 g/L)	Decrease	Anemias, iron deficiency, excessive fluid intake
	Female:	12–16 g/dL (115–155 g/L)	Increase	High altitude, burns, dehydration
	Athlete:	16–18 g/dL		
	Pregnancy:	11–12 g/dL		
	Child:	11–16 g/dL		
Hematocrit (proportion of packed cells in a given volume)	Male:	40%–54% (0.40–0.54)	Decrease	Anemias
	Female:	36%–46% (0.36–0.46)	Increase	Dehydration; diarrhea; drug influence: antibiotics
	Child:	36%–38% (0.36–0.38)		
RBCs	Male:	4.6–6.0 m/mm³ by 10–12/L	Decrease	Excessive fluid intake, intravascular hemolysis
	Female:	4.0–5.0		
	Child:	3.8–5.5	Increase	High altitude, dehydration
Blood volume	70–100 mL/kg of body weight		Increase	Response to regular strenuous exercise, altitudes
Plasma volume	30–50 mL/kg of body weight		Increase	Response to strenuous exercise
MCV[b]	Male:	80–98 μ³	Decrease	Excessive fluid intake > 80, iron deficiency anemia
	Female:	80–98 μ³		
	Child:	82–92 μ³	Increase	Dehydration > 98, pernicious anemias
Serum iron	Male:	80–480 μg/dL (14–32 μmol/L)	Increase	Excessive hemolysis (red blood cell destruction), drug influence: excessive iron supplements
	Female:	60–460 μg/dL (11–29 μmol/L)	Decrease	Blood loss, dietary deficiency

(Continued)

252

Test		Reference Value	Increase/Decrease	Clinical Significance
TIBC[c] (measures serum iron bound with transferrin)	Adult:	250–450 µg/dL (45–82 µmol/L) or 16% saturation	Increase	Iron deficiency anemia, acute and chronic blood loss
			Decrease	Pernicious anemia; drug influence: ACTH,[d] steroids
SGOT[e]	Adult:	5–40 µ/mL	Increase	Infections; strenuous exercise; vitamin dosage; drug influence: antibiotics, narcotics, antihypertensives cortisone, indomethacin
			Decrease	Aspirin use, salicylates
Haptoglobin	Adult:	30–160 mg/dL	Decrease	Hemolysis, pernicious anemias
Ferritin	Male:	18–300 µg/dL	Decrease	Bone marrow and liver storage of iron
	Female:	10–270 µg/dL or 60 µg/L < 12 depletion > 200 overload		
Serum cholesterol	Adult:	150–220 mg/dL (5.20–5.85 mmol/L)	Decrease	Increased fat oxidation, also in malnutrition, anemia
VLDL[f]		60 mg/dL	Decrease	
LDL[g]	Adult:	50–190 mg/dL (1.3–4.9 mmol/L)	Decrease	
Triglycerides	Adult:	> 150 mg/dL (< 1.80 mmol/L)	Decrease	Increased fat oxidation, protein malnutrition
	Child:	10–140 mg/dL	Increase	Hypertension: uncontrolled diabetes; high-carbohydrate diet; drug influence: estrogens, alcohol
HDL[h]	Male:	30–70 mg/dL (0.80–1.80 mmol/L)	Decrease	Steroid use
	Female:	30–90 mg/dL (0.80–2.35 mmol/L)	Increase	Increase in hepatic enzyme activity, increased production due to exercise or both
Bilirubin	Adult:	0.1–1.2 mg/dL (2–18 µmol/L)	Increase	RBC destruction; drug influence: steroids, increased vitamin A, C, and K, antibiotics
	Child:	0.2–0.8 mg/dL	Decrease	Iron deficiency, anemia, large amounts of caffeine, aspirin

(Continued)

253

TABLE E-1. (Continued)

Test		Normal Value	Response to Exercise	Rationale
Serum potassium	Adult:	3.5–5.0 mEq/L (mmol/L)	Decrease	Vomiting and diarrhea; dehydration; crash dieting; starvation; stress and trauma; injuries; burns; increased glucose ingestion; laxative abuse; drug influence: diuretics, thiazides, steroids, antibiotics, insulin, laxatives
	Child:	3.5–5.5 mEq/L	Increase	Acute renal failure, crushing injuries, and burns (with kidney shutdown)
Serum sodium	Adult:	135–145 mEq/L (or 135–145 mmol/L)	Increase	Dehydration; severe vomiting and diarrhea; congestive heart failure; drug influence: cough medicines, cortisones, antibiotics, laxatives
			Decrease	Vomiting, increased perspiration, reduced sodium in diet, burns, tissue injury, large amounts of water
Serum magnesium	Adult:	1.6–2.4 mEq/L	Decrease	Loss of gastrointestinal fluids, use of diuretics
Uric acid	Male:	3.5–7.8 mg/dL	Decrease	Folic acid deficiency; burns; drug influence: ACTH
	Female:	2.8–6.8 mg/dL		
	Child:	2.5–5.5 mg/dL	Increase	Dehydration; nitrogen catabolism; stress; increased protein; weight reduction diets; gout; drug influence: megadose of vitamin C, diuretics, thiazides, aspirin, ACTH
Fasting glucose	Adult:	65–110 mg/dL (3.9–6.1 mmol/L)	Decrease	Hypoglycemic response to excessive glucose/sucrose solutions, extended strenuous exercise
	Child:	60–100 mg/dL	Increase	Stress, crushing injury, burns, infections, hypothermia, mild exercise, dumping syndrome, diabetes

*a*RBC = red blood cell
*b*MCV = mean corpuscular volume
*c*TIBC = total iron-binding capacity
*d*ACTH = adrenocorticotropic hormone
*e*SGOT = serum glutamic oxaloacetic transaminase
*f*VLDL = very low-density lipoprotein
*g*LDL = low-density lipoprotein
*h*HDL = high-density lipoprotein

Reprinted with permission from Peterson M, Peterson K. Eat to Compete: A Guide to Sports Nutrition. Chicago, Ill: Year Book Medical Publishers, Inc; 1988:266–269. Adapted from Kee JL. Laboratory and Diagnostic Tests with Nursing Implications. New York, NY: Appleton-Century-Crofts; 1983; Monsen ER. The Journal adopts SI units for clinical laboratory values. J Am Diet Assoc. 1987;87:356; Tilkian SM, Conover MB, Tilkian AG. Clinical Implications of Laboratory Tests. St Louis, Mo: CV Mosby Co; 1979; Krebs PS, Scully BC, Zinkgraf SA. The acute and prolonged effects of marathon running on 20 blood parameters. Phys Sports Med. 1983;11:66; Martin DE, Vroom DH, May DF, et al. Physiological changes in elite male distance runners training. Phys Sports Med. 1986;14:152.

Vitamin and Mineral Recommended Dietary Allowances and Dietary Sources

Table F–1 may be used as a reference guide for comparing the various dietary sources and major functions of vitamins and minerals.

TABLE F–1. VITAMINS AND MINERALS: THEIR RECOMMENDED DIETARY ALLOWANCE/RECOMMENDED DAILY INTAKE, DIETARY SOURCES, MAJOR BODY FUNCTIONS, AND POSSIBLE ROLES IMPORTANT DURING EXERCISE

Vitamin or Mineral	RDA for Healthy Adult Men and Women (mg)[a]	Dietary Sources	Major Body Functions	Possible Roles Important During Exercise
WATER-SOLUBLE VITAMINS				
B₁ (thiamine)	1.5 1.1	Pork, organ meats, whole grains, legumes	Coenzyme (thiamine pyrophos-phate) in reactions involving removal of carbon dioxide	Energy release from carbohydrate; formation of hemoglobin; proper nervous system functioning
B₂ (riboflavin)	1.7 1.3	Widely distributed in foods	Constituent of two flavin nucleotide coenzymes involved in energy metabolism (FAD and FMN)	Energy release from carbohydrate and fat
Niacin	19 15	Liver, lean meats, grains, legumes (can be formed from tryptophan)	Constituent of two coenzymes involved in oxidation-reduction reactions (NAD and NADP)	Energy release from carbohydrate, both aerobic and anaerobic; inhibition of FFA release from adipose tissue
B₆ (pyridoxine)	2.0 1.6	Meats, vegetables, whole-grain cereals	Coenzyme (PLP) involved in amino acid metabolism	Energy release from carbohydrate; formation of hemoglobin and oxidative enzymes; proper nervous system functioning
Pantothenic acid	4–7 4–7	Widely distributed in foods	Constituent of CoA, which plays a central role in energy metabolism	Energy production from carbohydrate and fat
Folacin	0.2 0.18	Legumes, green vegetables, whole-wheat products	Coenzyme (reduced form) involved in transfer of single-carbon units in nucleic acid and amino acid metabolism	Red blood cell production
B₁₂	0.002 0.002	Muscle meats, eggs, dairy products (not present in plant foods)	Coenzyme involved in transfer of single-carbon units in nucleic acid metabolism	Red blood cell production

(Continued)

	Amount	Sources	Function	
Biotin	0.10–0.20 0.10–0.20	Legumes, vegetables, meats	Coenzyme required for fat synthesis, amino acid metabolism, glycogen (animal starch) formation	Carbohydrate and fat synthesis
C (ascorbic acid)	60 60	Citrus fruits, tomatoes, green peppers salad greens	Maintains intercellular matrix of cartilage, bone, dentine; important in collagen synthesis	Antioxidant; increased absorption of iron; formation of epinephrine; promotion of aerobic energy production; formation of connective tissue
FAT-SOLUBLE VITAMINS A (retinol)	1.0 0.8	Provitamin A (β-carotene) widely distributed in green vegetables; retinol present in milk, butter, cheese, fortified margarine	Constituent of rhodopsin (visual pigment); maintenance of epithelial tissues; role in mucopolysaccharide synthesis	Antioxidant; prevention of red blood cell damage
D	0.005–0.010 0.005–0.010	Cod-liver oil, eggs, dairy products, fortified milk, margarine	Promotes growth and mineralization of bones; increases absorption of calcium	Calcium transport in muscle
E (tocopherol)	10 8	Seeds, green leafy vegetables, margarines, shortenings	Functions as antioxidant to prevent cell membrane damage	Antioxidant; prevention of red blood cell damage; promotion of aerobic energy production
K (phylloquinone)	0.070–0.080 0.060–0.065	Green leafy vegetables; small amounts in cereals, fruits, and meats	Important in blood clotting (involved in formation of active prothrombin)	None determined
MINERALS Calcium	800–1200 800–1200	Dairy products dark green leafy vegetables, dried legumes	Bone and tooth formation; blood clotting; nerve transmission	Muscle contraction; glycogen breakdown
Phosphorus	800–1200 800–1200	Milk, cheese, meat, poultry, grains	Bone and tooth formation; acid-base balance	Formation of ATP and creatine phosphokinase; release of oxygen from red blood cells

(Continued)

TABLE F-1. (Continued)

Vitamin or Mineral	RDA for Healthy Adult Men and Women (mg)[a]	Dietary Sources	Major Body Functions	Possible Roles Important During Exercise
MINERALS				
Potassium	1875–5625	Meats, milk, many fruits	Acid-base balance; body water balance; nerve function	Nerve impulse transmission; muscle contraction; glycogen storage
Sodium	1100–3300	Common salt	Acid-base balance; body water balance; nerve function	Nerve impulse transmission; muscle contraction; water balance
Magnesium	350 280–300	Whole grains, green leafy vegetables	Activates enzymes; involved in protein synthesis	Muscle contraction; glucose metabolism in muscle cells
Iron	10 15	Eggs, lean meats, legumes, whole grains, green leafy vegetables	Constituent of hemoglobin and enzymes involved in energy metabolism	Oxygen transport by red blood cells; oxygen utilization in muscle cells
Zinc	15 12	Widely distributed in foods	Constituent of enzymes involved in digestion	Energy production in muscle cells
Chromium	0.05–0.20	Fats, vegetables, oils, meats	Involved in glucose and energy metabolism	Glucose and energy metabolism; normal blood sugar metabolism
Copper	2 2	Meats, drinking water	Constituents of enzymes associated with iron metabolism	Oxygen transport and utilization; close work with iron
Selenium	0.070 0.050–0.055	Seafood, meat, grains	Functions in close association with vitamin E	Antioxidant

[a]First values are for men.

Reprinted with permission from Berning JR, Steen SN. Sports Nutrition for the 90s: The Health Professionals Handbook. Gaithersburg, Md, copyright 1991, Aspen Publishers, Inc; pp 136–139. Data from Scrimshaw NS, Young VR. The requirements of human nutrition. Sci Am. 1976;235:50; Recommended Dietary Allowances, revised. Washington, DC: Food and Nutrition Board, NAS-NRC; 1989 (from the National Dairy Council); Williams MH. Beyond Training. Champaign, Ill: Human Kinetics Publishers, Inc; 1989; Anderson RA, Guttman HN. Trace minerals and exercise. In: Exercise, Nutrition and Energy Metabolism. New York, NY: Macmillan Publishing Co; 1988.

Appendix G
Organization Listings

The following is a list of organizations that can be used to obtain further information on exercise, fitness, health, nutrition, sports conditioning, sports medicine, therapy, and rehabilitation.

**Academy for Psychology of Sport—
  International**
2062 Arlington Ave.
Toledo, OH 43609

Academy for Sports Dentistry
12200 Preston Rd.
Dallas, TX 75230

**Amateur Athletic Union
  of the United States**
AAU House
Box 68207
Indianapolis, IN 46268

**American Academy of Occupational
  Medicine**
2340 Arlington Heights Rd.
Arlington Heights, IL 60005

**American Academy of Orthopaedic
  Surgeons**
222 S. Prospect
Park Ridge, IL 60068

American Academy of Pediatrics
P.O. Box 1034
Evanston, IL 60204

**American Academy of Pediatrics
Committee on Sports Medicine**
141 Northwest Point Blvd.
Box 927
Elk Grove Village, IL 60009-0927

**American Academy of Physical
  Medicine and Rehabilitation**
122 S. Michigan Ave.
Suite 1300
Chicago, IL 60603

**American Academy of Podiatric
  Sports Medicine**
1729 Glastonberry Rd.
Potomac, MD 20854

**American Alliance for Health,
  Physical Education, Recreation
  and Dance**
1900 Association Dr.
Reston, VA 22091

**American Anorexia/Bulimia
  Association**
418 East 76th St.
New York, NY 10021

**American Association
of Cardiovascular
and Pulmonary Rehabilitation**
7611 Elmwood Ave.
Middleton, WI 53562

**American Association of Osteopathic
Medicine**
4720 Montgomery Lane
Washington, DC 20014

**American Association for World
Health**
2001 S. St., NW
Washington, DC 20009

**American Athletic Trainers
Association and Certification
Board, Inc.**
660 W. Duarte Rd.
Arcadia, CA 91006

American Cancer Society
1599 Clifton Rd.
Atlanta, GA 30329

American Chiropractic Association
1916 Wilson Blvd.
Arlington, VA 22201

American College of Cardiology
9111 Old Georgetown Rd.
Bethesda, MD 20814

**American College of Occupational
Medicine**
55 W. Seegers Rd.
Arlington Heights, IL 60005

**American College of Preventive
Medicine**
1015 15th St., NW
Washington, DC 20005

American College of Sports Medicine
P.O. Box 1440
Indianapolis, IN 46206-1440

American Council on Exercise
6190 Cornerstone, Court East
San Diego, CA 92121-3773

American Dental Association
211 E. Chicago Ave.
Chicago, IL 60611

American Diabetes Association
4405 East West Highway
Bethesda, MD 20814

American Dietetic Association
216 W. Jackson Blvd.
Ste. 800
Chicago, IL 60606-6995

American Heart Association
7320 Greenville Ave.
Dallas, TX 75231

American Hospital Association
840 N. Lakeshore Dr.
Chicago, IL 60611

**American Industrial Hygiene
Association**
66 South Miller Rd.
Akron, OH 44313

American Institute of Nutrition
9650 Rockville Pike
Bethesda, MD 20014

American Lung Association
1740 Broadway
New York, NY 10019

**American Massage Therapy
Association**
1130 W. Lake Shore Dr.
Chicago, IL 60626

American Medical Association
535 N. Dearborn St.
Chicago, IL 60610

**American National Standards
Institute**
1430 Broadway
New York, NY 10018

American Nurses' Association
2420 Pershing Rd.
Kansas City, MO 64108

**American Occupational Therapy
Association, Inc.**
1383 Piccard Drive
P.O. Box 1725
Rockville, MD 20849

American Optometric Association
Sports Vision Section
243 N. Lindbergh Blvd.
St. Louis, MO 63141

American Orthopaedic Society
for Sports Medicine
70 West Hubbard St.
Chicago, IL 60610

American Orthotic and Prosthetic
Association
1444 N. St., NW
Washington, DC 20005

American Osteopathic Academy
of Sports Medicine
1551 NW 54th St.
Suite 200
Seattle, WA 98107

American Osteopathic Association
211 East Ohio St.
Chicago, IL 60611

American Physical Therapy
Association
1111 N. Fairfax St.
Alexandria, VA 22314

American Physiological Society
9650 Rockville Pike
Bethesda, MD 20814

American Podiatric Medical
Association
20 Chevy Chase Circle NW
Washington, DC 20015

American Psychological Association
1200 17th St., NW
Washington, DC 20036

American Public Health Association
1015 18th St., NW
Washington, DC 20036

American Red Cross
1730 E St., NW
Washington, DC 20006

American Society of Biomechanics
in Sports
2450 Lozana Rd.
Delmar, CA 92014

American Society for Clinical
Nutrition
9650 Rockville Pike
Bethesda, MD 20014

American Society for Testing
and Materials
1916 Race St.
Philadelphia, PA 19103

Aquatic Exercise Association
P.O. Box 497
Port Washington, WI 53074

Arthritis Foundation
3400 Peachtree Rd., NE
Atlanta, GA 30326

Association for Fitness in Business
310 N. Alabama
Indianapolis, IN 46204

Association of Physical Fitness
Centers
600 Jefferson St.
Rockville, MD 20852

Center for Occupational
and Environmental Health
University of California
2521 Channing Way
Berkeley, CA 94720

College of Health and Human
Performance
University of Florida
Gainesville, FL 32611

Commission on Accreditation
of Rehabilitation Facilities
101 North Wilmot Rd.
Tucson, AZ 85711

Consumer Product Safety
Commission
1111 18th St., NW
Washington, DC 20207

Federation of the Handicapped
211 W. 14th St.
New York, NY 10011

Food and Nutrition Board
National Research Council
National Academy of Sciences
2101 Constitution Ave. NW
Washington, DC 20418

Institute for Aerobics Research
12330 Preston Rd.
Dallas, TX 75230

International Center for Sports Nutrition
502 S. 44th St.
Omaha, NE 68131

International Chiropractic Association
1901 L St., NW
Washington, DC 20036

International Federation of Body Builders
2875 Bates Rd.
Montreal, Canada H3S1B7

International Federation of Sports Medicine
5800 Jeff Place
Edina, MN 55436

Joint Commission on Accreditation of Hospitals
875 North Michigan Ave.
Chicago, IL 60611

Library of Congress
Science and Technology Division
10 First St., SE
Washington, DC 20540

National Association of Governors' Councils on Physical Fitness and Sports
Pan American Plaza
201 S. Capitol Ave.
Indianapolis, IN 46225

National Association of the Physically Handicapped
76 Elm St.
London, OH 43140

National Athletic Trainers' Association
2952 Stemmens
Dallas, TX 75247

National Bureau of Standards
Route I-270 and Quince Orchard Rd.
Gaithersburg, MD 20899

**National Collegiate Athletic Association
Committee on Competitive Safeguards and Medical Aspects of Sports**
Box 1906
Mission, KS 66201

National Council Against Health Fraud
P.O. Box 1276
Loma Linda, CA 92354

National Environmental Health Association
720 S. Colorado Blvd.
Denver, CO 80222

National Health Council
350 5th Ave.
New York, NY 10017

National Institute for Occupational Safety and Health
Appalachian Laboratories
944 Chestnut Ridge Rd.
Morgantown, WV 26505-2888

National Institute for Occupational Safety and Health
Centers for Disease Control
1600 Clifton Rd.
Atlanta, GA 30333

National Institute for Occupational Safety and Health
Cincinnati Laboratories
4676 Columbia Parkway
Cincinnati, OH 45226

National Institutes of Health
9000 Rockville Pike
Bethesda, MD 20892

National Library of Medicine
8600 Rockville Pike
Bethesda, MD 20894

National Rehabilitation Association
633 S. Washington St.
Alexandria, VA 22314

National Safety Council
444 N. Michigan Ave.
Chicago, IL 60611

National Sporting Goods Association
1699 Wall St.
Mt. Prospect, IL 60056-5780

National Strength and Conditioning Association
300 Old City Hall Landmark
916 O St.
Box 81410
Lincoln, NE 68501

National Wheelchair Athletic Association
3617 Betty Dr.
Colorado Springs, CO 80917

Occupational Safety and Health Administration
Department of Labor
200 Constitution Ave.
Washington, DC 20210

President's Council on Physical Fitness and Sports
450 Fifth St., NW
Washington, DC 20001

Society for Nutrition Education
1736 Franklin St.
Oakland, CA 94612

Special Olympics
1701 K St., NW
Washington, DC 20006

Sports Physical Therapy Section
5915 Ponce deLeon Blvd.
5th Floor, Plumer Bldg.
Coral Gables, FL 33146

United Fresh Fruit and Vegetable Association
727 North Washington St.
Alexandria, VA 22314

United States Consumer Product Safety Commission
Office of Information and Public Affairs
Washington, DC 20207

United States Department of Health and Human Services
200 Independence Ave., SW
Washington, DC 20201

United States Food and Drug Administration
Office of Consumer Affairs
HFE-88
5600 Fishers Lane
Rockville, MD 20857

United States Government Printing Office
Washington, DC 20402

United States Olympic Committee
Division of Sports Medicine and Science
1750 East Boulder St.
Colorado Springs, CO 80909

United States Olympic Training Center
Sports Medicine
1776 Older Ave.
Colorado Springs, CO 80909-7760

United States Powerlifting Federation
(For Powerlifting)
1968 West, 6000 South
Roy, UT 84067

United States Sports Academy
1 Academy Dr.
Daphne, AL 36526-9552

United States Weightlifting Federation
(For Olympic Lifting)
1750 East Boulder St.
Colorado Springs, CO 80909

YMCA of the USA
101 North Wacker Dr.
Chicago, IL 60606

Journal Listings

The following is a list of journals that can be used to research areas in exercise, fitness, health, nutrition, sports conditioning, sports medicine, therapy, and rehabilitation.

BIOMECHANICS

Clinical Biomechanics
Journal of Biomechanics
International Journal of Sport Biomechanics

CARDIAC

American Heart Journal
American Journal of Cardiology
Circulation
Journal of the American College of Cardiology
Journal of Cardiac Rehabilitation
Journal of Cardiopulmonary Rehabilitation
Journal of Electrocardiology
Progress in Cardiovascular Diseases

HEALTH

American Journal of Epidemiology
American Journal of Preventive Medicine
American Journal of Public Health
Archives of Environmental Health
Health Education Quarterly
Holistic Medicine
Preventive Medicine

INDUSTRIAL AND OCCUPATIONAL MEDICINE

American Industrial Hygiene Association Journal
American Journal of Industrial Medicine
American Journal of Occupational Therapy
Applied Ergonomics
British Journal of Industrial Medicine
Ergonomics
Ergonomics Abstracts
European Journal of Applied Physiology and Occupational Physiology
Human Factors Journal
International Archives of Occupational and Environmental Health
Journal of Occupational Medicine
Occupational Health and Safety News
Occupational Therapy in Health Care

MEDICINE

American Journal of Medicine
Diabetic Medicine
Critical Reviews in Biomedical Engineering
Journal of the American Medical Association
Journal of Bone and Joint Surgery
Lancet
New England Journal of Medicine
Seminars in Arthritis and Rheumatism
Seminars in Orthopedics
Seminars in Spine Surgery
Spine
Stress Medicine

NUTRITION

American Journal of Clinical Nutrition
Critical Reviews in Food Science and Nutrition
International Journal of Obesity
International Journal of Sport Nutrition
Journal of the American College of Nutrition
Journal of the American Dietetic Association
Journal of Nutrition
Journal of Nutrition Education
Nutrition Action
Nutrition in Clinical Practice
Nutrition Reviews
Nutrition Today

PHYSIOLOGY AND ANATOMY

American Journal of Anatomy
American Journal of Physiology
European Journal of Applied Physiology
Journal of Applied Physiology
Journal of Physiology
Muscle and Nerve
Physiological Reviews

SPORT PSYCHOLOGY

International Journal of Sport and Exercise Psychology
Journal of Sports Psychology
Sport and Exercise Psychology
Sport Psychologist

SPORTS

International Olympic Lifter
Powerlifting U.S.A.

SPORTS MEDICINE

American Journal of Sports Medicine
Annals of Sports Medicine
Athletic Training
British Journal of Sports Medicine
Chiropractic Sports Medicine
Clinical Sports Medicine
International Journal of Sports Medicine
Journal of Orthopaedic and Sports Physical Therapy
Journal of Sports Medicine
Journal of Sports Medicine and Physical Fitness
Physician and Sportsmedicine
Sports Medicine
Sports Medicine Bulletin

SPORTS SCIENCE

Adapted Physical Therapy Quarterly
Canadian Journal of Sport Sciences
Exercise and Sport Science Reviews
Human Movement Science
Isokinetics and Exercise Science
Journal of Applied Physiology, Respiration, Environmental and Exercise Physiology
Journal of Applied Sport Science Research
Journal of Human Movement Studies
Journal of Human Muscle Performance
Journal of Physical Education, Recreation and Dance
Medicine and Science in Sports and Exercise
National Strength and Conditioning Association Journal
Pediatric Exercise Science
Research Quarterly
Research Quarterly in Exercise and Sport
Scandinavian Journal of Sports Science
Sport Science Review
Women in Sport and Physical Activity

THERAPY AND REHABILITATION

Adapted Physical Activity Quarterly
American Corrective Therapy Journal
American Journal of Physical Medicine and Rehabilitation
Archives of Physical Medicine and Rehabilitation

Chiropractic Technique
Clinical Management in Physical Therapy
Critical Reviews in Physical and Rehabilitation Medicine
Foot and Ankle
Journal of Chiropractic
Journal of Manipulative and Physiological Therapeutics
Journal of Manual Medicine
Journal of Physical and Medical Rehabilitation
Journal of Physical Medicine
Journal of Rehabilitation
Journal of Rehabilitation Research and Development
Journal of Sport Rehabilitation
Orthopedic Clinics of North America
Orthopedic Product News
Pediatric Physical Therapy
Pediatric Research
Pediatrics
Physical and Occupational Therapy in Geriatrics
Physical and Occupational Therapy in Pediatrics
Physical Therapy
Physical Therapy Bulletin
Physical Therapy in Health Care
Physical Therapy Practice
Physical Therapy Reviews
Physical Therapy Today
Physiotherapy
Rehab Management, The Journal of Therapy and Rehabilitation

REFERENCES

1. Adams GM. *Exercise Physiology Laboratory Manual*. Dubuque, Iowa: Wm C Brown Publishers; 1990.
2. American Association of Cardiovascular and Pulmonary Rehabilitation. *Guidelines for Cardiac Rehabilitation Programs*. Champaign, Ill: Human Kinetics Publishers, Inc; 1991.
3. American College of Sports Medicine. *Guidelines for Exercise Testing and Prescription*. 4th ed. Philadelphia, Pa: Lea & Febiger; 1991.
4. American College of Sports Medicine. Information for authors. *Med Sci Sports Exerc.* 1991;23(1):i–v.
5. American College of Sports Medicine. Policy statement regarding the use of human subjects and informed consent. *Med Sci Sports Exerc.* 1991;23(1):vi.
6. American Heart Association. *The Exercise Standards Book* (reprinted from *Circulation.* 1979;59:421A; *Circulation.* 1979;59:849A; *Circulation.* 1979;59:1084A; *Circulation.* 1980; 62:699A). Dallas, Tex: American Heart Association; 1980.
7. American Heart Association. AHA Medical/Scientific Statement: Exercise standards—A Statement for Health Professionals from the American Heart Association. *Circulation.* 1990;82(6):2286–2322.
8. Åstrand P-O. *Work Tests with the Bicycle Ergometer*. Varberg, Sweden: Monark-Crescent AB; (undated).
9. Åstrand P-O, Rodahl K. *Textbook of Work Physiology: Physiological Bases of Exercise*. 3rd ed. New York, NY: McGraw-Hill Book Co; 1986.
10. Backus RDH, Reid DC. Evaluating the health status of the athlete. In: MacDougall JD, Wenger HA, Green HJ, eds. *Physiological Testing of the High-Performance Athlete*. 2nd ed. Champaign, Ill: Human Kinetics Publishers, Inc; 1991.
11. Blair SN, Painter P, Pate RR, et al, eds. *Resource Manual for Guidelines for Exercise Testing and Prescription* (American College of Sports Medicine). Philadelphia, Pa: Lea & Febiger; 1988.
12. Block G. A review of validations of dietary assessment methods. *Am J Epidemiol.* 1982;115:492.

13. Brannon FJ, Geyer MJ, Foley NW. *Cardiac Rehabilitation*. Philadelphia, Pa: FA Davis Co; 1988.

14. Brown TL, LeMay HE. *Chemistry: The Central Science*. 2nd ed. Englewood Cliffs, NJ: Prentice-Hall; 1981.

15. Chung EK. *Exercise Electrocardiography: Practical Approach*. 2nd ed. Baltimore, Md: Williams & Wilkins; 1983.

16. Dubin D. *Rapid Interpretation of EKG's*. 3rd ed. Tampa, Fla: Cover Publishing; 1974.

17. Dunne LJ. *Nutrition Almanac*. 3rd ed. New York, NY: McGraw-Hill Book Co; 1990.

18. Garg A, Chaffin DB, Herrin GD. Prediction of metabolic rates for manual materials handling jobs. *Am Ind Hyg Assoc J*. 1978;39:661–674.

19. Goldberger AL, Goldberger E. *Clinical Electrocardiography: A Simplified Approach*. St. Louis, Mo: CV Mosby Co; 1986.

20. Halliday D, Resnick R. *Fundamentals of Physics*. 2nd ed. New York, NY: John Wiley & Sons, Inc; 1986.

21. Herbert DL. *Legal Aspects of Sports Medicine*. Canton, Ohio: Professional Reports Corporation; 1990.

22. Herbert DL, Herbert WG. *Legal Aspects of Preventive and Rehabilitative Exercise Programs*. 2nd ed. Canton, Ohio: Professional Reports Corporation; 1989.

23. Herbert WG, Herbert DL. Legal considerations. In: Blair SN, Painter P, Pate RR, et al, eds. *Resource Manual for Guidelines for Exercise Testing and Prescription* (American College of Sports Medicine). Philadelphia, Pa: Lea & Febiger; 1988.

24. Heyward VH. *Designs for Fitness: A Guide to Physical Fitness Appraisal and Exercise Prescription*. Minneapolis, Minn: Burgess Publishing Co; 1984.

25. Heyward VH. *Advanced Fitness Assessment and Exercise Prescription*. 2nd ed. Champaign, Ill: Human Kinetics Publishers, Inc; 1991.

26. Karam C. *A Practical Guide to Cardiac Rehabilitation*. Gaithersburg, Md: Aspen Publishers, Inc; 1989.

27. Keys A. Dietary survey methods. In: *Nutrition, Lipids and Coronary Heart Disease* (*Nutrition in Health and Disease*). New York, NY: Raven Press; 1979;1.

28. Kibler WB. *The Sport Preparticipation Fitness Examination*. Champaign, Ill: Human Kinetics Publishers, Inc; 1990.

29. Koeberle BE. *Legal Aspects of Personal Fitness Training*. Canton, Ohio: Professional Reports Corporation; 1990.

30. Krause MV, Mahan KL. *Food, Nutrition and Diet Therapy*. 7th ed. Philadelphia, Pa: WB Saunders Co; 1984.

31. Kreighbaum E, Barthels KM. *Biomechanics: A Qualitative Approach for Studying Human Movement*. Minneapolis, Minn: Burgess Publishing Co; 1981.

32. McArdle WD, Katch FI, Katch VL. *Exercise Physiology: Energy, Nutrition and Human Performance*. 3rd ed. Philadelphia, Pa: Lea & Febiger; 1991.

33. Moran MJ, Shapiro HN. *Fundamentals of Engineering Thermodynamics*. New York, NY: John Wiley & Sons, Inc; 1988.

34. Özişik MN. *Heat Transfer: A Basic Approach*. New York, NY: McGraw-Hill Book Co; 1985.

35. Page DM, ed. Dietary assessment. In: *Manual of Clinical Nutrition*. Pleasantville, NJ: Nutrition Publications; 1983.

36. Peterson M, Peterson K. *Eat to Compete: A Guide to Sports Nutrition*. Chicago, Ill: Year Book Medical Publishers, Inc; 1988.

37. Pollock ML, Wilmore JH. *Exercise in Health and Disease: Evaluation of Prescription for Prevention and Rehabilitation*. 2nd ed. Philadelphia, Pa: WB Saunders Co; 1990.

38. Powers SK, Howley ET. *Exercise Physiology: Theory and Application to Fitness and Performance*. Dubuque, Iowa: Wm C Brown Publishers; 1990.

39. Ross RM, Jackson AS. *Exercise Concepts, Calculations and Computer Applications*. Carmel, Ind: Benchmark Press; 1990.

40. Sale DG. Testing strength and power. In: MacDougall JD, Wenger HA, Green HJ, eds. *Physiological Testing of the High-Performance Athlete*. 2nd ed. Champaign, Ill: Human Kinetics Publishers, Inc; 1991.

41. Stein J, ed. *The Random House College Dictionary*, revised ed. New York, NY: Random House; 1984.

42. Thoden JS. Testing aerobic power. In: MacDougall JD, Wenger HA, Green HJ, eds. *Physiological Testing of the High-Performance Athlete*. 2nd ed. Champaign, Ill: Human Kinetics Publishers, Inc; 1991.

43. Thomas CL, ed. *Taber's Cyclopedic Medical Dictionary*. 15th ed. Philadelphia, Pa: FA Davis Co; 1985.

44. Tippens PE. *Applied Physics*. 3rd ed. New York, NY: McGraw-Hill Book Co; 1985.

45. Wasserman K, Hansen JE, Sue DY, et al. *Principles of Exercise Testing and Interpretation*. Philadelphia, Pa: Lea & Febiger; 1987.

46. White FM. *Fluid Mechanics*. 2nd ed. New York, NY: McGraw-Hill Book Company; 1986.

47. Whitney EN, Hamilton EMN. *Understanding Nutrition*. 2nd ed. St Paul, Minn: West Publishing Co; 1981.

48. Yule JD, ed. *Concise Encyclopedia of the Sciences*. New York, NY: Facts on File; 1978.

49. Zigon ST. *How to Use the American College of Sports Medicine Metabolic Equations*. Canton, Ohio: Professional Reports Corporation; 1990.

Glossary

In addition to defining various terms and concepts found throughout the book, this glossary has also been referenced and, therefore, can be used as a supplement for those clinicians seeking additional information on exercise testing, prescription, and rehabilitation–related topics. The terms and concepts used in this glossary have generally been represented as they appear in the original source.

Note: *Syn* = synonym

Absolute. Units of work, power, or energy that are not adjusted for body size, gender, or fitness differences; non-weight-bearing activities are measured in absolute units (eg, kg·min^{-1}, watts, L · min^{-1}).[10]

Absolute $\dot{V}O_2$. The amount of oxygen consumed over a given time period; expressed as liters · min^{-1}.[63]

Acceleration. The change in velocity (speed and/or direction) per unit of time.[48]

Accessory Movement. Movement within a joint and surrounding soft tissues that is necessary for normal range of motion but cannot be voluntarily performed. Terms that relate are component motions and joint play.[45]

Acclimatization. The ability of the body to undergo physiologic adaptations so that the stress of a given environment, such as high environmental temperature, is less severe over time.[87]

Accommodating Resistance Training. A form of training in which the resistance is varied in a systematic manner in an attempt to match the force-producing capabilities of the muscle or muscle group (eg, Hydra-Gym).[62] *See* Isokinetic

Active-Assistive Range of Motion. A type of active range of motion in which assistance is provided by an outside force, either manually or mechanically, because the prime mover muscles need assistance to complete the motion.[45]

Active Inhibition. A stretching maneuver to inhibit tonus in a tight muscle.[45]

Active Range of Motion. Movement, within the unrestricted range of motion for a segment, that is produced by an active contraction of the muscles crossing that joint.[45]

Active Stretching. Accomplished by the client using his or her own muscles and without any assistance from an external force (eg, the client slowly and deliberately lifts one leg while in a standing position to its end range without holding that position for any specific length of time).[2]

Activities of Daily Living. The self-care, communication, and mobility skills required for independence in everyday living (eg, gait, sitting, standing, dressing).[80] *Syn:* independent living skills, daily living skills[80]

Acute-Onset Muscle Soreness. Related to an impedence of circulation, causing muscular ischemia. Lactic acid and potassium collect in the muscle and stimulate pain receptors. This occurs immediately after exercise and is resolved when exercise has ceased.[12]

Adenosine Diphosphate (ADP). The two-phosphate product of ATP breakdown; it is formed when ATP releases its stored energy.[82]

Adenosine Triphosphate (ATP). The major energy carrier that transfers chemical potential energy from one molecule to another; energy is transferred to ATP during its formation from ADP and phosphate as a result of the catabolism of carbohydrates, fat, and protein. It is released to perform work by the cell during the subsequent breakdown of ATP into ADP and phosphate.[82]

Adipose Tissue. Tissue that is composed largely of fat-storing cells.[82]

Aerobic. Relating to the energy processes that occur in the presence of oxygen.[87]

Aerobic Energy. Energy that results from the breakdown of carbohydrates, fats, and protein within the Krebs cycle and the electron transport system. Oxygen is required in this type of energy transformation.[10]

Aerobic Exercise. 1. Exercise during which the energy needed is supplied by the oxygen inspired.[80] 2. Submaximal, rhythmic, repetitive exercise of large muscle groups, during which the needed energy is supplied by inspired oxygen.[45]

Aerobic Fitness. The ability to sustain prolonged endurance activities that use the oxygen energy system.[87] *Syn:* cardiovascular fitness, cardiovascular endurance[87]

Aerobic Metabolism. Catabolism of energy substrates with the utilization of oxygen; energy transfer resulting from involvement of electron transport and the accompanying oxidative phosphorylation.[19]

Aerobic Power. The maximal volume of oxygen consumed per unit of time.[35] *Syn:* maximal oxygen uptake, maximal oxygen consumption

Aerobic Threshold. A 2-mM concentration of lactic acid in blood plasma; theorized to be the intensity of work where aerobic metabolism is the major contributor of energy for muscular work.[10]

Aerobic Walking. Rapid walking designed to elevate the heart rate so a training effect will occur; more strenuous than ordinary leisure walking.[87]

Afterload. The workload applied to the heart during systole by the resistance of the systemic vasculature.[42]

Age-Predicted Maximal Heart Rate. Estimated attainable highest number of ventricular contractions, computed by subtracting one's age from 220. It is considered a fairly accurate estimate of a sample's true maximal heart rate and generally within 10 to 15 beats of an individual's actual maximal heart rate and is frequently used to prescribe target heart-rate ranges.[10]

Agility. Ability to change direction quickly while maintaining control of the body.[75]

Agonist Muscle. 1. A muscle that causes a motion (prime mover).[48] 2. A muscle that contributes to the desired movement by its concentric contraction.[35]

All or None Law. A phenomenon whereby a motor unit contracts either maximally or not at all under similar environmental conditions.

Alpha Motor Neurons. Nerves that cause skeletal muscle fibers (extrafusal fibers) to contract.[35]

Amount of a Substance. That amount of the particular substance containing the same number of particles as there are in 12 grams (1 mole) of the nuclide ^{12}C (units: mole or millimole). For respiratory gases, one mole of the gas at STPD is equal to 22.4 liters.[6]

Anabolism. The building up of the body substance; the constructive phase of metabolism by which a cell takes from the blood the substances required for repair and growth.[80]

Anaerobic. Relating to the energy processes that occur in the absence of oxygen.[07]

Anaerobic Capacity. The ability to persist at the maintenance or repetition of strenuous muscular contractions that rely substantially on anaerobic mechanisms of energy supply.[35]

Anaerobic Exercise. Exercise during which the energy needed is provided without utilization of inspired oxygen.[80]

Anaerobic Fitness. Ability to perform high-intensity, all-out exercise.[10]

Anaerobic Metabolism. Catabolism of energy substrates without the utilization of oxygen; energy transfer that does not require oxygen.[19]

Anaerobic Power. The maximal rate at which energy can be produced for short periods of time.[35]

Anaerobic Threshold. The work rate at which blood lactate concentration starts to increase during graded exercise (ie, onset of blood lactate accumulation); the work rate at which metabolic acidosis and associated changes in respiratory gas exchange occur during graded exercise.[19] *Syn:* lactate threshold

Anatomic Position. The upright body position in which all joints are extended and the palms are facing forward.[48]

Angle of Projection. The angle at which an object or body is projected at release or takeoff; measured in relation to a stated frame of reference, usually the horizontal.[48] *Syn:* angle of release, angle of takeoff

Antagonistic Muscle. 1. A muscle that can cause the joint movement opposite to the movement being done by an agonist.[48] 2. A muscle that causes a movement opposite the desired movement. Resistance to the desired movement would occur if it were to contract.[35]

Anthropometry. 1. Measurement of human body characteristics, such as size, breadth, girth, and distance between anatomic points. It also includes segment masses, the centers of gravity of body segments, and the ranges of joint motion.[65] 2. Anthropometry is a practical and less expensive alternative to estimating body composition. Anthropometry is the science dealing with the measurement of size, weight, and proportions of the human body. It includes measures such as skinfolds, circumferences, diameters, height, and weight.[5,62]

Apnea. Lack of breathing.[42]

Archimedes' Principle. A body that is partially or totally immersed in a fluid will experience an upward buoyant force that is equal to the weight of the volume of fluid displaced by that body.[48]

Arrhythmia. An irregular rhythm of the heart rate.[87]

Arteriosclerosis. Thickening of the walls of the arterioles with loss of elasticity and contractility.[80]

Arteriovenous Oxygen Difference (a-$\bar{v}O_2$ difference). The difference in oxygen content between the blood entering and that leaving the pulmonary capillaries.[19]

Arthritis. Inflammation of the structures of a joint.[45]

Assessment. 1. Measurement, quantification, or placing a value or label on something; assessment is often confused with evaluation; an assessment results from the act of assessing.[9] 2. To determine the importance, size, or value. Clinically, a judgment or interpretation.[40]

Assisted Training. Strength training technique characterized by helping the exerciser perform a few additional repetitions after muscle failure has occurred with the selected resistance.[85]

Assistive Device. Appliance that aids, facilitates, or compensates for ambulation, stability, correction of deformities, immobilization, or amplification to enhance functional ability.[10]

Asthma. An obstructive lung disease seen in young patients, associated with a hypersensitivity to specific allergens and resulting in bronchospasm and difficulty in breathing.[45]

Atherosclerosis. A form of arteriosclerosis characterized by a variable combination of changes of the intima (ie, innermost coat of a structure) of arteries, not arterioles, consisting of the focal accumulation of lipids, complex carbohydrates, blood and blood products, fibrous tissue, and calcium deposits and associated with changes in the media of the arteries.[80]

Athlete. A person trained to compete in contests involving physical agility, stamina or strength; a trained competitor in a sport, exercise, or game requiring physical skill.[78]

Athletic Trainer. An individual who is responsible for the prevention (ie, performing preseason physical evaluations, taping, and bracing), recognition and evaluation (ie, evaluation of injured athletes), management and treatment (ie, administering standard approved techniques of first aid), and rehabilitation (ie, utilizing appropriate therapeutic modalities and exercise) of athletic-related injuries. It should be noted that the above is only a partial listing of the responsibilities and duties of an athletic trainer.[46,56]

ATP-CP System. The metabolic pathway involving muscle stores of ATP and the use of creatine phosphate to rephosphorylate ADP. This pathway is used at the onset of exercise and during short-term, high-intensity work.[63]

Atrophy. Reduction in size and/or mass of cells and tissues.[15]

Auscultation. Listening with a stethoscope.[42]

Axis of Rotation. The imaginary line or point about which a body or segment rotates.[48]

Balance. Ability to maintain equilibrium while in motion.[75]

Ballistic (Dynamic) Stretching. 1. A rapid stretching movement (eg, bobbing to touch toes).[63] 2. A dynamic or ballistic-type stretching technique performed by the client using the momentum of his or her own moving body segments (ie, the leg or arm). Ballistic-type stretching techniques involve bobbing, bouncing, rebounding, and rhythmic-type movements.[2] 3. The final position or end range of ballistic stretching is not held.[74] 4. Progressive Velocity Flexibility Program (PVFP) takes an athlete through a series of stretching exercises in which the velocity and range of lengthening are combined and controlled on a progressive basis. The PVFP allows an athlete to progress from an environment of control to activity simulation, from slow-velocity methodical activity to high-velocity functional activity.[88]

Basal Metabolic Rate. Measurement of energy expenditure in the body under resting, postabsorptive conditions; indicative of the energy needed to maintain life under these basal conditions.[87]

Basal Metabolism. The amount of energy needed for maintenance of life when the subject is at digestive, physical, and emotional rest.[80]

Base of Support (BOS). The region bounded by body parts in contact with some resistive surface that exerts a counterforce against the body's applied force. For example, the outline of the foot defines one's base of support when standing on one foot, or if one is hanging by both hands from a horizontal bar, the area enclosed between the outer limits of the fingers forms the base of support.[48]

Bayes' Theorem. Concerned with analyzing the probability that a patient may be considered to have a certain diagnosis or disease when it is known that the patient has certain attributes such as an abnormal test. It is usually known how frequently that particular attribute is present in the population considered to have the specific disease.[34,80]

Benefit/Risk Ratio. The relationship of health benefits to be received versus the risks associated with certain behaviors and actions.[87]

Biomechanics. The area of study wherein knowledge and methods of mechanics are applied to the structure and function of the living human system.[48]

Biopsy. The extraction of small pieces of tissue for chemical and/or histologic analysis and study.[15]

Blood Pressure (BP). The pressure exerted by the blood against the walls of blood vessels (unit: mm Hg).[19]

Body Builders. Persons who use strength training as a means for achieving a better muscular appearance, especially with regard to muscle size, shape, definition, and proportion.[85]

Body Composition. Body composition is a component that falls within kinanthropometric testing parameters. Body composition can be defined as the quantification of the various components of the body (especially fat, water, and muscle).[80] It can be measured by various methods including hydrostatic weighing (criterion measure), anthropometry (eg, skinfolds, circumferences), and other methods such as radiographic analysis, ultrasound techniques, electrical conductance, and computerized tomography.

Body Density. Density of the human body expressed as g/cc. The higher the proportion of the body weight that is lean body weight, the higher the body density.[66]

Body Weight Exercises. Exercises in which one's body weight serves as the resistance (eg, push-ups and sit-ups).[85]

Bone. Osseous tissue, a specialized form of dense connective tissue consisting of bone cells (osteocytes) embedded in a matrix made up of calcified intercellular substance. Bone provides shape and support for the body of vertebrates, serves as a storage site for mineral salts, and plays an important role in providing in the marrow a site for the formation of blood cells.[80]

Bounding. Exercises that exaggerate the normal running stride in order to stress a specific aspect of the stride cycle. Typically used to improve stride length and frequency.[25]

Bradycardia. Slow heart action; usually defined as a heart rate under 60 beats per minute.[19]

Break Tests. The tester exerts a force against the tested person's limb segment until the tested person's effort is overcome and the part gives way.[21]

Bulk-Up Method. A method of weight training designed to increase muscle mass.[85]

Buoyant Force. The upper force exerted on an immersed body by the water beneath it.[48]

Cable Tensiometer. Measures the pulling force of a muscle during a static or isometric contraction.[44]

Cadence. The number of steps taken per minute.[60]

Calisthenics. An exercise program that emphasizes development of gracefulness, suppleness, and range of motion and the strength required for such movement.[80]

Calorie. The unit in which heat energy is measured. The amount of heat needed to change the temperature of one gram of water one degree centigrade.[82]

Calorimetry. Determination of heat loss or gain; a means of determining energy expenditure of an animal by direct measurement of its heat production or indirect measurement of respiratory gas exchange.[19]

Cardiac Cycle. One contraction–relaxation episode of the heart.[82]

Cardiac Output. 1. The volume of blood pumped by each ventricle per minute (not the total output pumped by both ventricles).[82] 2. The product of heart rate and stroke volume.[63]

Cardiac Rehabilitation. Process by which the person with cardiovascular disease, including but not limited to patients with coronary heart disease, is restored to and maintained at his or her optimal physiological, psychological, social, vocational, and emotional status.[3]

Cardiovascular Endurance. The ability of the cardiovascular system to provide sufficient energy to sustain aerobic exercise for prolonged periods of time.[87]

Catabolism. The destructive phase of metabolism, the opposite of anabolism. Catabolism includes all the processes in which complex substances are converted into simpler substances, usually with a release of energy.[80]

Cellulite. A commercially created name given to the ''lumpy'' fat that often appears in the thigh and hip regions of women. It is simply normal fat in small compartments formed by connective tissue.[87]

Center of Gravity. That point at which all the body's mass seems to be concentrated; the balance point of the body; the point around which the sum of all torques of the segmental weights is equal to zero. The point of application of gravity's force on a mass; the center of mass.[48]

Center of Mass. Theoretical point at which all of a body's mass is considered to be concentrated.[10]

Central Training Effects. Training effects that can be measured by changes in cardiac function.[42]

Certified Strength and Conditioning Specialist (CSCS). The purpose of the certification examination given by the National Strength and Conditioning Association is to improve the level of knowledge and skills possessed by those who design and implement strength and conditioning programs and to identify those who have acquired the appropriate levels of expertise to be recognized as Certified Strength and Conditioning Specialists. The certification is designed to ensure a minimum level of competence among practitioners and to create a better awareness among the public of the nature and purpose of the profession and the need for industry guidelines for the safe and effective strength training and conditioning of athletes.[59]

Circadian Rhythm. A physical measurement, such as body temperature of a chemical response (eg, the excretion of catecholamines) that varies periodically over 24 hours.[65]

Circuit Training. 1. A method of training involving activities or weight stations that are accomplished in sets during which the participant moves from one activity to another with little rest between sets.[40] 2. Refers to work performed on a number of exercise modalities (eg, cardiovascular and resistance training equipment) with or without relief sessions between the exercise modalities.[5]

Closed-Circuit Spirometry. 1. A method in which a person breathes and rebreathes from a prefilled container or spirometer of oxygen.[54] 2. The method of estimating metabolic rate of the body using a spirometer to measure air taken into and expelled from the lungs.[35]

Closed Kinetic Chain. Exists when the distal segment of an extremity is fixed (eg, when the foot is in contact with the ground and the individual is performing a squatting-type motion).[50,60]

Cocontraction. A simultaneous contraction of agonistic and antagonistic muscle groups about a joint.[40]

Complex Training. Alternating weight training and plyometrics within the same workout session (eg, combining strength movement exercises like squats with speed movements like the standing triple jump).[25]

Component Motions. Motions that accompany active motion but are not under voluntary control (eg, upward rotation of the scapula and clavicle that occur with shoulder flexion).[45] *Syn:* accessory movement

Concentric Muscle Contraction. A dynamic action in which the ends of the muscle (bony attachments) are moved closer together and movement of the skeleton occurs.[47] *Syn:* shortening, miometric, positive work[47]

Conditioning. An augmentation of the energy capacity of the muscle through an exercise program.[45]

Conduction. Process of body heat movement into the molecules of cooler objects in contact with the body.[63]

Continuous Training. 1. Activity in which the heart rate is increased to a predetermined level and maintained at that level for the duration of the training session.[49] 2. A steady-paced exercise performed at either moderate or high aerobic intensity (60% to 80% max $\dot{V}O_2$) for a sustained duration.[54]

Contraction. Development of tension within a muscle or muscle group with or without changes in its overall length.[40]

Contracture. 1. A shortening of connective tissue that results in decreased range of motion in the corresponding joint.[40] 2. Shortening or tightening of the skin, fascia, muscle, or joint capsule that prevents normal mobility or flexibility of that structure.[45]

Contraindication. Any symptom or circumstance indicating the inappropriateness of a form of treatment otherwise inadvisable.[80]

Controlled Movement Speed. A weightload is raised and lowered in a slow and controlled manner to provide consistent application of force throughout the exercise movement.[85]

Convection. The transmission of heat from one object to another through the circulation of heated molecules.[63]

Cool-Down. Post-performance exercise used to dissipate heat, maintain blood flow, and aid recovery of muscles.[75] *Syn:* warm-down

Coordination. Using the right muscles at the right time with correct intensity. Coordination is the basis of smooth and efficient movement, which often occurs automatically.[45]

Coronary Risk Factors. The behaviors (eg, smoking) or body properties (eg, cholesterol levels) that may predispose an individual to coronary heart disease.[87]

Creatine Phosphate (CP). A compound found in skeletal muscle used to resynthesize ATP from ADP.[63]

Cross Training. 1. Regularly performing more than one aerobic activity to exercise different muscle groups and provide variety.[29] An example of cross training may include the interchanging of weight-supported activities (eg, cycling, rowing, swimming) with weight-bearing activities (eg, walking, jogging, stair climbing) and can also incorporate circuit weight training and calisthenic-type activities. 2. Chronic exercise program incorporating activities that may synergistically support overall physical fitness; fitness probably results from some central physiological adaptations without peripheral over-training.[10] 3. Encompasses a complex training prescription in which two or more sports are combined into either a single workout or a long-term cyclical program. It allows for the simultaneous training of multiple physiological variables (eg, aerobic and anaerobic power, muscular strength and endurance).[61] 4. The training effect that occurs in one side of the body as a result of exercising the opposite side of the body.[35]

Cryostretching. A technique where stretching is combined with cold application for the purpose of lengthening connective tissue structures and/or increasing the range of joint motion. Cryostretching may be used when the therapeutic goal is to tear connective tissue (such as adhesions), rather than stretch it; when the affected body area is so painful that without cold induced analgesia, no range of motion therapy could be attempted; when muscle spasticity significantly interferes with the proper performance of range of motion therapy.[72]

Cycle Ergometer. A stationary cycle used to regulate power output, which is regulated by placing more resistance on the flywheel and/or pedaling at a faster rate.[66]

Deceleration. The decrease in velocity per unit time.[48]

Deconditioning. A change that takes place in cardiovascular, neuromuscular, and metabolic functions as a result of prolonged bed rest or inactivity.[45]

Dehydration. Excessive loss of body fluid.[15]

Delayed-Onset Muscle Soreness (DOMS). The cause of DOMS apparently is sublethal and lethal damage to a small group of recruited muscle fibers. The perception of soreness is caused by the activation of free nerve endings around skeletal muscle fibers. DOMS is severe muscular discomfort, which occurs 24 to 48 hours after exercise and may increase in intensity for 2 to 3 days until it has completely disappeared within 7 days. The type of activity that causes the most soreness is eccentric exercise. Muscle fibers may take as long as 12 weeks to repair.[12,23,33,37]

Density. The mass per unit volume of an object or body (mass density); or weight per unit volume (weight density).[48]

Depth Jump. Jumps that use the athlete's body weight and gravity to exert force against the ground. They are performed by stepping out from a box and dropping to the ground, and then attempting to jump back up to the height of the box (emphasizing a "touch and go" action off the ground).[25]

Detraining. A deconditioning process that affects performance because of diminished physiologic activity.[35,36]

Diabetes Insipidus. A disease resulting from defective antidiuretic hormone (ADH) control of urine concentration; marked by great thirst and excretion of a large volume of urine.[82]

Diabetes Mellitus. 1. A disease in which the hormonal control of plasma glucose is defective because of an absolute or relative deficiency of insulin.[82] 2. Type I diabetics are insulin dependent, whereas Type II are not.[63]

Diastolic Pressure. The minimum blood pressure during the cardiac cycle, that is, the pressure just prior to ventricular ejection.[82]

Direct Calorimetry. Assessment of the body's metabolic rate by direct measurement of the amount of heat produced.[63]

Double Product. The product of the heart rate and the systolic blood pressure.[66] *Syn:* rate pressure product (RPP)

Duration of Exercise. The number of minutes per exercise session.[66]

Dynamic Exercise. Alternate contraction and relaxation of a skeletal muscle or group of muscles causing partial or complete movement through a joint's range of motion.[19]

Dynamometer. 1. Instrument used to measure the force or torque of a selected muscular contraction.[10] 2. Operates by a spring device, which when compressed moves a pointer. Therefore, by knowing how much force is required to move the pointer a particular distance, the clinician can then determine exactly how much external "static" force has been applied to the dynamometer.[54]

Dyspnea. Shortness of breath or labored breathing.[63]

Eccentric Muscle Contraction. A dynamic action in which the ends of the muscle (bony attachments) are moved further apart by external force.[47] *Syn:* lengthening, pliometric, negative work[47]

Eccentrics. A type of muscle loading that involves an external force application with resultant tension increase during physical lengthening of the musculotendinous unit.[1] *Syn:* negative work, negatives, deceleration, shock absorbers[1]

Ectomorphy. The category of somatotype that is rated for linearity of body form.[63]

Efficiency. Relating to human movement, the ratio of work accomplished to energy expenditure. In general, during exercise, efficiency of the human body is approximately 20% to 30%.[10]

Ejection Fraction. The proportion of end-diastolic volume that is ejected during a ventricular contraction.[63]

Elastic Stretch. A temporary increase in the length of a tissue that returns to its original length when the stress is removed. High-force, short-duration stretching favors recoverable, elastic tissue deformation.[20,72]

Electrocardiogram (ECG, EKG). A record of the electrical activity of the heart; shows certain waves called P-, Q-, R-, S-, and T- waves. The P-wave is caused by depolarization and contraction of the atrial muscle tissues, and the remaining waves are related to depolarization and contraction of the ventricles.[19]

Electrolyte. A substance that ionizes in solution and is capable of conducting an electrical current.[15]

Electron Transport Chain. A series of cytochromes in the mitochondria that are responsible for oxidative phosphorylation.[63]

Elftman Proposal. This principle states that optimal force production of different modes of contraction are arranged in the following predictable hierarchy:[1,32] Eccentric → Isometric → Concentric

End-Feel. The sensation imparted to the hands of the clinician at the end-point of the available range of movement. This varies according to the limiting structure or tissue.[40]

Endomorphy. The somatotype category that is rated for roundness (fatness).[63]

Endorphin. A neuropeptide produced by the pituitary gland having pain-suppressing activity.[63]

Endurance. 1. The time limit of a person's ability to maintain either a specific isometric force or a specific power level involving combinations of concentric or eccentric muscular contractions.[6] 2. The ability to continue performance of a movement activity.[48] 3. The ability to resist fatigue.[45]

Energy. 1. The capability of producing force, performing work or generating heat (units: joule or kilojoule).[6] 2. Energy is manifested in various forms: motion (kinetic energy), position (potential energy), light, heat, ionizing radiation, or sound. Changes in energy may be physical or chemical or both.[80]

Energy Expenditure. The power used during activity or rest. It is usually expressed in watts, in kilocalories per minute or hour, or in millimeters of oxygen per kilogram of body weight per minute.[65]

Equilibrium. The state of a system whose motion is not being changed, accelerated, or decelerated.[48]

Ergogenic. Tending to increase work output or performance.[15]

Ergogenic Aids. 1. Anything that helps increase work performance above levels that might be obtained under normal conditions. Ergogenic aids may be categorized by the mode in which they facilitate performance, and the typical categories include pharmacological (eg, anabolic steroids, amphetamines), nutritional (eg, protein supplements, carbohydrate loading), physiological (eg, blood doping, oxygen rebreathing, alkaline salts), psychological (eg, visualization, hypnosis), mechanical (eg, sport-specific specialty clothing, sport-specific specialty equipment, weightlifting belt), and restorational (eg, whirlpool therapy).[71] 2. Any substance or technique apart from actual physical or mental training that improves athletic performance by either delaying fatigue or increasing work capacity.[10]

Ergolytic Substances. Substances that tend to impair work output or performance (eg, alcohol, marijuana, smokeless tobacco, cocaine, diuretics, caffeine).[11,30,31]

Ergometer. An instrument to measure work and power output.[15]

Ergometry. Measurement of work and power; utilizing standardized equipment to measure work and power output during exercise.[19]

Ergonomics. The science that is concerned with the problem of how to fit a job to a person's anatomical, physiological, and psychological characteristics in such a way as to enhance human efficiency and well-being.[80]

Evaluation. 1. A judgment based on a measurement; often confused with assessment and examination; evaluations are judgments of the value or worth of something.[9] 2. An examination and corresponding judgment (diagnosis or assessment).[40]

Evaporation. The change of water from a liquid form to a vapor form. Results in the removal of heat.[63]

Examination. A test or a group of tests used for the purpose of obtaining measurements or data.[9]

Exercise. 1. Any and all activity involving generation of force by the activated muscle(s) that results in a disruption of a homeostatic state. In dynamic exercise, the muscle may perform shortening (concentric) contractions or be overcome by external resistance and perform lengthening (eccentric) contractions. When the muscle force results in no movement, the contraction should be termed static or isometric.[6] 2. Any and all activity involving generation of force by the activated muscle(s). Exercise can be quantified mechanically as force, torque, work, power, or velocity of progression.[47]

Exercise Cost Tables. Tables that express the typical exercise intensity of various physical activities.[66]

Exercise Epidemiology. The study of diseases associated with physical inactivity.[66]

Exercise Load. The amount of weight used as resistance during an exercise.[45]

Exercise Physiologist. 1. An independent research scientist who has earned a doctoral degree with an emphasis in the life sciences and has a primary research interest in physical exercise.[4] 2. May be classified as either a research exercise physiologist (ie, doctoral level) or a clinical exercise physiologist (ie, masters or doctoral level).

Exercise Physiology. 1. The science that deals with the study of muscular activity and the associated functional responses and adaptations.[4] 2. The study of human and animal acute and chronic response to various forms of exercise.[66]

Exercise Prescription. 1. An exercise schedule usually for the purpose of increasing the state of physical fitness. Individual components of the exercise prescription consist of intensity, duration, frequency, and the mode of exercise.[80] 2. An individual program of exercise based on an individual's level of fitness and health status.[10]

Exercise Science. The study of humans during exercise.[66]

External Respiration. Movement of gas in and out of the lungs (pulmonary ventilation).[63] *See* Ventilation

False Negative Exercise Test. Graded exercise stress test that is interpreted as normal but the individual actually has coronary heart disease. Thus, the ability of a graded exercise test to diagnose coronary heart disease is not 100% accurate.[10]

False Positive Exercise Test. Graded exercise stress test that indicates myocardial ischemia (eg, significant S-T segment depression) but as further evaluation shows, the individual does not have significant coronary heart disease.[10]

Fartlek Training. 1. Involves a combination of techniques such that continuous, interval, and repetition training are used in a single session. Fartlek is a Swedish term meaning "speed play" and denotes that the various intensities of work are selected by the athlete on an unstructured basis.[49] 2. A free form of training that involves alternate fast- and slow-pace variations (at the participant's discretion) over a varied terrain (eg, flat, uneven, hilly).[12,54]

Fast-Twitch Glycolytic Fiber (FG). Large skeletal muscle fiber innervated by alpha-I motor neuron and characterized by a fast contraction time and low oxidative (aerobic) and high glycolytic (anaerobic) metabolic capacity. These fibers are recruited primarily for high-intensity contractions such as utilized in short distance sprinting or power lifting. Also called Type IIB fiber.[10]

Fast-Twitch Oxidative Glycolytic Fiber (FOG). Large skeletal muscle fiber innervated by alpha-I motor neuron and characterized by fast contraction time and medium oxidative (aerobic) and high glycolytic (anaerobic) metabolic capacity. These fibers are recruited primarily for high-intensity contractions such as middle distance running events. Also called Type IIA fiber.[10]

Fat. Adipose tissue of the body. Serves as a source of energy, provides an insulating layer that inhibits heat loss, acts to support and protect certain organs such as the eye and kidney, provides essential fatty acids necessary for normal growth and development, and in foods is a vehicle for natural fat-soluble vitamins.[80]

Fat-Free Weight. The component of the body consisting of muscle, bone, blood, and other organs.[66] *Syn:* lean body weight

Fatigue. Diminished work capacity, usually short of true physiologic limits.[75]

Fat Weight. Proportion of body weight that is fat or adipose tissue.[66]

Fiber Type Composition. The makeup of a muscle that allows for classification into three types of muscle fiber (Type I, Type IIa, Type IIb). Classifications are based on enzymatic and protein composition, mechanical characteristics, contraction rate, and metabolic capabilities.[10]

Fick Equation. This equation, under conditions of maximal exercise, expresses the relationship between oxygen uptake, oxygen transport, and oxygen utilization:[34]

$$\dot{V}O_2 \text{ max} = (\text{max HR} \times \text{max SV}) \times (\text{max } CaO_2 - \text{min } C\bar{v}O_2),$$

where $\dot{V}O_2$ max = mL $O_2 \cdot \text{min}^{-1}$; when normalized for body weight, it is expressed as mL $O_2 \cdot \text{kg}^{-1} \cdot \text{min}^{-1}$

$$
\begin{aligned}
\text{max HR} &= \text{maximal heart rate (bpm)} \\
\text{max SV} &= \text{maximal stroke volume (mL} \cdot \text{beat}^{-1}) \\
\text{max } CaO_2 &= \text{maximal arterial oxygen content (mL } O_2/\text{mL blood)} \\
\text{min } C\bar{v}O_2 &= \text{minimal mixed venous oxygen content}
\end{aligned}
$$

Fick Principle. A restatement of the law of conservation of mass used in making indirect measurements, for example, of cardiac output: the amount of blood traversing the pulmonary capillaries per unit of time is a measure of cardiac output and, because gas diffusion across the pulmonary alveolar walls depends on pulmonary blood flow, the cardiac output (liters per minute) equals O_2 absorption (cc per minute) divided by the arterial O_2 minus the mixed venous O_2 (cc per liter).[34,38]

Field Tests. A test of physical performance performed in the field (outside the laboratory).[63]

Fine Motor Skill. Type of skill performed by the small musculature, particularly of the hands and fingers.[10]

Fitness. One's capacity to perform work (exercise) of a specific intensity and duration, which may be aerobic, anaerobic, or muscular.[10]

Flexibility. 1. Range of motion possible in a joint or series of joints.[19] 2. The ability of muscle and other soft tissue to yield to a stretch force.[17,45] 3. The term flexibility is sometimes used interchangeably with extensibility.[45]

Force. 1. That which changes or tends to change the state of rest or motion in matter (preferred SI unit: newton).[6] 2. The product of mass times acceleration.[48] 3. A weight is a force and it is a mass undergoing gravitational acceleration [typical units: pounds (lb), newtons (N), kiloponds (kp), kilograms (kg)]. A kilogram is really a unit of mass; however, in common usage it is used as a weight.[5]

Frank-Starling Mechanism. Force of the ventricular contraction during systole is a direct function of the resting end diastolic fiber length. The greater the ventricular filling, the greater the stretch on the ventricular cardiac fibers and, thus, the greater the force of ventricular contraction.[10]

Free Weight. An object of determined mass used for physical conditioning and competitive lifting.[47]

Frequency of Exercise. The number of days of exercise per week.[66]

Friction. The force that resists the sliding of one surface upon another.[48]

Functional Assessment. An evaluation of a person's ability levels using task-specific tests that involve the whole body versus single-joint testing.[40] *Syn:* functional capacity assessments, physical capacity evaluations, worker assessments, functional capacity evaluations, worker capacity evaluations

Generalized Equations. Body composition equations that estimate body density from the sum of skinfolds and age. The equations are termed "generalized" as contrasted from "population specific" because they can be validly applied to men and women varying greatly in terms of body composition and age.[66]

Goniometer. An apparatus used to measure joint movements and angles.[80]

Graded Exercise Stress Test (GXT). Used either as a diagnostic tool or to evaluate the functional capacity of the cardiovascular system. It usually involves continuous incremental exercise performed on a bicycle ergometer or treadmill where the electrocardiogram and blood pressure (occasionally oxygen consumption) are monitored.[10]

Gravity. The attraction of two objects with a force proportional to the product of their masses and inversely proportional to the squared distance between them (law of gravitation).[10]

Gross Efficiency. A simple measure of exercise efficiency defined as: work performed/energy expended × 100%.[63]

Gross Motor Skill. Motor task either requiring large musculature or moving the body in space.[10]

Handling. Lifting, lowering, conveying, pushing, pulling, or sliding an object in order to move it from one place to another. If the motion is powered by a person's muscles, it is termed manual handling.[65]

Health Risk Appraisal. A method of assessing cardiovascular disease risk with self-report questionnaires.[66]

Heart Rate (HR). The number of contractions of the heart per minute (unit: beats per minute).[82]

Heat Cramps. Acute painful spasms of voluntary muscles following hard work in a hot environment without adequate fluid and salt intake.[80]

Heat Exhaustion. A state of very definite weakness produced by the excess loss of normal fluids and sodium chloride in the form of sweat. The skin is cool, clammy, and with profuse diaphoresis.[80]

Heat Stress. Temperature–humidity combination that leads to heat disorders such as heat cramps, heat exhaustion, or heat stroke.[75]

Heatstroke. A condition or derangement of the heat-control centers due to exposure to the rays of the sun or very high temperatures. Loss of heat is inadequate or absent. The skin is hot, dry, and characterized by a cessation of sweating.[80]

Heat Syncope. Fainting caused by excessive heat exposure.[87]

Hemodynamic. Relating to the forces involved in circulating blood through the body.[19]

Hitting the Wall. Used to describe the phenomenon of depletion of muscle glycogen stores with a concomitant increased reliance on fat as a fuel source. This typically occurs in marathoners at about the 19- or 20-mile mark and results in a decrement in performance.[10]

Homeostasis. The maintenance of relatively stable internal physiologic conditions in higher animals under fluctuating environmental conditions.[10]

Hydrostatic Densitometry. Criterion measure for estimating body fat percentage by measuring body density. It is based on Archimedes' principle where the body is weighed in air and then weighed fully submerged in water. The underwater weight is corrected for residual volume, gastrointestinal air, and water temperature. Percent fat is then calculated using body density in either the Brozek or Siri equation.[10] *Syn:* underwater weighing

Hyperplasia. Increase in the number of cells.[15]

Hypertension. Higher than normal arterial blood pressure; often defined as a resting blood pressure greater than 140/90 mm Hg.[19]

Hyperthermia. An above-normal increase in body temperature.[63]

Hypertrophy. Increase in the size or mass of body tissue.[15]

Hypokinetic Diseases. Illness caused by or associated with a lack of physical exercise, such as cardiovascular disease, obesity, and osteoporosis.[10]

Hypothermia. A condition in which heat is lost from the body faster than it is produced.[63]

Hypoxia. Low oxygen content; lack of adequate oxygen in inspired air, as occurs at high altitude.[19]

Indirect Calorimetry. Estimation of heat or energy production on the basis of oxygen consumption, carbon dioxide production, and nitrogen excretion.[63]

Individual Differences Principle. Adapting training and rehabilitation programs to specifically meet the individual's needs and capacities.[54]

Inertia. A state in which a body remains at rest or in uniform motion until acted on by an outside force.[40]

Instrument. A machine, a questionnaire, or any device that is used as part of, or as a test to obtain, measurements.[9]

Intensity of Exercise. 1. A specific level of muscular activity that can be quantified in terms of power (energy expenditure or work performed per unit of time), the opposing force (eg, by free weight or weight stack) employed in strength training, isometric force sustained, or velocity of progression.[6,47] 2. The difficulty of exercise. It is usually represented by a percentage of maximal.[66]

Intermittent Work. Exercises performed with alternate periods of rest, as opposed to continuous work.[45]

Internal Ventilation. Refers to the utilization of oxygen at the mitochondria where ATP is produced; distinguished from external respiration, in which atmospheric air is brought into the lungs.[63]

Interval Training. 1. Alternating periods of work (high-intensity activity) and periods of relief (low intensity activity).[77] 2. Repeated series of exercise or work intervals interspersed with rest periods or relief intervals.[54]

Ischemia. Local deficiency of blood, usually due to the constriction or partial occlusion of arterial blood vessels.[19]

Isoinertial. Measures the ability of a person to overcome the initial static resistance by measuring the maximal amount of weight he or she can handle and move to an assigned point at a freely chosen speed. The actual speed of movement does vary within the specified range of movement.[16]

Isokinetic Dynamometer. Contains a speed-controlling mechanism that accelerates to a preset speed when any force is applied. Once constant speed is attained, the isokinetic loading mechanism accommodates automatically to provide a counterforce equal to the force generated by the muscle. Maximum force or any percentage of maximum effort can be applied during all phases of the movement at a constant velocity.[44]

Isokinetic Exercise. 1. A concentric or eccentric contraction that occurs at a set speed and uses a resistance that accommodates to the force produced at all points in the range of motion.[40] 2. There is usually no eccentric component (although new equipment does allow for this) in the return movement but rather a "double-concentric" principle exists, in which the return movement is accomplished by a concentric contraction of the antagonist muscle group (eg, concentric contraction of the quadricep in knee extension and a concentric contraction of the hamstrings in knee flexion).[27] *Syn:* accommodating resistance exercise

Isokinetics. 1. A preset fixed speed (0° to 500° per second) with resistance that accommodates to the individual at every point in the range of motion.[86] 2. Constant speed or isokinetic movements do not generally occur naturally; however, the advantage of constant speed testing is that a body segment is allowed to generate its maximum force or torque production throughout the range of motion tested.[41]

Isometric Exercise. A concentric muscular contraction of agonistic and antagonistic muscle groups about a joint in which there is no perceptible joint motion.[40]

Isotonic Exercise. 1. Concentric or eccentric contractions of variable speed using a set weight or resistance throughout the full range of motion.[40] 2. Isotonic exercise may be divided into concentric and eccentric phases and further subdivided into constant resistance (ie, weight does not change through the range of movement and thus is limited by the inherent weak points on the strength curve of the exercising muscle) and variable resistance (ie, an attempt is made through equipment design utilizing cams, levers, pulleys, etc to vary the resistance experienced by the working muscle through its range of motion, attempting to match its strength curve).[27]

Job Demands. The physiological, psychological, and perceptual requirements of a job that determine the suitability of a given workload for the potential work force.[65]

Job Site Analysis. The measurement of factors (eg, environment, postures and positions, motions and movements, tools and applications) at a given location that influence job task performance.[40]

Job Task Analysis. An analysis of the components (eg, weights and measures, heights and distances, cycles and repetitions) of performing a worker's job through observation and measurement.[40]

Joint Mobilization. Passive traction and/or gliding movements applied to joint surfaces that maintain or restore the joint play normally allowed by the capsule, so that the normal roll-slide joint mechanics can occur as a person moves.[45]

Joint Play. Capsular laxity or elasticity that allows movements of the joint surfaces. The movements include distraction, sliding, compression, rolling, and spinning.[45]

Kilogram·meter (kg·m). A unit of work that is equal to the energy required to lift 1 kg (2.2 lb) vertically a distance of 1 m (3.3 ft).[39] *See* Kilopond·meter

Kilopond (kp). 1. A unit of force defined as the weight of a 1-kg mass.[69,70] 2. One kilopond = one kilogram (mass) undergoing unit gravitational acceleration. Typically, they are written as "1 kp = 1 kg", and they are often used interchangeably.[5]

Kilopond·meter (kp·m). 1. Braking power (kp) set by adjusting belt tension (on a cycle ergometer), multiplied by a distance pedaled (m), gives the amount of work in kilopond·meters (kp·m). Thus, if the distance is expressed per minute, then the rate of work in kp·m per minute will be obtained.[14] 2. Oftentimes kp·m (also abbreviated as kp-m and kpm) is used interchangeably with kg·m (also abbreviated as kg-m and kgm).[63]

Kinanthropometry. Kinanthropometry is the quantitative interface between anatomy and physiology or between structure and function. Kinanthropometry is an emerging scientific specialization that employs measurements to appraise human size (eg, height, weight), shape (eg, somatotypes), proportion (eg, proportionality), body composition (eg, hydrostatic weighing, electrical conductance, ultrasound techniques, and anthropometric methods such as skinfolds and circumferences), maturation (eg, skeletal age, menarche, genitalia assessment), and gross function (eg, strength, flexibility, endurance). It explores problems related to growth, exercise, performance, and nutrition.[67, 68]

Kinesiology. The study of human movement from an anatomic and/or mechanical perspective.[48]

Kinesthesia. A perception of movement obtained from information about the position and rate of movement of the joints.[63]

Krebs Cycle. Metabolic pathway in the mitochondria in which energy is transferred from carbohydrates, fats, and amino acids to NAD for subsequent production of ATP in the electron transport chain.[63]

Lactate Threshold. A point during a graded exercise test (GXT) when the blood lactate concentration increases abruptly.[63]

Lactic Acid. 1. An acidic metabolite that is the end product of anaerobic glycolysis.[19] 2. An end product of glucose metabolism in the glycolytic pathway; formed in conditions of inadequate oxygen and in muscles with few mitochondria.[63]

Lactic Acid System. The energy system that produces ATP anaerobically by the breakdown of glycogen to lactic acid.[87] *Syn:* anaerobic glycolytic system

Length–Tension Relationship. The relationship between the length of the muscle and the tension produced by the muscle. It states that higher tensions are developed the closer the length of the muscle is to its resting length.[10]

Load. Force exerted on the muscle by an object.[82]

Make Tests. 1. A dynamometer is held stationary by the examiner while the tested person exerts a maximum effort against it.[21] 2. The clinician may attempt to hold his or her hand stationary while the client exerts a maximum force against it.

Manipulation. A passive movement using physiologic or accessory motion, which may be applied with a thrust or when the person is under anesthesia. The client cannot prevent the motion.[45]

Manual Muscle Testing. In manual muscle testing the demands are to perform antigravity movement and to hold against resistance. Observation of the quality and measurement of the quantity of performance is the basis of establishing a rating of the muscle's ability to contract, produce movement, or respond to resistance. It does not measure the ability of the muscle to function as a part of a movement pattern.[52]

Manual Resistance Exercise. A type of active exercise in which resistance is provided by a clinician for attaining either a dynamic or a static muscular contraction.[45]

Mass. 1. A quantity of matter of an object, a direct measure of the object's inertia (note: mass = weight/acceleration due to gravity; units: gram or kilogram).[6]

Materials Handling. The movement of parts, raw supplies, chemicals, subassemblies, finished products, or other materials between sections of a manufacturing system or through distribution systems to the customer or client. The movement may be done by hand, as in lifting cases and pushing hand trucks and carts, or with automated equipment or aids, as in using forklifts, trucks, storage and retrieval systems, or conveyors.[65]

Maximal Aerobic Power (MAP). The maximal amount of oxygen that an organism can be stimulated to extract from the atmosphere and then transport to and use in tissue.[79] *Syn:* peak aerobic power, maximal voluntary oxygen consumption, aerobic work capacity, endurance capacity

Maximal Oxygen Consumption ($\dot{V}O_2$ max). 1. The greatest rate of oxygen consumption attained during exercise at sea level; usually expressed in liters per minute ($L \cdot min^{-1}$) or milliliters per kilogram body weight per minute ($mL \cdot kg^{-1} \cdot min^{-1}$).[19] 2. Greatest rate of oxygen uptake by the body measured during severe dynamic exercise, usually on a cycle ergometer or a treadmill; dependent on maximal cardiac output and the maximal arteriovenous oxygen difference.[63] *Syn:* maximal oxygen uptake, maximal aerobic capacity

Maximal Voluntary Contraction. A condition in which a person attempts to recruit as many fibers in a muscle as possible for the purpose of developing force.[47]

Measurement. The numeral assigned to an object, event, or person or the class (category) to which an object, event, or person is assigned according to rules.[9]

Mechanical Resistance Exercise. A type of active exercise in which resistance is applied through the use of equipment or a mechanical apparatus.[45]

Mesomorphy. The somatotype category that characterizes the muscular form or lean body mass aspect of the human body.[63]

MET. 1. A metabolic equivalent unit; a unit used to estimate the metabolic cost of physical activity; one MET is approximately equal to 3.5 milliliters of oxygen consumed per kilogram of body weight per minute.[19] 2. An expression of the rate of energy expenditure at rest.[63] 3. Is a multiple of the resting rate of oxygen consumption. A MET represents the approximate rate of oxygen consumption of a seated individual at rest. A person exercising at 5 METs is consuming oxygen at 5 times the resting rate.[5]

Metabolic Acidosis. An acidosis (any situation in which the hydrogen-ion concentration of arterial blood is elevated) due to a metabolic production of acids other than carbon dioxide, for example, the production of lactic acid during severe exercise or of ketones in diabetes mellitus.[82]

Metabolic Alkalosis. An alkalosis (any situation in which the hydrogen-ion concentration of arterial blood is reduced) resulting from the removal of hydrogen ions from the body by mechanisms other than the respiratory removal of carbon dioxide, for example, the loss of hydrogen from the stomach with persistent vomiting.[82]

Metabolic Rate. 1. The total energy expenditure of the body per unit time.[82] 2. The energy expended in order to maintain all physical and chemical changes occurring in the body.[87]

Metabolism. The sum of all physical and chemical changes that take place within an organism; all energy and material transformations that occur within living cells.[80]

Minute Ventilation. The volume of air breathed per minute; the product of tidal volume and breathing frequency.[19]

Mobility. The ease with which an articulation or a series of articulations is allowed to move before being restricted by the surrounding structures.[48]

Mobilization. Passive stretching movements performed by a therapist at a speed slow enough that the client can stop the movement. The technique may be applied with oscillatory motions or with sustained stretches using physiologic or accessory movements.[45,53]

Modality. Method of application of, or the employment of, any therapeutic agent; limited usually to physical agents (eg, hydrotherapy, ultrasound, cryotherapy).[38]

Mode of Exercise. A type of exercise (eg, walking, jogging, cycling, playing sports, swimming, etc).[66]

Momentum. A system's resistance to change in its state of motion (inertia) multiplied by its velocity.[48]

Motor Unit. A single motor nerve cell and its branches, with associated muscle fibers; the smallest functional unit of muscular contraction.[48]

Muscle. A type of tissue composed of contractile cells or fibers that affects movement of an organ or part of the body. The outstanding characteristic of muscular tissue is its ability to shorten or contract and also possesses the properties of irritability, conductivity, and elasticity. Three types of muscle differentiated on the basis of histologic structure occur in the body, namely, smooth, striated (skeletal), and cardiac.[80] The human body contains over 600 skeletal muscles, which taken all together comprise the largest tissue in the body, accounting for 40% to 45% of the total body weight.[82]

Muscle Balance. Maintaining a natural strength ratio between opposing muscle groups and training for overall muscular development, rather than specializing on particular muscles or exercises.[85]

Muscle Contraction. The active state of muscle. The attempt of a muscle cell or muscle tissue to shorten along the longitudinal axis of the muscle cell(s) when activated.[47]

Muscle Cramps. A tonic muscle cramp is a constant muscle contraction that lasts for a period of time and is caused by the body's depletion of essential electrolytes or an interruption of synergism between opposing muscles. A clonic muscle cramp is an involuntary muscle contraction marked by alternate contraction and relaxation in rapid succession and stems from nerve irritation.[12]

Muscle Energy Techniques. 1. Techniques that are active in nature and may be likened to proprioceptive neuromuscular facilitation contract-relax techniques, except that they employ submaximal rather than maximal contractions. The techniques may be isotonic (with the counterforce less than the force of the patient's muscular contraction, producing motion into or toward the motion barrier); isometric (with the counterforce meeting the force of the patient's muscular contraction, producing no joint motion); and isokinetic (with the counterforce increasing during contraction to meet changing contraction forces as the muscle shortens and its force increases).[55,73] 2. A term suggested by Fred L. Mitchell, DO, to describe a form of osteopathic manipulative technique in which the patient uses his muscles, on request, from a precisely controlled position, in a specified direction, against a distinctly executed operator counterforce.[7]

Muscle Fatigue. A decrease in the mechanical response of muscle with prolonged stimulation.[82]

Muscle Pump. High-intensity training that saturates the target muscle tissue with blood and temporarily increases the cross-sectional area.[85]

Muscle Setting Exercise. A form of isometric exercise but one not performed against any appreciable resistance; gentle static muscle contractions used to maintain mobility between muscle fibers and to decrease muscle spasm and pain (eg, quadricep and hamstring set).[45]

Muscle Stiffness. Occurs when a group of muscles have been worked hard for a long period of time. The fluids that collect in the muscles during and after exercise are absorbed into the bloodstream at a very slow rate. As a result, the muscle becomes swollen, shorter, and thicker and therefore resists stretching.[12]

Muscle Tension. The force exerted by a contracting muscle on an object.[82]

Muscle Tone. The small amount of tension produced by skeletal muscles under resting conditions in the body as a result of a low-frequency discharge of the motor neurons.[82]

Muscular Endurance. 1. The ability of a muscle or group of muscles to perform repeated contractions against an immovable object (isometric), against gravity (isotonic), and against a preset speed.[40] 2. The time limit of a person's ability to maintain either an isometric force or a power level involving combinations of concentric or eccentric muscular contractions or both.[47] 3. Usually measured as the number of repetitions completed against 50% to 60% of the maximal resistance.[19]

Muscular Fitness. The strength, muscular endurance, and flexibility needed to carry out daily tasks and avoid injury.[75]

Muscular Strength. The maximal force or tension generated by a muscle or muscle group.[19]

Myocardial Infarction. An area of cardiac muscle tissue that undergoes necrosis after cessation of blood supply through a segment of the coronary arterial system.[19]

Myocardial Ischemia. A condition in which the myocardium experiences an inadequate blood flow; sometimes accompanied by irregularities in the electrocardiogram (arrhythmias and ST-segment depression) and chest pain (angina pectoris).[63]

Negative Work. The work done on a muscle group by an external force as the muscles act eccentrically in opposition to the external force.[10]

Nicotinamide Adenine Dinucleotide (NAD). Coenzyme that transfers hydrogen and the energy associated with those hydrogens; in the Krebs cycle, NAD transfers energy from substrates to the electron transport chain.[63]

Norms. Performance standards based on the scores of a group of people.[18]

Obesity. An excessive accumulation of body fat; usually reserved for individuals who are 20% to 30% or more above the average weight for their size.[87]

Objectivity. The degree to which multiple scorers agree on the magnitude of scores.[18]

Occupational Therapy. The health profession that uses work-related skills to treat or train the physically or emotionally ill, to prevent disability, to evaluate behavior, and to restore disabled persons to health, social, or economic independence.[80]

Olympic Lifters. 1. Persons who train with weights in order to lift heavier weightloads in their competitive events, the clean and jerk and the snatch.[85] 2. The clean and jerk is a lift in which the barbell is lifted from a platform to a temporary position at the shoulders, which is termed the "clean," followed by the bar being thrust in one continuous motion from the shoulders to an overhead hold with outstretched arms, which is termed the "jerk." The snatch is a lift in which the barbell is lifted from a platform in one continuous forceful motion to an overhead position with both arms evenly extended overhead.[81]

One-Repetition Maximum (1-RM). The heaviest weightload a person can lift one time.[85]

Open-Circuit Spirometry. 1. Indirect calorimetry procedure in which either inspired or expired ventilation is measured and oxygen consumption and carbon dioxide production is calculated.[63] 2. Method in which a person does not rebreathe from a container of oxygen as in the closed-circuit method but, instead, inhales ambient air that has a constant composition of 20.93% oxygen, 0.03% carbon dioxide, and 79.04% nitrogen.[54] 3. The process of estimating metabolic rate by collecting and analyzing expired air.[35]

Open Kinetic Chain. Exists when the distal segment of an extremity is free (eg, when a person is not bearing weight on an extremity and is performing seated leg extensions).[50,60]

Optimal Flexibility. The required amount of flexibility or range of motion at the joint that will allow for maximal performance of the defined activity while protecting the joint from acute or chronic injury.[20]

Orthostatic Hypotension. Lower than normal arterial blood pressure occurring when an individual assumes an erect posture.[19]

Osteoarthritis (Degenerative Joint Disease). A chronic degenerative disorder primarily affecting the articular cartilage with eventual bony overgrowth at the margins of the joints.[45]

Osteoporosis (Bone Atrophy). A condition of bone that leads to a loss of bone mass, a narrowing of the bone shaft, and widening of the medullary canal.[45]

Overload Principle. 1. Describes the need to increase the load (intensity) of exercise to cause a further adaptation of a system.[63] 2. A training stimulus consisting of intensity, frequency, and duration that exceeds normal physical exertion levels in order to enhance physiological capacity.[54]

Overstretch. A stretch beyond the normal range of motion of a joint and surrounding soft tissues.[45]

Overtraining. Constant severe training that does not provide adequate time for recovery. Symptoms include an increased frequency of injury, irritability, increased resting and exercise heart rate, altered appetite, apathy, loss of sleep, and decreased performance.[10,35] *Syn:* burnout, staleness

Overuse Syndrome. Injury resulting from continual low-level stress placed on a body part.[10]

Overweight. Body weight greater than that which is considered normal.[87]

Oxidative Phosphorylation. Mitochondrial process in which inorganic phosphate (Pi) is coupled to ADP as energy is transferred along the electron transport chain in which oxygen is the final electron acceptor.[63]

Oxygen Consumption. The rate at which oxygen is utilized by the body in aerobic metabolism; usually expressed as liters of oxygen consumed per minute ($L \cdot min^{-1}$) or milliliters of oxygen consumed per kilogram body weight per minute ($mL \cdot kg^{-1} \cdot min^{-1}$).[19] *Syn:* oxygen uptake

Oxygen Debt. The elevated post-exercise oxygen consumption; related to the replacement of creatine phosphate, lactic acid resynthesis to glucose, and elevated body temperature, catecholamines, heart rate, breathing, and so on.[63]

Oxygen Deficit. A measure of the energy production not provided by oxidative phosphorylation in the transition from rest to exercise; ATP provided by high-energy phosphates and anaerobic glycolysis.[63]

Oxygen Dissociation Curve. Oxygen combines with hemoglobin to a greater or lesser extent depending upon the oxygen gas tension (PO_2) in the blood. The relationship describing this is known as the oxygen dissociation curve.[66]

Oxygen Pulse. The oxygen uptake divided by the heart rate. Hence, it is the amount of oxygen extracted by the tissues of the body over a single beat of the heart or of a stroke volume.[84]

Oxygen System. The energy system that produces ATP via the oxidation of various food-stuffs, primarily fats and carbohydrates.[87]

Oxygen Uptake. *See* Oxygen consumption

Parcours. A modification of the circuit training concept. A parcours is, essentially, a graded jogging trail along which exercise stations have been erected.[49]

Passive Range of Motion. Movement, within the unrestricted range of motion for a segment, that is produced entirely by an external force. There is no voluntary muscle contraction.[45]

Passive Stretching. A type of mobility exercise in which manual, mechanical, or positional stretch is applied to soft tissues and in which the forces are applied opposite to the direction of shortening.[45]

Perceived Exertion. A psychophysical measure of the amount of effort required for a given action or task.[65]

Percent Grade. A measure of the elevation of the treadmill; calculated as the sine of the angle.[63]

Periodization. 1. In athletics, periodization is used to refer to two training concepts: periodization of the annual plan, or its division into phases of training in order to allow a program to be set into smaller and more manageable segments, with the ultimate goal being to reach peak performance at the main competition(s) of the year; and periodization of the dominant motor abilities (strength, speed, and endurance), which refers to the methodical sequence of developing the same.[22] 2. The organization of training into a cyclic structure to attain the optimal development of an athlete's performance capacities. It consists of changes of objectives, tasks, and content of training. Periodization can also be defined as a division of the training year to meet two specific objectives: preparation for optimal improvement in performance and preparation for a definite climax to the competitive season.[58] *Syn:* cycle training

pH. A measure of the acidity of a solution; calculated as the negative $\log_{10}$ of the $[H^+]$ in which 7 is neutral. Values that are greater than 7 are basic and less than 7 are acidic.[63]

Phasic. Intermittent activity.[82]

Physical Activity. Characterizes all types of human movement; associated with living, work, play, and exercise.[63]

Physical Agents. Techniques and devices that employ heat, cold, sound, and various categories of the electromagnetic spectrum, such as light and electricity.[40] *Syn:* modality

Physical Fitness. 1. A broad term describing healthful levels of cardiovascular function, strength, and flexibility.[63] 2. The ability to carry out daily tasks with vigor and alertness, without undue fatigue, and with ample energy to enjoy leisure-time pursuits and meet unforeseen emergencies.[80]

Physical Therapy. The health profession that is concerned with health promotion, prevention of physical disabilities, and rehabilitation of persons disabled by pain, disease, or injury; and that is involved with evaluating patients and with treating through the use of physical therapeutic measures as opposed to medicines, surgery, or radiation.[8]

Physical Work Capacity (PWC). The maximal level of work an individual is able to perform, often at a specified heart rate such as 150 or 170 bpm, and may be used as a measure of aerobic fitness.[10]

Physiologic Movement. Movement that a person normally can do, such as flexion, extension, rotation, abduction, and adduction.[45]

Plastic Stretch. A permanent increase in the length of a tissue that remains elongated after the stress is removed. Low-force, low-elongation stretching enhances permanent, plastic deformation.[20,72]

Plyometric Contraction. Eccentric contraction of a muscle followed immediately by a concentric contraction.[47] *Syn:* stretch-shortening cycle[47]

Plyometrics. 1. Exercises characterized by powerful muscular contractions in response to rapid, dynamic loading or stretching of the involved muscles.[64] 2. A quick powerful movement involving a prestretching or countermovement that activates the stretch-shortening cycle. The purpose of plyometric training is to heighten the excitability of the nervous system for improved reactive ability of the neuromuscular system. Any exercise that utilizes the natural elastic components of muscle and the myotatic reflex to produce a more powerful muscular response.[83] *See* Stretch shorten cycle

Positive Work. The work done by a muscle group as it acts concentrically. When the signs of the net muscle movement and the angular velocity at the joint are the same, positive work is done.[10]

Power. 1. The rate of performing work; the derivative of work with respect to time; the product of force and velocity (preferred SI unit: watt). Other related processes such as energy release and heat transfer should, when expressed per unit of time, be quantified and presented in watts.[6] 2. The rate of doing work or dissipating energy, which is force times linear displacement divided by time. A measure of rotary motion, power is equated to torque times angular displacement divided by time.[40] 3. Typical units of power are $kp \cdot m \cdot min^{-1}$, $kg \cdot m \cdot min^{-1}$, $J \cdot min^{-1}$, and watts (W). The metabolic equivalent of power is the rate of energy expenditure ($\dot{E}$) that occurs in response to the imposed mechanical work rate or power. Typical units of $\dot{E}$ are METs and $\dot{V}O_2$. Nonweight-bearing activities (eg, cycle ergometry) are measured in units of absolute power. Measures of absolute mechanical power include $kp \cdot m \cdot min^{-1}$, $kg \cdot m \cdot min^{-1}$, and watts (W). Absolute measures of $\dot{E}$ are $kcal \cdot min^{-1}$, $L\ O_2 \cdot min^{-1}$, and $mL\ O_2 \cdot min^{-1}$. Weight-bearing activities (eg, jogging) are measured in units of relative power. Relative measures of $\dot{E}$ include MET and $mL\ O_2 \cdot (kg\ body\ weight)^{-1} \cdot min^{-1}$, which is usually written as $mL \cdot kg^{-1} \cdot min^{-1}$. It should be noted that relative measures of $\dot{E}$ are all expressed as "per kg body weight."[5]

Powerlifters. Persons who train with weights in order to lift heavier weightloads in their competitive events, the squat, deadlift, and the bench press.[85]

Preload. The volume of blood in the left ventricle just before systole, the end-diastolic volume.[42]

Premature Atrial Contraction (PAC). Early contraction of the atria originating at some ectopic site outside of the sinoatrial node.[19]

Premature Ventricular Contraction (PVC). Early contraction of the ventricle resulting from initiation of an impulse either within or at some ectopic site outside of the conduction system.[19]

Pressure. 1. The ratio of force to the area over which the force is applied.[48] 2. Stress or force exerted on a body, as by tension, weight, or pulling.[80]

Primary Risk Factor. A sign (eg, high blood pressure) or a behavior (eg, cigarette smoking) that is directly related to the appearance of certain diseases independent of other risk factors.[63]

Progressive Resistance Exercise (PRE). 1. A training program in which the muscles must work against a gradually increasing resistance; an implementation of the overload principle.[63] 2. An approach to exercise whereby the load or resistance to the muscles is applied by some mechanical means and is quantitatively and progressively increased over time.[45]

Proprioceptive Neuromuscular Facilitation (PNF). A form of exercise in which accommodating resistance is manually applied to various patterns of movement for the purpose of strengthening and retraining the muscles guiding joint motion.[40]

Proprioceptors. Sensory receptors located in and around joints and muscles that respond to changes in position, length, tension, and acceleration of the host tissues.[48]

Pulse Pressure. The difference between the systolic and diastolic blood pressures.[84]

Radiation. Process of energy exchange from the surface of one object to the surface of another that is dependent on a temperature gradient but does not require contact between the objects.[63]

Range of Motion (ROM). 1. The amount of motion allowed between any two bony levers.[45] 2. The total amount of angular displacement through which two adjacent segments may move.[48]

Rate-Pressure Product. Heart rate multiplied by systolic blood pressure. A clinical indicator of myocardial oxygen demand.[42]

Rating of Perceived Exertion (RPE). 1. A psychophysical method of rating exercise intensity.[66] 2. Numerical scale devised by Borg to describe the subjective feeling of effort required at varying levels of exercise intensity. Originally designated as a 6-20 scale and recently revised to a 0-10 scale.[10]

Recommended Dietary Allowances (RDA). Standards of nutrition associated with good health for the majority of people. Standards exist for protein, vitamins, and minerals for children and adults.[63]

Regression Equation. A statistical method of estimating one variable from another. For example, VO_2 max can be estimated from maximal treadmill time or percent body fat can be estimated from skinfold measurements.[66]

Rehabilitation. The processes of treatment and education that lead the disabled individual to attainment of maximal function, a sense of well-being, and a personally satisfying level of independence.[80]

Relative $\dot{V}O_2$. Oxygen uptake (consumption) expressed per unit body weight (eg, $mL \cdot kg^{-1} \cdot min^{-1}$).[63]

Reliability. 1. The degree of consistency with which a test measures what it measures.[18] 2. Refers to the amount of variation that occurs in test results between trials in one testing session or in the results between two or more different days of testing.[70] 3. Factors that may affect reliability include device calibration, joint axis alignment, client positioning, joint stabilization, testing protocol utilized, testing order, clinician procedures, client cooperation, and client fatigue.[41] *Syn:* reproducibility

Repetition Maximum (RM). 1. The greatest amount of weight a muscle can move through the range of motion a specified number of times in a load-resisting exercise routine.[45]

Repetition Minimum. The least amount of weight required to help a client lift a body part against gravity a specified number of times.[45]

Repetitions. The number of times an exercise is performed in succession.[85]

Repetition Training. Differs from interval training only in intensity of exercise during the work and recovery phases. The work phase of repetition training is almost maximal and the recovery phase almost complete.[49]

Residual Volume (RV). The air remaining in the lung after a maximal expiration.[66]

Resistance Exercise. Any form of active exercise in which a dynamic or static muscular contraction is resisted by an outside force.[45]

Respiration. The consumption of molecular oxygen during metabolism; the exchange of gas between the cells of an organism and the external environment.[82]

Respiratory Acidosis. Lower than normal blood pH secondary to pulmonary insufficiency resulting in retention of carbon dioxide; can be caused by hypoventilation.[19]

Respiratory Alkalosis. Higher than normal pH of blood and other body fluids in association with reduced blood carbon dioxide level; can be caused by hyperventilation.[19]

Respiratory Exchange Ratio (R or RER). 1. The ratio of carbon dioxide produced to oxygen consumed as measured at the mouth; computed as $\dot{V}CO_2/\dot{V}O_2$.[19,35] 2. Indicative of substrate utilization during steady-state exercise in which a value of 1.0 represents 100% carbohydrate metabolism and 0.7 represents 100% fat metabolism.[63] 3. Often used as a synonym for respiratory quotient (RQ) even though R may reflect processes other than foodstuff metabolism (ie, carbohydrate, fat, and protein), for example, hyperventilation due to acidosis.[35] 4. Respiratory exchange ratio is the VCO_2/VO_2 at the lungs, measured by open circuit spirometry.[5]

Respiratory Quotient (RQ). 1. The ratio of carbon dioxide produced to oxygen used at the tissue level.[35] 2. Respiratory quotient describes metabolism as it occurs at the cellular level.[5]

Rest Interval. The time period between bouts in an interval training program.[63]

Resultant. A single vector, often representing a force or velocity, equivalent to two or more other such vectors, being their vector sum.[78]

Reversibility Principle. The loss of physiologic capacity (detraining) that results from significant reductions in exercise workloads.[54]

Rheumatoid Arthritis. A chronic joint disease, which is often systemic; characterized by inflammation of the synovial membrane, with periods of exacerbation and remission.[45]

Runner's High. Euphoric sensation in which the runner feels a heightened sense of well-being, enhanced appreciation of nature, and loss of self-consciousness.[10]

Scalar. A quantity that has magnitude only; that is, no direction is associated with it.[48]

Screening. The process of examining a population (usually a high-risk population) for a given state or disease.[40]

Secondary Risk Factor. A characteristic (age, gender, race, and body fatness) or behavior (inactivity) that increases the risk of coronary heart disease when primary risk factors are present.[63]

Second Wind. A phenomenon characterized by a sudden transition from an ill-defined feeling of distress or fatigue during the early portion of prolonged exercise to a more comfortable, less stressful feeling later in the exercise.[15]

Set. The number of separate exercise bouts performed.[85]

Skill. Refined movement requiring coordination, agility, balance, timing, and speed.[45]

Skinfold Technique. A technique used to compute an individual's percentage of body fat; various skinfolds are measured and a regression formula is then used to compute the body fat.[87]

Slow-Twitch Oxidative Fiber (SO). Small skeletal muscle fiber innervated by alpha-2 motor neuron and characterized by a slow contraction time and high oxidative (aerobic) and low glycolytic (anaerobic) metabolic capacity. These fibers are recruited primarily for low-intensity endurance-type activities. Also called Type I fiber.[10]

Somatotype. Body type classification method used to characterize the degree to which an individual's frame is linear (ectomorphic), muscular (mesomorphic), or round (endomorphic).[63]

Specificity Principle. 1. Indicates that the adaptation of a tissue is dependent on the type of training undertaken.[63] 2. Specific physiologic adaptations as a result of specific training and rehabilitation programs that consist of energy source specificity (ie, aerobic or anaerobic), contraction specificity (ie, isometric, concentric, eccentric), muscle group specificity (ie, upper versus lower extremity, flexor versus extensor, fast twitch versus slow twitch), and speed specificity (ie, specific training velocities).[36]

Speed. 1. Total distance traveled per unit of time (unit: meter per second).[6] 2. The magnitude of a body's displacement per unit of time without regard to direction.[48] 3. The product of stride frequency and stride length.[57]

Spirometry. Measurement of various lung volumes.[63]

Sport. An athletic activity requiring skill or physical prowess and often of a competitive nature.[78]

Sports Medicine. The study of the physiological, biomechanical, psychosocial, and pathological phenomena associated with exercise and athletics and clinical application of the knowledge gained from the study to the improvement and maintenance of functional capacities for physical labor, exercise, and athletics and to the prevention and treatment of disease and injuries related to exercise and athletics.[51]

Sports Physical Therapy. The practice involving injury prevention, performance enhancement, recognition and management of acute athletic injuries, and treatment and rehabilitation of athletic injuries.[76]

Spot Reducing. The theory that exercising a specific body part, such as the thighs, will facilitate the loss of body fat from that spot.[43,87]

Spotter. A training partner who gives assistance with an unsuccessful lifting attempt, adds resistance during an exercise, provides encouragement and feedback, and otherwise helps the exerciser train in a safe and effective manner.[85]

Sprain. An injury to the joint capsule or the supporting ligaments or both resulting from overstress, which causes some degree of damage to the fibers and their attachments. First degree: some disruption of fibers with little or no loss of function. Second degree: some portion of the ligament/capsule is torn with some loss of function. Third degree: a complete tear and therefore total loss of function.[40]

Stability. The ability of an articulation to absorb shock and withstand motion without injury to the joint; also, the resistance to disturbance of a body's equilibrium.[48]

Stance Phase. It begins at the instant the heel of one extremity contacts the ground (heel strike) and ends when only the toe of the same extremity is on the ground (toe off).[60]

Static Exercise. The contraction of a skeletal muscle or group of muscles without movement of a joint.[19]

Static Stretching. 1. Stretching procedure in which a muscle is stretched and held in a stretched position for a specified time.[63] 2. A static stretching technique is performed by the client applying a small torque to a muscle after it is positioned at its end range of motion.

Steady State. 1. Describes the tendency of a controlled system to achieve a balance between an environmental demand and the response of a physiological system to meet that demand to allow the tissue (body) to function over a period of time.[63] 2. A level of metabolism, usually during exercise, when the oxygen consumption satisfies the energy expenditure and an individual is performing in an aerobic state.[87] 3. If the level of exercise is submaximal, a stage is reached where the major hemodynamic parameters plateau and, except for minor variations, remain relatively constant for up to several hours.[42] 4. During exercise, the heart rate initially increases rapidly but then tends to plateau over a period of time (usually between 3 to 5 minutes). When performing the YMCA bicycle ergometer test, steady state is said to have occurred when the heart rate is 5 or fewer beats per minute.[39] 5. A condition in which the supply of oxygen to tissues is equal to the demand of oxygen.[35]

Steady-State Threshold. The intensity level of exercise in which the production of energy appears to shift rapidly to an anaerobic mechanism, such as a rapid rise in lactic acid. The oxygen system will still supply a major portion of the energy, but the lactic acid system begins to contribute an increasing share.[87]

Step Duration. The amount of time spent during a single step. Measurement usually is taken in seconds per step.[60]

Step Length. The linear distance between two successive points of contact of opposite extremities. It is usually measured from heel strike of one extremity to the heel strike of the opposite extremity.[60]

Sticking Point. The point in which the body has the least biomechanical advantage in moving a weight.

STPD. Standard Temperature and Pressure, Dry. Gas volume at 0°C, 760 mm Hg total pressure, and partial pressure of water at zero, that is, dry.[80]

Strain. An overexertion trauma to a portion of the contractile musculotendinous unit or its attachment to the bone.[40]

Strength. 1. The maximal force a muscle or muscle group can generate at a specified velocity.[47] 2. The peak force of torque developed during a maximal voluntary contraction (MVC) under a given set of conditions (eg, contraction type and velocity).[70] *Syn:* resistance

Strength Curve. The peak force that can be developed by a muscle or muscle group varies through a range of movement, and this variation in peak force is called a strength curve.[70]

Stress. In medicine, the result produced when a structure, system, or organism is acted upon by forces that disrupt equilibrium or produce strain. In health care, the term denotes the physical (gravity, mechanical force, pathogen, injury) and psychologic (fear, anxiety, crisis, joy) forces that are experienced by individuals.[80]

Stress Test. 1. A medical diagnostic procedure for identifying patients who may have heart disease.[66] 2. Method of evaluating cardiovascular fitness. While exercising, usually on a treadmill or a bicycle ergometer, the individual is subjected to steadily increasing levels of work, while at the same time the amount of oxygen consumed is being determined and an electrocardiogram is being monitored.[80] *Syn:* graded exercise test (GXT), exercise tolerance test

Stretching. Describes any therapeutic maneuver designed to lengthen (elongate) pathologically shortened soft-tissue structures and thereby to increase range of motion.[17,45]

Stretch Shorten Cycle. The primary volitional movement is preceded by the opposite or antagonistic movement in a rapid manner producing a subsequently greater magnitude of contractile force due to the addition of potential energy transferred from the series elastic component.[1,13,24] *See* Plyometrics

Stretch Weakness. A clinical term denoting the effect on muscles from prolonged immobilization in a lengthened position, in other words, beyond the neutral or physiological rest point.[40]

Stride. The length of one stride is traveled during one gait cycle. The gait cycle includes the activities that occur from the point of initial heel contact of one lower extremity to the point at which the heel of the same extremity contacts the ground again. During one gait cycle each extremity passes through two phases, a single stance phase and a single swing phase. Therefore, each gait cycle consists of two stance and two swing phases.[60]

Stride Duration. The amount of time it takes to accomplish one stride.[60]

Stride Length. The linear distance between two successive events that are accomplished by the same lower extremity during gait. Generally, stride length is determined by measuring the distance from the point of heel strike of one lower extremity to the next heel strike of the same extremity.[60]

Stride Rate. The sum of the time for ground contact and the time one is in the air.[26]

Stroke Volume. The volume of blood ejected by a ventricle during one beat of the heart.[82]

Summation. Repeated stimulation of a muscle that leads to an increase in tension compared to a single twitch.[63]

Swing Phase. It begins as soon as the toe of one extremity leaves the ground and ceases just prior to heel strike of the same extremity.[60]

Syncope. Sudden, but transient, unconsciousness.[42]

Synergy. The cooperative effort of two or more muscles contracting to accomplish a single movement.[48]

Système International D'Unités (SI). An internationally standardized system of units.[80]

Systolic Pressure. The maximal blood pressure reached during the cardiac cycle.[82]

Tachycardia. Abnormal rapidity of heart action, usually defined as a heart rate over 100 beats per minute.[19]

Target Heart Rate. A predetermined heart rate to be obtained during exercise.[45]

Target Heart Rate (THR) Range. The range of heart rates describing the optimum intensity of exercise consistent with making gains in maximal aerobic power.[63]

Ten-Repetition Maximum (10-RM). The heaviest weight load an exerciser can lift 10 times in succession.[85]

Test. 1. A procedure or set of procedures that is used to obtain measurements (data); the procedures may require the use of instruments.[9] 2. An examination. Method to determine the presence or nature of a substance or the presence of a disease.[80] 3. A form of examination for evaluating the performance capabilities, traits, or achievements of an individual.[78]

Tetanus. Highest tension developed by a muscle in response to a high frequency of stimulation.[63]

Therapeutic Exercise. Bodily movements prescribed to restore or alter favorably specific functions in an individual following an injury.[28]

Tidal Volume. The volume of air moved during a single respiratory cycle (inhalation or expiration).[19]

Tightness. A nonspecific term referring to mild shortening of an otherwise healthy musculotendinous unit. May sometimes be used to describe a mild transient contracture.[45]

Tight Weakness. The weakening of a muscle that has been kept in a habitually shortened position. It may test strong in the shortened position but test weak as it is lengthened.[45]

Tonic. Continuous activity.[82]

Tonus. Low level of muscle activity at rest.[63]

Torque. 1. The effectiveness of a force to produce rotation about an axis (unit: newton·meter).[6] 2. The product of force and the perpendicular distance from the line of action of the force to the axis of rotation.[47]

Total Lung Capacity. The total amount of air in the lungs; the vital capacity plus the residual volume.[45]

Training. The process of acquiring fitness specific to a sport or activity.

Training Effect. 1. Describes physiologic changes and adaptations that result from participation in a structured exercise program. 2. Improvements in test performance based solely on familiarity with testing techniques.[28]

Triple Product. The product of the heart rate, systolic blood pressure, and ejection time.[66]

True Negative Test. Stress test that accurately diagnoses no coronary heart disease in patients free of heart disease.[66]

True Positive Test. Stress test that accurately diagnoses coronary heart disease in patients with heart disease.[66]

Twitch. The tension-generating response following the application of a single stimulus to muscle.[63]

Underwater Weighing. *See* Hydrostatic densitometry

US RDA. Nutritional information on foods that expresses the degree to which the food meets the adult RDA value for various nutrients.[63]

Validity. 1. The degree to which a useful (meaningful) interpretation can be inferred from a measurement.[9] 2. The degree to which a test measures what it is supposed to measure.[18]

Valsalva's Maneuver. An attempt to exhale forcibly with the glottis closed; causes increased intrathoracic pressure, slowed pulse rate, decreased venous return, and increased venous pressure.[19]

Variable Resistance Training. A form of dynamic contraction in which the resistance is altered throughout the range of motion (eg, Nautilus).[62]

Vasoconstriction. A decrease in the diameter of a blood vessel (usually an arteriole) resulting in reduction of blood flow to the area supplied by the vessel.[15]

Vasodilation. An increase in the diameter of a blood vessel (usually an arteriole) resulting in an increased blood flow to the area supplied by a vessel.[15]

Vector. A quantity having both magnitude and direction.[48]

Velocity. 1. Displacement per unit of time. A vector quantity requiring that direction be stated or strongly implied (units: meter per second or kilometer per hour).[6] 2. The speed and direction of a body.[48]

Velocity Spectrum Rehabilitation. A rehabilitation program that uses strength training at multiple speeds of movement, from slow to fast.[40]

Ventilation. The movement of air into or out of the lungs (eg, pulmonary or alveolar ventilation).[63] *Syn:* external respiration

Vital Capacity (VC). The maximal amount of air that can be breathed in or out.[66]

Volume. 1. A space occupied, for example, by a quantity of fluid or a gas (unit: liter or milliliter). Gas volumes should be indicated as ATPS, BTPS, or STPD.[6] 2. The three-dimensional space occupied by a body (length, width, and height).[48]

V̇O₂ Max. *See* Maximal oxygen consumption

Warm-up. A preperformance activity used to increase muscle temperature and to rehearse skills.[75]

Weight. The force with which a quantity of matter is attracted toward Earth by normal acceleration of gravity (traditional unit: kilogram of weight).[6]

Wellness. A conscious and deliberate approach to an advanced state of physical, psychologic, and spiritual health.[75]

Work. 1. Force expressed through a distance but with no limitation on time (preferred SI unit: joule or kilojoule). Quantities of energy and heat expressed independently of time should also be presented in joules. The term "work" should not be employed synonymously with muscular exercise.[6] 2. A measure of the amount of energy required to produce a physical displacement of matter.[82] 3. The force applied to a body multiplied by the distance through which that force is applied.[48] 4. Typical units of work are kp·m, kg·m, ft·lb, N·m, and J. The metabolic equivalent of work is the total energy expended (E) in performing the mechanical work [typical unit of E is kcal (calories)].[5]

Work Capacity. The ability to achieve work goals without undue fatigue and without becoming a hazard to oneself or co-workers.[75]

Work Hardening. A complete program of treatment designed to place an injured worker back into the preinjury job or occupation.[40]

Work Interval. The duration of the work phase of each work-to-rest interval.[63]

Workout. A complete exercise session, ideally consisting of an initial warm-up period followed by aerobic, strength, and flexibility exercises, and concluded with a cool-down period.

REFERENCES

1. Albert M. *Eccentric Muscle Training in Sports and Orthopaedics.* New York, NY: Churchill Livingstone; 1991.
2. Alter MJ. *Sport Stretch.* Champaign, Ill: Human Kinetics Publishers, Inc; 1990.
3. American Association of Cardiovascular and Pulmonary Rehabilitation. *Guidelines for Cardiac Rehabilitation Programs.* Champaign, Ill: Human Kinetics Publishers, Inc; 1991.
4. American College of Sports Medicine. *What Is an Exercise Physiologist?* Indianapolis, Ind: American College of Sports Medicine; (undated).
5. American College of Sports Medicine. *Guidelines for Exercise Testing and Prescription*, 4th ed. Philadelphia, Pa: Lea & Febiger; 1991.

6. American College of Sports Medicine. Information for authors. *Med Sci Sports Exerc.* 1991;23(1):i–v.

7. American Osteopathic Association. Glossary of osteopathic terminology. *J Am Osteo Assoc.* 1981;80(8):552–566.

8. American Physical Therapy Association. Letter to the authors. January 10, 1991.

9. American Physical Therapy Association (Task Force on Standards for Measurement in Physical Therapy). Standards for tests and measurements in physical therapy practice. *Phys Ther.* 1991;71(8):589–597.

10. Anshel MH, ed; Freedson P, Hamill J, et al., *Dictionary of the Sport and Exercise Sciences.* Champaign, Ill: Human Kinetics Publishers, Inc; 1991.

11. Armstrong LE, Costill DL, Fink WJ. Influence of diuretic-induced dehydration on competitive running performance. *Med Sci Sports Exerc.* 1985;17:456–461.

12. Arnheim DD. *Modern Principles of Athletic Training.* 7th ed. St Louis, Mo: Times Mirror/Mosby College Publishing; 1989.

13. Asmussen E, Bonde-Peterson F. Storage of elastic energy in skeletal muscles in man. *Acta Physiol.* 1974;91:385.

14. Åstrand P-O. *Work Tests with the Bicycle Ergometer.* Varberg, Sweden: Monark-Crescent AB; (undated).

15. Åstrand P-O, Rodahl K. *Textbook of Work Physiology: Physiological Bases of Exercise.* 3rd ed. New York, NY: McGraw-Hill Book Co; 1986.

16. Ayoub MM, Mital A. *Manual Materials Handling.* New York, NY: Taylor & Francis; 1989.

17. Basmajian JV, Wolf SL, eds. *Therapeutic Exercise.* 5th ed. Baltimore, Md: Williams & Wilkins; 1990.

18. Baumgartner TA, Jackson AS. *Measurement for Evaluation in Physical Education and Exercise Science.* 4th ed. Dubuque, Iowa: Wm C Brown Publishers; 1991.

19. Blair SN, Painter P, Pate RR, et al, eds. *Resource Manual for Guidelines for Exercise Testing and Prescription* (American College of Sports Medicine). Philadelphia, Pa: Lea & Febiger; 1988.

20. Blanke D. Preseason conditioning: Flexibility. In: Mellion MB, Walsh WM, Shelton GL, eds. *The Team Physician's Handbook.* Philadelphia, Pa: Hanley & Belfus, Inc; 1990.

21. Bohannon RW. Muscle strength testing with hand-held dynamometers. In: Amundsen LR, ed. *Muscle Strength Testing: Instrumented and Non-Instrumented Systems.* New York, NY: Churchill Livingstone; 1990.

22. Bompa TO. Periodization of strength: The most effective methodology of strength training. *Nat Strength Condit Assoc J.* 1990,12(5):49–52.

23. Byrnes WB, Clarkson PM. Delayed onset muscle soreness and training. In: Katch FI, Freedson PS, eds. *Clinics in Sports Medicine.* Philadelphia, Pa: WB Saunders Co; 1986;5.

24. Cavagna GA, Saibene FP, Margaria R. Effect of negative work on the amount of positive work performed by an isolated muscle. *J Appl Physiol.* 1965;20:157.

25. Chu DA. *Jumping into Plyometrics.* Champaign, Ill: Leisure Press; 1992.

26. Dintiman GB. *How to Run Faster.* West Point, NY: Leisure Press; 1984.

27. DiNubile NA. Strength training. In: DiNubile NA, ed. *The Exercise Prescription* [Clinics in Sports Medicine 10(1)]. Philadelphia, Pa: WB Saunders Co; 1991.

28. Drez D, ed. *Therapeutic Modalities for Sports Injuries.* Chicago, Ill: Year Book Medical Publishers, Inc; 1989.

29. Editors of the University of California, Berkeley, Wellness Letter. *The Wellness Encyclopedia: The Comprehensive Family Resource for Safeguarding Health and Preventing Illness.* Boston, Mass: Houghton Mifflin; 1991.

30. Eichner ER. Ergolytic drugs. *Sports Sci Exchange.* 1989;2:1–4.

31. Eichner ER. Ergolytic drugs. *Internal Medicine for the Specialist.* 1990;11(1):74–80.

32. Elftman H. Biomechanics of muscle. *J Bone Joint Surg.* 1966;48:363.

33. Evans WJ. Exercise-induced skeletal muscle damage. *Physician Sportsmed.* 1987;15(1):89.

34. Fardy PS, Yanowitz FG, Wilson PK. *Cardiac Rehabilitation, Adult Fitness and Exercise Testing.* 2nd ed. Philadelphia, Pa: Lea & Febiger; 1988.

35. Fisher AG, Jensen CR. *Scientific Basis of Athletic Conditioning.* Philadelphia, Pa: Lea & Febiger; 1990.

36. Fleck SJ, Kraemer WJ. *Designing Resistance Training Programs.* Champaign, Ill: Human Kinetics Publishers, Inc; 1987.

37. Francis KT. Delayed muscle soreness: A review. *J Orthop Sports Phys Ther.* 1983;15:10.

38. Friel JP, ed. *Dorland's Illustrated Medical Dictionary*. 26th ed. Philadelphia, Pa: WB Saunders Co; 1981.

39. Golding LA, Myers CR, Sinning WE, eds. *Y's Way to Physical Fitness: The Complete Guide to Fitness Testing and Instruction*. 3rd ed. Champaign, Ill: Human Kinetics Publishers, Inc; 1989.

40. Gould JA, ed. *Orthopaedic and Sports Physical Therapy*. 2nd ed. St Louis, Mo: CV Mosby Co; 1990.

41. Hageman PA, Sorensen TA. Eccentric isokinetics. In: Albert M. *Eccentric Muscle Training in Sports and Orthopaedics*. New York, NY: Churchill Livingstone; 1991.

42. Irwin S, Tecklin JS. *Cardiopulmonary Physical Therapy*. 2nd ed. St Louis, Mo: CV Mosby Co; 1990.

43. Katch FI, Clarkson PM, Kroll W, et al. Effects of sit up exercise training on adipose cell size and adiposity. *Res Q Exerc Sport*. 1984;55(3):242–247.

44. Katch FI, Katch VL, McArdle WD. Physiologic fitness: The basis of sports medicine. In: Grana WA, Kalenak A, eds. *Clinical Sports Medicine*. Philadelphia, Pa: WB Saunders Co; 1991.

45. Kisner C, Colby LA. *Therapeutic Exercise: Foundations and Techniques*. 2nd ed. Philadelphia, Pa: FA Davis Co; 1990.

46. Knight KL. *Clinical Experiences in Athletic Training*. Champaign, Ill: Human Kinetics Publishers, Inc; 1990.

47. Knuttgen HG, Kraemer WJ. Terminology and measurement in exercise performance. *J Appl Sports Sci Res*. 1987;1(1):1–10.

48. Kreighbaum E, Barthels KM. *Biomechanics: A Qualitative Approach for Studying Human Movement*. Minneapolis, Minn: Burgess Publishing Co; 1981.

49. Kulund DN. *The Injured Athlete*. 2nd ed. Philadelphia, Pa: JB Lippincott Co; 1988.

50. Lemkuhl LD, Smith LK. Mechanical principles: Kinematics. In: Lemkuhl LD, Smith LK. *Brunnstrom's Clinical Kinesiology*. 2nd ed. Philadelphia, Pa: FA Davis Co; 1983.

51. Lombardo JA. Sportsmedicine: A team effort. *Physician Sportsmed*. 1985;13(4):12–81.

52. Lynch L. Manual muscle strength testing of the distal muscles. In: Amundsen LR, ed. *Muscle Strength Testing: Instrumented and Non-Instrumented Systems*. New York, NY: Churchill Livingstone; 1990.

53. Maitland GD. *Peripheral Manipulation*. 3rd ed. Stoneham, Mass: Butterworth-Heinemann; 1991.

54. McArdle WD, Katch FI, Katch VL. *Exercise Physiology: Energy, Nutrition and Human Performance*. 3rd ed. Philadelphia, Pa: Lea & Febiger; 1991.

55. Mitchell F, Moran P, Pruzzo N. *An Evaluation and Treatment Manual of Osteopathic Muscle Energy Procedures*. Valley Park, Mich: Mitchell, Moran and Pruzzo Assoc; 1979.

56. National Athletic Trainers' Association, Board of Certification, Inc. *Role Delineation Validation Study for the Entry-Level Athletic Trainers' Certification Examination*. Dallas, Tex: National Athletic Trainers' Association, Inc; 1990.

57. National Strength and Conditioning Association. Roundtable—Speed development. *Nat Strength Condit Assoc J*. 1984;5(6):12.

58. National Strength and Conditioning Association. Roundtable—Periodization (Part 1). *Nat Strength Condit Assoc J*. 1986;8(5):12–22.

59. National Strength and Conditioning Association. *Certified Strength and Conditioning Specialist Examination Sites* (Suppl). Lincoln, Neb: National Strength and Conditioning Association; 1991.

60. Norkin C, Levangie P. *Joint Structure and Function: A Comprehensive Analysis*. Philadelphia, Pa: FA Davis Co; 1983.

61. O'Shea P. The science of cross-training: Theory and application for peak performance. *Nat Strength Condit Assoc J*. 1990;12(6):40–44.

62. Pollock ML, Wilmore JH. *Exercise in Health and Disease: Evaluation of Prescription for Prevention and Rehabilitation*. 2nd ed. Philadelphia, Pa: WB Saunders Co; 1990.

63. Powers SK, Howley ET. *Exercise Physiology: Theory and Application to Fitness and Performance*. Dubuque, Iowa: Wm C Brown Publishers; 1990.

64. Radcliffe JC, Farentinos RC. *Plyometrics: Explosive Power Training*. 2nd ed. Champaign, Ill: Human Kinetics Publishers, Inc; 1985.

65. Rodgers SH, ed. *Ergonomic Design for People at Work*. New York, NY: Van Nostrand Reinhold; 1986;2.

66. Ross RM, Jackson AS. *Exercise Concepts, Calculations and Computer Applications*. Carmel, Ind: Benchmark Press; 1990.

67. Ross WD, Marfell-Jones MJ. Kinanthropometry. In: MacDougall JD, Wenger HA, Green HJ, eds. *Physiological Testing of the High-Performance Athlete*. 2nd ed. Champaign, Ill: Human Kinetics Publishers, Inc; 1991.

68. Ross WD, McKin DR, Wilson BD. Kinanthropometry and young skiers: An introduction and research prospectus. In: Taylor AW, ed. *Application of Science and Medicine to Sport*. Springfield, Ill: Charles C Thomas Publisher; 1975.

69. Sale DG. Testing strength and power. In: MacDougall JD, Wenger HA, Green HJ, eds. *Physiological Testing of the High-Performance Athlete*. 2nd ed. Champaign, Ill: Human Kinetics Publishers, Inc; 1991.

70. Sale DG, Norman RW. Testing strength and power. In: MacDougall JD, Wenger HA, Green HJ, eds. *Physiological Testing of the Elite Athlete*. Ithaca, NY: Mouvement Publications, Inc; 1982.

71. Sanders B. *Sports Physical Therapy*. Norwalk, Conn: Appleton & Lange; 1990.

72. Sapega AA, Quedenfeld TC, Moyer RA, et al. Biophysical factors in range-of-motion exercise. *Physician Sportsmed*. 1981;9(12):57–65.

73. Saunders HD. *Evaluation, Treatment and Prevention of Musculoskeletal Disorders*. Eden Prairie, Minn: Educational Opportunities; 1985.

74. Schultz P. Flexibility: The day of the static stretch. *Physician Sportsmed*. 1979;7:109–117.

75. Sharkey BJ. *Physiology of Fitness*. 3rd ed. Champaign, Ill: Human Kinetics Publishers, Inc; 1990.

76. Sports Physical Therapy, Brochure of the Sports Physical Therapy Section, American Physical Therapy Association, 1989.

77. Stamford B. What is interval training? *Physician Sportsmed*. 1989;17(9):193.

78. Stein J, ed. *The Random House College Dictionary*, revised ed. New York, NY: Random House; 1984.

79. Thoden JS. Testing aerobic power. In: MacDougall JD, Wenger HA, Green HJ, eds. *Physiological Testing of the High-Performance Athlete*. 2nd ed. Champaign, Ill: Human Kinetics Publishers, Inc; 1991.

80. Thomas CL, ed. *Taber's Cyclopedic Medical Dictionary*. 15th ed. Philadelphia, Pa: FA Davis Co; 1985.

81. United States Weightlifting Federation. The clean and jerk lift and the snatch lift. Colorado Springs, Colo: United States Weightlifting Federation; undated.

82. Vander AJ, Sherman FH, Luciano DS. *Human Physiology: The Mechanisms of Body Function*. 3rd ed. New York, NY: McGraw-Hill Book Co; 1980.

83. Voight ML, Draovitch P. Plyometrics. In: Albert M. *Eccentric Muscle Training in Sports and Orthopaedics*. New York, NY: Churchill Livingstone; 1991.

84. Wasserman K, Hansen JE, Sue DY, et al. *Principles of Exercise Testing and Interpretation*. Philadelphia, Pa: Lea & Febiger; 1987.

85. Westcott WL. *Strength Fitness: Physiological Principles and Training Techniques*. 3rd ed. Dubuque, Iowa: Wm C Brown Publishers; 1991.

86. Wilk K. Dynamic muscle strength testing. In: Amundsen LR. *Muscle Strength Testing: Instrumented and Non-Instrumented Systems*. New York, NY: Churchill Livingstone; 1990.

87. Williams MH. *Lifetime Fitness and Wellness: A Personal Choice*. 2nd ed. Dubuque, Iowa: Wm C Brown Publishers; 1990.

88. Zachazewski JE. Flexibility for sports. In: Sanders B, ed. *Sports Physical Therapy*. Norwalk, Conn: Appleton & Lange; 1990.

Index

Letters after page numbers indicate figures (*f*) and tables (*t*).

A

Abbreviations, 229*t*–230*t*
Abdominal curl-up isotonic exercise, 155*f*
Absolute, 271
Absolute one-repetition maximum
    method, 31
Absolute VO$_2$, 271
ACC, cognitive skills for exercise testing,
    39–40*t*
Acceleration, 271
Accessory movement, 271
Acclimatization, 271
Accommodating resistance training, 271
ACLS (Advanced Cardiac Life Support),
    7
ACP, cognitive skills for exercise testing,
    39–40*t*
ACSM. *See* American College of Sports
    Medicine (ACSM)
Active-assistive range of motion, 271
Active inhibition, 125–126, 271
Active range of motion, 271
Active stretching, 125*t*, 272
Activities of daily living (ADL), 27, 272
Acute-onset muscle soreness, 272
Adenosine diphosphate (ADP), 272
Adenosine triphosphate (ATP), 272
Adipose tissue, 272
ADL (activities of daily living), 27, 272
ADP (adenosine diphosphate), 272
Advanced Cardiac Life Support (ACLS),
    7
Aerobic, 272

Aerobic energy, 272
Aerobic exercise, 272
Aerobic fitness, 272
Aerobic metabolism, 272
Aerobic power, 89, 90*t*, 272
Aerobic threshold, 272
Aerobic walking, 272
Afterload, 272
Age-predicted maximal heart rate, 272
Agility
  balance and, 189
  definition of, 272
  testing, 97, 97*t*
Agonist muscle, 272
AHA. *See* American Heart Association
    (AHA)
All or none law, 272
Alpha motor neurons, 272
American College of Cardiology,
    cognitive skills for exercise testing,
    39–40*t*
American College of Physicians,
    cognitive skills for exercise testing,
    39–40*t*
American College of Sports Medicine
    (ACSM)
  guidelines for exercise testing and
    participation, 40, 41*t*
  specialty certifications of, 5*t*
American Heart Association (AHA)
  cognitive skills of exercise testing,
    39–40*t*
  specialty certifications of, 5*t*
American Occupational Therapy
    Association, 4

N

National Athletic Trainers' Association, 4
National Strength and Conditioning
    Association (NSCA), specialty
    certifications of, 5t
Naughton protocol, modified, 53t
Negative work, 287
Niacin, 256t
Nicotinamide adenine dinucleotide
    (NAD), 287
Norms, 287
NSCA (National Strength and
    Conditioning Association),
    specialty certifications of, 5t
Nutrition, suggested readings, 216–217
Nutritional factors, affecting exercise
    prescription, 13
Nutrition assessment form, 247f–248f

O

Ober's test, 22
Obesity, 217–218, 287
Objectivity, 287
Occupational therapy, 287–288
Olympic lifters, 288
Olympic lifting world records, 100t
One-repetition maximum, 32, 288
Open-circuit spirometry, 288
Open kinetic chain, 288
Optimal flexibility, 288
Organizations, 259–263
Orthostatic hypotension, 288
Osteoarthritis, 288
Osteoporosis, 218, 288
Overload principle, 288
Overstretch, 288
Overtraining, 288
Overuse syndrome, 288
Overweight, 288
Oxford protocol, for isotonic training,
    146t
Oxidative phosphorylation, 288
Oxygen consumption, 288
Oxygen debt, 288–289
Oxygen deficit, 289
Oxygen dissociation curve, 289
Oxygen pulse, 289
Oxygen system, 289
Oxygen uptake, 289

P

PAC (premature atrial contraction), 290
Pain management, suggested readings,
    222

Palpation method, for heart rate
    measurement, 48
Pantothenic acid, 256t
Parcours, 289
Partial abdominal sit-up isotonic exercise,
    156f
Passive range of motion, 289
Passive stretching, 125t, 289
Pectoralis minor tightness test, 22
Pelvic tilt isometric exercise, 153f
Perceived exertion, 289
    cardiovascular endurance exercise
        prescription and, 171
    scales, rating of, 51t
Percent grade, 289
Performance, suggested readings,
    207–208
Periodization, 189–190t, 289
Personal factors, affecting exercise
    prescription, 12
Personnel, in exercise testing, 4t
pH, 289
Phasic, 289
Phosphorus, 257t
Phylloquinone, 257t
Physical activity, 289
Physical agents, 289
Physical assessment form, 244f–246f
Physical demand levels of work, 116t
Physical education, suggested readings,
    218–219
Physical fitness, 289
Physical science formulas, 235t–237t
Physical therapy, 289–290
Physical work capacity (PWC), 290
Physiological factors, affecting exercise
    prescription, 13
Physiologic calculations, suggested
    readings, 219
Physiologic movement, 290
PILE (Progressive Isoinertial Lifting
    Evaluation), 28
Piriformis tightness test, 22
Plasma volume, 252t
Plastic stretch, 290
Plyometric contraction, 290
Plyometrics, 290
PNF (proprioceptive neuromuscular
    facilitation), 291
Positive work, 290
Posterior shoulder isometric exercise,
    151f
Posterior shoulder lateral raise isotonic
    exercise, 160f
Post-test responsibilities, of clinician, 6
Potassium, 254t, 258t
Power, 290
    intensity, frequency and duration, 189
    modes of training, 189
Powerlifters, 290
Powerlifting records, 99t

Other Books of Interest
from
Appleton & Lange

Hayes
Manual for Physical Agents
Fourth Edition

Minor & Minor
Patient Care Skills: Positioning, Transfers, Range of Motion, Ambulation
nd Edition

Nelson & Currier
Clinical Electrotherapy
Second Edition

Portney & Watkins
Clinical Research

Shurr & Cook
Prosthetics and Orthotics

Somers
Spinal Cord Injury: Functional Rehabilitation